LAURA ROBINSON OATMAN

WHOLE EARTH DIET

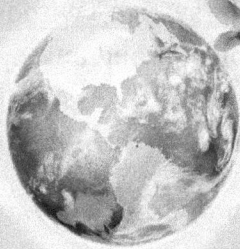

**HEALTHY BODY. HAPPY LIFE.
PEACEFUL WORLD.**

Whole Earth Diet

by Laura Robinson Oatman

Cover Design by Melodye Hunter
Typesetting: Zonoiko Arafat
Cover Design by Melodye Hunter

Copyright © 2015 by Laura Robinson Oatman

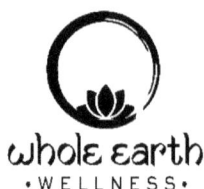

whole earth
•WELLNESS•

ISBN: 978-0-9964269-2-3

Crescendo Publishing, LLC
300 Carlsbad Village Drive
Ste. 108A, #443
Carlsbad, California 92008-2999
www.CrescendoPublishing.com
GetPublished@CrescendoPublishing.com

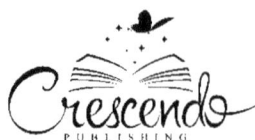

A Message from the Author

Click on the link to hear a personal message from Laura Robinson Oatman, author of *Whole Earth Diet*.

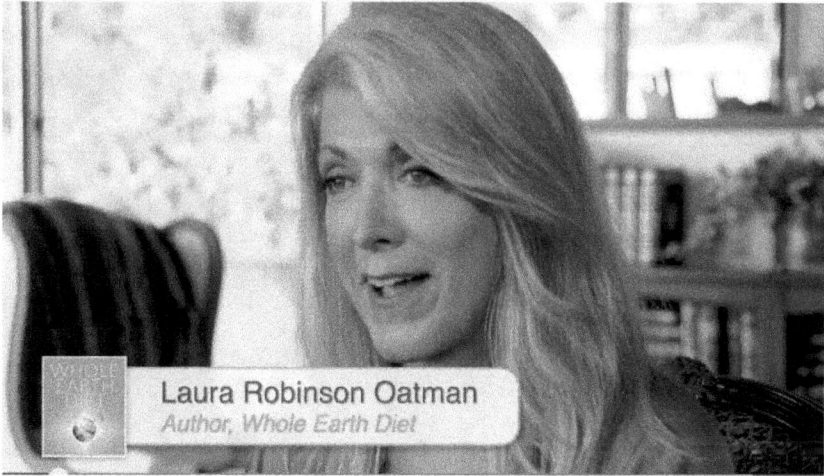

Laura Robinson Oatman
Author, Whole Earth Diet

www.youtube.com/watch?v=qQm1fZYjtRQ

This book is dedicated to our beautiful Earth and all the

earthlings—two-legged or four, furry, scaled, or feathered—

who dwell here.

What People Are Saying About

Laura Robinson Oatman

"The Whole Earth Diet is an immensely practical guide to the best of healthful eating. The most effective way to promote good health is to eat a vegan diet—our clinical research studies at the Physicians Committee have shown time after time that this is the case. And eating plants is not only the best way to take care of your own health and wellness, it is also the best way to eat sustainably for the Earth. No matter where you stand right now, transitioning toward a vegan diet should be your next step. Let Laura help lead the way, and enjoy the benefits of eating and living in a way that benefits the whole Earth. You'll be so glad that you did!

~**Neal Barnard, M.D.,** President, Physicians Committee for Responsible Medicine; Professor George Washington University School of Medicine, Washington, DC

"Starting with how to simply make breakfast and ending with how to simply save the world, Whole Earth Diet is just the thing this planet has been waiting for."

~**Kim Barnouin,** Author, *Skinny Bitch*

"This book is guaranteed to change the life of any one who reads it. Laura Oatman brings a fresh new perspective on the necessity of a plant-based diet for an individual's health. Health benefits of plant based diet are well documented with good references. In fact many cardiologists started recommending plant based diet for their patients."

~**Mohammad Kanakriyeh, M.D.**, Pediatric Cardiologist, Loma Linda University, Loma Linda, CA

"Read this book and lean into a whole new world of health and happiness. Eating plant-based is a game changer - for you, and for the world."

~**Kathy Freston**, *New York Times* best-selling author *Veganist, The Lean, Quantum Wellness*

"Laura Oatman's perspective on plant-based nutrition is both personal and universal in scope. Her integrative approach took us (myself and my husband, both 9 year veterans of plant-based eating) to a whole new level. We are healthier, lighter in weight, and delighted to have found a sense of belonging in her Rainbow Warrior Tribe! Her book is unique amongst diet books for its insight and truthfulness into how we eat contributes to creating a peaceful and wholesome planet for all. Even If you have many books about plant-based nutrition, you need this one. If you have never read a book on plant-based nutrition, read this one first."

~**Kathy Fullmer**, certified in Plant Based Nutrition by the T. Colin Campbell Foundation, B.S. in Microbiology, Montana State University, member of the Physicians' Committee for Responsible Medicine, Perryville, MO

"As someone who has benefited enormously from Laura Robinson Oatman's professional health coaching services, I would like to add my own endorsement of the value of her services. I came to see Laura only because I was forcefully "nudged" by my internist to see a nutritionist and not because I felt excited about making changes to my lifestyle or eating habits. I am skeptical by nature and quite honestly approached my first few appointments with a "show me" attitude, and that is exactly what Laura did. After working with her for three months I've slowly become more educated about the impact my diet has on my health and well being. I've willingly given up some foods I thought I'd never be able to live without, achieved my weight loss goals, and measurably improved my energy level. Best of all, I feel better than I have in years."

~**Lynn Multari**, Newport Beach, CA

"Love the power of community. I have lost some of my belly and an inch of my waist. I still do not weigh myself. I actually feel good. I will continue to eat this way. I may still add the fiber most days. I am a vegan. I claimed that years ago before I knew what it was. So even when I am not perfect, this is my path. I feel so good today."

~**Teri Sewell Huff**, Denver, CO

"I recently started my next step in my journey to honor myself and my body in a more clean and natural way. Changing habits can be difficult and sometimes seem to have a life of their own. Having a coach to help you thru the good times and bad is so helpful for me. Making the adjustments to going totally vegetarian takes some education and training and Laura is so helpful in pointing me in the right directions. I am focusing on maintaining a plant based diet, making exercise a more routine part of my day and with Laura's help moving towards where I really want to be, free from foods/chemicals and habits that rob me of my joy and peace of mind. I am so grateful for the service Laura and her company provide. I highly recommend these services to others also on the road to fully honoring their body/mind and spirit. Thank You Laura!"

~Julie Russell RN, Ladera Ranch, Ca

"Laura, thank you for your program! Last year I was so depressed and didn't know how to start changing my life but knew I had too. In a matter of three years I was laid-off, lost my marriage, my best friend passed away due to an illness, and lost my house due to the economy. I gained over sixty pounds and was pushing a size 14. When I started your program I didn't know what to expect but I knew I had to do something because my health was declining! I remember sitting down with you at our first meeting and you asked me a simple question, "If you could change your life, how would you see it?" Oh that was easy! I want a job and to be thin again! We set our meetings and goals up and began the process. You were there with me every step of the way, setting realistic changes in my diet, educating me on making better choices with food, text motivating messages, and during our meetings you lifted my spirits even when I slipped. With out your support and commitment to me I wouldn't be where I am today! Eight months later I was working again and approaching a size 8! I don't take antidepressants anymore and I eat well. I feel happy and my complexion shows it! I never knew the food I was eating was slowly killing me. It doesn't sound funny to me any more that YOU ARE WHAT YOU EAT!"

~DeeAnn Gray, Newport Beach, CA

"Laura is a wonderful coach. We worked together for 6 months and the results were very close to my goals: my blood pressure is lower, I lost close to what we set up as a goal and I have a new appetite for life in general. I was and still am impressed with her knowledge, her personal approach and understanding of who I am and WHY I wanted to change. She has a wide-ranging and far-reaching approach and she is meticulous and flexible at the same time. I felt she was completely on "my team" and that my success was her success. If you want to gradually change your life and feel 10 years younger give her a call. You will be glad you did!"

~**Christina R**, Mission Viejo, CA

"When I joined Whole Earth Wellness on their retreat, I had never before spent a full weekend solely focused on my health. It felt so indulgent! I learned so much. I felt supported by those on the trip and there were amazing results."

~**Jan Henderson**, Mission Viejo, CA

"I did the bikini cleanse. Thank goodness they don't make a guy like me put one on after the program! I've learned so much through the Whole Earth Diet and courses, especially around choosing whole foods. I was on a pizza and diet coke path. Now I am thinking differently about food. You wouldn't run your car on jello — why is your body any different? During the whole process, I continuously noticed a difference:my energy increased, I was dropping weight, my whole body felt in sync, and my attitude changed. I was looking at my life circumstance in a whole new way."

~**Gregg Goodrich**, Tucson, AZ

"I'm passionate about making more environmentally sustainable choices. I was learning about sustainability and became more and more interested in reducing meat consumption. This program was a great start for learning how to live and thrive on a plant-based diet."

~**Erin Hoffer**, Boston, MA

"I thought I was a pretty healthy eater, but I wanted to do more. What I loved about the programs is that I can transition to a plant-based diet at my own pace. For me, it has been a gradual process and I am able to really commit each step of the way. There's no judgment with Laura; she helps you get where you want to be."

~**Christy Peterson**, Chicago, IL

"It was hard being in my 20s and facing health issues, but the 1:1 coaching program was the support I needed to get healthy. They taught me how to make real changes in my lifestyle and eating. I've done a 360 in the way I feel — both physically and emotionally. Now, my friends and family look to me for advice about food."

~**Kali Poulos**, Huntington Beach, CA

"Greg used to be on red rice yeast and a ton of other natural supplements for his cholesterol. Went off all of it and just did vegan. His family has high cholesterol...all the men have stents...so you know he is always told 'here take this pill, it's a genetic issue.' Cholesterol went down from 280 to 211...since we have been vegan. The MD believes that if he now just exercises his HDL will lower and his cholesterol will be below 200...I love you for all you have done!"

~**Kelly Higdon**, Oceanside, CA

"I really wanted to take a quick moment to thank you for all your love, kindness, and support. Your program is amazing, and now that I've moved and am only working 36-40hrs/wk, my life has completely changed. I'm eating healthier, and am losing real weight with very little effort. I'm eating a 100% whole foods diet without oils. I'm actually eating fruits and vegetables, and even enjoy them. I'm back to going to Church again, and I've even signed up to be a Big Sister. Thank you, I couldn't have done it without you. I'm so excited to begin this amazing chapter in my life."

~**Christina Hartshorn RN**, Mansfield, OH

"I can always count on Laura for inspiration and the latest information in support of my plant based diet. Her research and insight is truly compelling."

~**Val Riley**, Newport Beach, CA

"Laura taught me, without judgment or force, to desire that which feeds my body, soul, and spirit. I am cleaner, happier, and way healthier. I weigh less without trying. Seriously owe my life to this gifted and beautiful woman. So many are unaware of the risks eating food from our store shelves puts us at—learn and LIVE."

~**Joanne Miller**, Newport Beach, CA

"If you want to be part of the solution, if your heart is full of abundant love, if you want to walk toward the light, then lend an ear to Laura Robinson Oatman who exudes beauty, grace, love, honor, and friendship. And she knows a thing or two."

~**Rickie Makimoto**, Costa Mesa, CA

A Brief Note to the Reader

It is my greatest wish that this book will change your life dramatically for the better. It is with deepest conviction that I express to you that the only way to heal your body, your mind, your heart, and your soul—and heal this Earth in the process—is with a total transition to the Whole Earth Diet. But before we begin, I need to say just a couple things:

Before you begin to make any changes to diet or exercise, please get a complete physical health evaluation done, and let your doctor know about the changes you will be making, in particular if you have any current health conditions. This is not because these diet and lifestyle recommendations are dangerous—quite the contrary! If anything, this will prove to be a measuring stick against which you can compare your current numbers to your numbers six months from now and see the dramatic and objective results in weight, body measurements, and blood pressure, as well as with blood testing, C-reactive protein, triglycerides, glucose, and blood cholesterol levels.

However, if you are taking medications, particularly for diabetes, high blood pressure, or blood thinners for heart conditions, you will want to check with your doctor about adjustments to medications as you go. When you switch to a plant-based diet, very often you will be able to start to decrease and eventually discontinue your medications altogether, BUT do not do this on your own. Work with your medical doctor on the monitoring, reduction, and/or elimination of your current prescription drug regimen.

Talk to your doctor before you begin to exercise as well, particularly if you have been a couch potato for years, have a great deal of weight to lose, and/or are over forty.

Don't expect change to happen overnight, and don't expect it to be easy. This shift will take time, and you must stick with it to see results. But move at your own pace. Some of you will want to go "all the way" with this right away, and some of you will be more comfortable going gradually. It is all good! Let's begin.

Acknowledgements

It is with utmost gratitude that I thank:

Homer Oatman, for being my best friend and love of my life, and for supporting me as I pursue my dream to spread this message to the whole earth;

Ted and Jean Robinson, for giving me life, showing me the world, and giving me roots to value family history and traditions;

Erik, Annalise, Dane, Scott, and Brett Oatman, for giving my life purpose, and giving me the vision to see into a hopeful, awakened future;

My brother Kurt, for being the vegetarian trailblazer for our family, long before the rest of us figured this out;

Mohini Bhatia, for being my soul sister, who shares the Whole Earth vision and poured her heart and soul into the concept stages of this project with me;

My lifelong BFFs: my childhood BFF Carol Botdorf who was and still is the closest thing to a sister that I will ever have; my younger self BFF Michele Swift Chodos who can go for years without talking and always pick up right where we left off; and my "golden years" BFF Peta Paladin, for being my morning exercise buddy, and for supporting and encouraging me throughout these last few crazy years.

For the trailblazers who have been the real tip of the spear in this movement: Dr. Neal Barnard, Rory Freedman, Kim Barnouin, Dr. Caldwell Esselstyn, Will Tuttle, Mimi Kirk, Tanya Petrovna, Jenny Ross, Philip Wollen, Harold Brown, Howard Lyman, Seba Johnson, Matthew Scully, Gene Baur, Nathan Runkle, Bruce Friedrich, Dr. Dean Ornish, Dr. Joel Fuhrman, Dr. T. Colin Campbell, John Robbins, Dr. John McDougall, Melanie Joy, Kathy Freston, Ingrid Newkirk, Joaquin Phoenix, and Sam Simon—eternal gratitude to all of you.

For my mentors, coaches, and teachers who helped me find my most authentic self: Denise Brown, Lisa Bollow, Robbin Simons, JuliAnn Stitick, Starla Fortunato, Tracey Trottenberg, Lisa Walker, Ann Bennett and Narelle Sheehan.

For my fearless fellow vegan health coaches who are not afraid to take a stand, most of whom have supported my programs from the start: Patti Woods, Fran Batzer, Teri Sewell Huff, Karin Olsen, Deniece Young, Katrina LaPointe Anotado, Cherie Oden, Susan Yeoman, Steven Todd Smith, Lisa Fallon Mindel, Bonnie Furman, Lois Rosenberg Brown, Eileen Elam Sabolcik, Gretchen Brooks Nassar, Ashley Neese, Rebecca Turner, Karen Dwire, Kerry Myers, Tara Crawford, Whitney Werner Fretham, Danielle Marggraf, Christine Ronchin Icardo, Teena Jamieson AbuHamdeh, Neader Williams, Rebecca Ruhsam Reinbold, Laraine Broschinsky, Natalie Meadows, Bonnie Damitz Crutcher, Lisa Hartman Matricardi, Christina Tangney, Hope Carson Pickard, Trish Wooten, Victoria Moran, Kim Jones, Dominique Hoffman, Barbara Bhavani Cooper, Debra Libby, Lois Niven, Eve Beili, Lauren Washer-Whitman, Christie Norris, Ashley Sue Paulson, Ken Pataky, Thelma Tabiolo, Sadiya Wims, Carley Lang—never give up! You guys are my inspiration every day.

For my amazing Power Partner Spice Girls who have the cleanest digestive tract in town: Rickie Makimoto, Jane Shafron, Don Phravorachith, Marni Ellison Smith, Kimberly Gerber, Mahyar Ghassemian, Laura Hall, Linda Kang, Diana Perna, Jane Khalaf, and Mary Neil!

For my dearest Swinettes who have been so supportive even when they think I have gone completely nuts: Carol Chun Craddock, Irina Chiose, Deirdre Vouziers, Rosa Balsera, Sandra Bye, Peggy Minger-McCants, Marj Griggs-Hoover, Fran Henderson Reiner, and DeeAnn Grey.

And all my Warriors for Peace: Jennifer Bonnell O'Connor, Val Riley, Susan Green, Catherine Biggers, Joanne Miller, Christina Hartshorn, Christen King, Lynn Gardner, Kali Poulos, Gregg Goodrich, Tina Sanchez, Mark & Lauren Benson Button, Monique Leimel, Mohammed & Cindy Kanakriyeh, Alexis Autenrieth, Annette Reeves, Anjana Menon, Lisa Grundhoffer, Azeem & Zeena Dhalla, Patrick Fetzer, Erin Hoffer, Emily Laine, Maureen Sauerman, Lycette Irving, Louise McDermott, Robert Gonzalez, Karie Gibbons, Kelly Kovacs, DeNell Todd, Gail Slaughter, Julie Hamett Kaufman, Wes Johnson, Cheryl Gaines, Ashley Edwards, Tami Herbert, Terre Patterson, Ashley Christianson, Nanci Masada-Okawa, Stephanie Hodal, Julie Russell, Laura Sanchez, Harold Lee, Terry Loftus, Annie Stathakis, Melissa Daubert, Vic Martin, Kathy Fullmer, Dan Reichert, Julie Diebolt-Price, Mariana Bomfim Magness, Tonja Indseth, Liz Clayton, Colleen Gehlbach, Bhuvnesh Ojha Pukaar, Jordi Salomon, Barbara Becker, Lynn Brown, Jan Henderson, Kelly Higdon, Kathleen Kane, Midori Kimata, Vera Martinovic, Louise McDermott, Laurie Perez, Phuong Phu, Mary Pickhardt, Suzanne Robinson, Janice Salmon, Shirley & Rochelle Zubcov, Melody Chong, Bozena Kloda-Urbanski, Toni Tartamella, Robin Krall

Richter, Janice Salmon, Jodi LaBossiere, Shaila Mistry, Anshu Mohan, Mary Jane Feldmeier O'Brien, Kris Hess, Kate Azar, Elaine Wilson, and Lorrie Kazan.

Last but certainly not least - all the good folks at Peet's Coffee in Newport Beach who always knew my drink without asking – my Large Matcha Green Tea Latte with almond milk and a pump of peppermint – thank you to Christiana, Ashley, Josh, Courtney, Savannah and Angel for filling my cup! This was the fuel I used to write this book.

Table of Contents

PART ONE:

HEALTHY BODY ~ THE WHOLE EARTH DIET

PART TWO:

HAPPY LIFE ~ THE WHOLE EARTH LIFESTYLE

PART THREE:
PEACEFUL WORLD ~ THE WHOLE EARTH VISION

Introduction

━━━━━•●•━━━━━

"When the earth is ravaged and the animals are dying, a new
tribe shall come onto the Earth, from many colors, classes
and creeds,
and who by their actions and deeds shall make the Earth
green again.
They shall be known as the Rainbow Warriors."

~A Native American Prophesy

Are you sick and tired of being fat, sick, and tired? Or following the latest trendy diets that leave you unsatisfied and unsuccessful again? Then whatever you do, do NOT put this book back on the shelf. Take it home. Read it tonight. Maybe you picked this up out of curiosity, thinking you would like to lose a little weight. But it's so much more important than that. Your life is about to dramatically change for the better. "How?" you ask.

You will never have to diet again.

You are going to start on a journey to live your best, happiest life.

You are about to become the tip of the spear of something big, an earth-changing paradigm shift that you will one day share with your grandchildren ... AND

You will not have to do it alone.

You can do this, and I am here to support you every single step of the way.

This book is going to change the world, starting with you. Yes, you. Because you, my friend, are a fellow Warrior for light, for peace, for truth, for justice, a defender of the weak and the voiceless, and you have just found your Tribe. You don't know it yet, but I do. You were meant to pick up this book and read it. You are already a fellow Warrior of the Rainbow, and we are in this together. So welcome—but hurry up. Get on your mighty steed. We don't have a lot of time left to save the world, so let's ride!

Okay, okay, I feel you hesitating. *"This lady is just plain crazy, obviously. ... What kind of a cult is this? Holy crap."* Okay, I'll calm down a bit. This is not a cult, I promise. Just give me a few pages and you'll start to see.

Let's start at the beginning. I know why you picked this book up. It was the word "diet," right? I know what you're looking for. I've been where you are, standing in your shoes, overweight, unhappy, and seeking real change, but not quite sure how to get there or even where I wanted to go or why. I wanted an easy solution, someone to just tell me what to do, or a magical diet pill, while at the same time I was thinking that all the "baggage" of extra weight I was carrying around with me was all my fault—for being lazy, for lacking willpower, for eating too much, for not exercising. I know how physically, mentally, and emotionally exhausting it feels to be overweight.

How many diets have you already tried that just haven't worked for you? High-protein, low-carb, low-fat? High-carb, low-protein, no-fat? This "guaranteed, big-name diet program," or that "heavily advertised weight-loss program," one after the next, assaulting your senses on the television. Maybe you have tried these programs and lost weight, but you gained it all back when you returned to your "normal" way of eating. Maybe you have just never been successful with weight loss, ever.

Maybe you have just decided to lose weight because, darn it, you want to look and feel good again ... or maybe your doctor told you that your health is in serious risk unless you lose some weight. Maybe you've already been diagnosed with diabetes, heart disease, or cancer, or maybe you have high blood pressure or high cholesterol or suffer from an autoimmune disorder? Or maybe you just picked up this book because you feel like a steaming pile of dog doo and are sick and tired of looking like crap.

Folks, this is serious business, and it is not all about how good you look in a bathing suit (though that is definitely the icing on the cake!). We are here to talk about the cake itself. And if you're wondering if you can have your cake and eat it too, the answer is "yes." *Yes*, now I've got you back with me— with the promise that I won't take your cake away! So let's start.

But first, who am I?

My story

My name is Laura Robinson Oatman. I was born in LA on Halloween in 1959 on my mother's birthday. Back then I was Lorre Jean Robinson. I grew up in the sixties, way up in the wild hills of Beverly Hills, attended Beverly Hills Catholic School, and spent all my free time hiking those still-rustic canyons, always looking for coyotes and foxes, raccoons and rattlesnakes. In the seventies I was the typical California teenager, an animal lover, a beach lover, eating a vegetarian diet and practicing yoga and Transcendental Meditation with the Maharishi Mahesh Yogi. I attended Marymount High School with the daughters of celebrities and millionaires, but I was never one of those popular girls. I spent most of my time studying, and attended college courses at UCLA across the street while still in high school and still too young to drive. Like an alien from another planet, I had an insatiable hunger to learn about the history of our Whole Earth.

In 1976, the summer after my high school graduation, our family went on an amazing trip around the world. I mention it because it was such a milestone moment in my life that forever altered my worldview. Growing up in LA and attending private schools, I was sheltered, to say the least. I grew up with the idea that people from different cultural backgrounds were segregated into different hoods, and were just ... different. But on our trip around the world, I saw the world as it really was and is—an amazing watercolor painting as one country, one culture, one people who blend into the next without any distinct division ... a million different shades of the rainbow. There was no black or white, brown or yellow. And the many cultures were so fascinating and so beautiful to me, not to mention the foods and the music and the people, all of it. It was a remarkable highlight of my life. 1976. It was that summer that I fell in love, with the Whole Earth.

When we returned from that trip, our family moved to Newport Beach in Orange County, one hour south of LA. I studied social sciences at UC Irvine, then architecture in graduate school at UCLA, and married a fellow architecture student, Homer Oatman, in 1984. Settling down in the OC and being the good Catholics that we were, we had five babies in five years, four boys and a girl. Though I did take fourteen years off to be a stay-at-home mom when the kids were little, I worked as an architect for many years for WATG, a large firm whose specialty is designing hotels around the world. In 2006, I went to work for a hotel developer whose office was in downtown LA, thus beginning my daily round-trip commute of more than three hours for three years. I was a project director there, and I had a comfortable six-figure income with lots of international travel that had me working on beaches (literally) in Mexico, the Caribbean, Miami, and Southeast Asia. And I was getting paid for it. On the surface, we had it all—a wonderful marriage, two fantastic incomes, five wonderful kids, and a job that had me traveling all over the Whole Earth that I loved.

But underneath all that I was a mess. The young girl that was once a meditating vegetarian yogi of the 1970s had become a carnivorous, junk-food-eating, stressed-out corporate executive of the 2000s. I had really lost touch with who I was. I was making good money, but I was thirty pounds heavier than I am today. I was under constant stress and owned by my Blackberry 24/7 no matter the time zone. I had no time for my husband or my kids who, even though they were teenagers, still wanted Mom around once in a while for birthdays or hockey tournaments. We never went to church—who had time for that? The stress from work led me to eating all sorts of junk food, drinking too much and "social smoking" on business trips. I had no time to cook, so I picked up fast food, ate on the run, and put on weight. I was constantly coughing, sneezing or congested, never sure if it was a cold or allergies or asthma or usually a combination of all three. One of my last business trips to Anguilla was a doozy; I returned home with both a torn retina in my left eye and a mysterious insect bite on my right leg that turned into a flesh-eating-bacteria-type rash that stumped the dermatologists and didn't heal for over two years. Everything looked good on the surface, but underneath I was hiding a physical, mental, emotional, and spiritual mess.

Then, in 2008 the economy crashed. In October, I lost my job when the design and construction division were no longer part of their corporate plan. Three months later, my husband's residential architecture firm also went through a bloody downsizing, as the custom home division was no longer a part of their corporate plan. So there we were in early 2009, thrown to the curb, stunned, both suddenly unemployed. I was almost fifty, he was almost sixty, and neither of us had any hope of being rehired anywhere. Not with architecture firms downsizing all around us and the market being flooded with tech-savvy young architects willing to work for a lot less money, even interning for free. At that time we were supporting three of our kids living away from home at college, with a junior and senior in high school wondering if they would still be able to go to college too. It really couldn't have hit us at a worse time.

In a state of shock and without skipping a beat, we immediately formed "Oatman Architects," suddenly becoming very familiar again with our church pews. With my hospitality and his custom home design background, we hung out our shingle: "Designing homes that feel like resorts and hotels that feel like home." Homer was blessed with a nice custom home project right away that kept us off the streets that first year, but there wasn't a lot of work on the luxury hotel side (the understatement of the year). So I went through a bit of a midlife crisis, though in retrospect it wasn't a crisis at all but a revelation and a transformation.

It started with the thought that maybe it wasn't so wise to have two architects under one roof when the economy goes into a death spiral, which it always does from time to time (though this one was by far the worst we had ever seen!). The only thing that was certain was that both Mom and Dad being economically-at-risk architects wasn't safe or smart with our five young adult children relying on us for financial support; we needed to "diversify our portfolio." Homer's custom home design started to take off, but aside from a couple fun winery concept designs in Northern California, my hotel design career seemed dead in the water. Maybe it was time to reconsider who I was and what I really wanted to be when I grew up. I wasn't sure what that was, but I did know that I needed to start by picking myself back up, losing my excess weight, and regaining my physical health.

So I picked up a little book that I thought might be a good place to start, *Skinny Bitch*, with this cool cartoon character skinny model on the cover. It promised a quick-and-easy way for me to become a skinny bitch too and start looking fabulous! Well, okay, why not? Little did I know what was about to happen. By the time I finished reading the book, two hours later, my world had been rocked. I would never, ever touch meat and dairy again. The inner me, the real me, the authentic animal-loving vegetarian me was reawakened—which led to my current life journey. It all began with food, with a transition to a 100 percent whole-foods plant-based vegan diet!

Wait, don't put the book down yet, my meat-loving friends! Hear me out.

Once I lost the meat and dairy, I lost the weight, I felt better than I had in years, and I started to follow my passion instead of a paycheck. Not only did my physical health improve, but my emotional, mental and spiritual life improved, as I went back to yoga and meditation and church on Sundays. I was now completely inspired to learn more about health, wellness and holistic nutrition. I learned that there was more to this than just removing the meat and dairy, though that was huge. I also learned about all the processed crap we are eating, the evil trifecta of salty/sweet/fat tastes that are produced in laboratories to keep us all addicted and fat. There was big money in an unhealthy America. I was hooked on learning more.

I went back to school at the Institute for Integrative Nutrition in New York and received my certification as a Holistic Health Coach. Then I dove deeply into the two areas of health and wellness that resonated most deeply with me – the vegan diet, and the ancient lifestyle techniques of Ayurveda from India. I became a Certified Plant-Based Nutritionist through eCornell, and then a Certified Ayurvedic Educator through the California College of Ayurveda. With those certifications under my belt, I then studied with Physicians Committee for Responsible Medicine (PCRM) in Washington DC to deepen my knowledge around the health benefits of a plant-based diet with their Food For Life Program, and my young company, Whole Earth Wellness, became an "Educational Alliance Partner" with PCRM.

In March 2011, I started coaching individual clients, leading group programs and hosting wellness retreats, teaching and supporting a vegan diet and a holistic lifestyle, not just as a path toward individual health, but as a path toward health for the Whole Earth. The sixteen-year-old vegetarian, meditating, animal-loving, Whole-Earth-loving beach girl had finally come full circle to who she was so many years ago, to who she really is deep down at the core of her being. I had finally found my purpose, at age fifty, at the halftime of my life.

That's a brief outline of my story. Now let's get down to business.

What's the big deal if everyone is a little "bigger"?

I have noticed lately, as the nation's waistlines are increasing, that there is more and more of a tendency to say, "It's okay. Love yourself and feel comfortable in your own skin no matter how chubby." Plus-sized models are featured on the cover of *Sports Illustrated*. "Big is beautiful" and "Embrace your size" are the recurring messages—as they feed you the commercials on TV for this new diabetic pill, or that medical scooter, or this sampler box of fun, free, colorful catheters! Being heavy would be fine if extra weight was only a superficial issue, and it wouldn't bother me at all if I didn't know what I know. This is not about self-esteem or looking good. This is not about "accepting yourself." This is a national health crisis of unprecedented proportion.

Did you know that worldwide obesity has doubled since 1980 (1)? Two-thirds of our population is overweight, and one-third is morbidly obese (2). (And they don't call it "morbidly obese" because they are worried about how you look.) More than 40 million kids under the age of five were overweight or obese in 2010 (3), so we are passing this trend on as fast as we can to our next generation. Obesity is directly linked to our biggest killer diseases: heart disease, cancer, and diabetes (4). For the first time, our children have a lower life expectancy than their parents (5). And with all the advances in medicine, we cannot blame this on the doctors or hospitals. Regarding our biggest killers—obesity, heart disease, diabetes, cancer—we are feeding these deadly, chronic diseases with a slow drip of poison, slowly but surely killing ourselves with what we eat, with what we have been brainwashed to believe is "normal food."

What's more, the cost of the medical care required to deal with these diseases is straining our global economies, not to mention individual households. Each year, 100 million people slide into poverty as a result of medical care payments (6). Another 150 million people are forced to spend nearly half their income on medical expenses (7), and most of these illnesses stem from obesity—which is entirely preventable.

We are never educated about the prevention of obesity, the cause of these chronic, killer diseases. It is as if these things were beyond our control, as if these boogey-monster diseases come like lightning strikes from out of nowhere to slay otherwise healthy folks without warning. We are led to believe that these chronic diseases are normal, that everyone should take multiple medications daily, that everyone sooner or later will end up in a motorized wheelchair. Look how fun they make it all look in those television advertisements for this drug or that! I can't keep them all straight anymore, but man, those people taking those drugs on TV are all living the good life, right?

This is all wrong.

I am now fifty-five while writing this book, and my husband is sixty-five, and we go to as many funerals for friends in our age group as my parents do now in their eighties. Our "Baby Boomer" friends in their fifties and sixties are suddenly dropping dead from heart attacks or strokes or deep vein thrombosis; or being diagnosed with colon cancer or breast cancer and undergoing the devastating effects of chemotherapy and radiation; or they are simply taking handfuls of medications daily to deal with their high blood pressure, their high cholesterol, their blood sugar levels, their ongoing depression, their inability to sleep, and one side effect leads to another medication leads to another side effect leads to another medication, and on and on it goes. The frustrating thing for me is that everyone acts as if this is normal. This is not right; everyone deserves to live a long, healthy life, and I see my friends' lives being stolen away from them far too soon, and it is not their fault. They just didn't know.

In addition to the decline in our physical health, there are other holistic wellness issues at work against us — the current global economic recession that has many out of work and finances out of whack. Beyond health and the economy, all you have to do is flip between TV stations to see the deep, bitter cultural divide in our country, and really around the world. All of this fighting, bickering, and stress have created a spiritual crisis, which has no doubt had an impact on achieving sustained well-being. And at the extreme end of all of this, our world in some places seems to be spiraling out of control with violence, terrorism, and war. We should be evolving beyond all this by now. There is something terribly wrong with this picture.

And the kicker?

All of this is preventable. And the beautiful thing is this. The simple solution is the same, no matter the disease, no matter the social issue, and the real beauty is that it starts with you. **You** can be that change. Sound crazy? Trust me. You'll get it by the end. It is a diet and lifestyle that benefits both yourself personally and the world at large because at the end of the day, it is all the same. We are sick because the Earth is sick, and the Earth is sick because we are sick. It is a vicious downward spiral.

So here I am in California, and there you are wherever you are on this Earth, and we are both going to start throwing the pebbles of truth into the pond while others everywhere will do the same. And we are going to do this together. The pebbles will turn into rocks, the rocks into boulders, the ripples into waves, and we will change this world by spreading the news about a whole-foods, plant-based, vegan diet, combined with holistic wellness. In this book, we're also tapping into centuries-old principles of health and well-being, holistic wellness guidelines that are accessible to everyone, no matter where you're standing on Earth or what century you are in! This is why the book that you have just picked up is called the *Whole Earth Diet*. It starts with real, Whole foods for you, the individual. The recipes and guidelines come from around the Whole Earth. And it ends with the healing of the Earth, that is once again Whole and peaceful. It is holistic in the broadest and deepest sense of the word.

Remember, though, that it all starts with you. This book is going to help YOU finally lose that weight and keep it off. This book is going to help and support YOU to live your healthiest, happiest, best life possible … and in the process,

YOU can help change the world for the better! Sound good? Are you in? How could you not be??

Let's get started.

What is the Whole Earth Diet, and what makes it different?

The Whole Earth Diet is not a diet in the traditional sense of the word. There are not a lot of strict rules on eating less to help you lose weight. We all know *those* diets. They. Just. Don't. Work! If you are eating restricted calories, or if you are eating only the frozen meals that a particular diet program sells to you, sure, you will lose weight, at first. But I promise you, you will gain it all back. Why? Because you didn't learn to completely rethink nutrition in a much larger context. You were probably taught to eat something similar to what you have been eating all along, using the USDA Food Pyramid as your nutritional guide. Just eat less! Oh, and don't forget to exercise like crazy! If you don't lose weight, you're just not trying hard enough!

With the Whole Earth Diet, you will learn all about plant-based nutrition, and rethink everything you thought you knew about food. You will be eating real, whole, plant-based, organic, seasonal, locally grown foods. Food that grew gently out of the ground instead of violently out of a slaughterhouse. All the fruits, veggies, whole grains and beans that you want - cooked, raw, or sprouted. You can also enjoy healthy fats, nuts, and seeds, as you work towards eventually eliminating meat, dairy, and processed foods. The recipes are simple, easy and familiar, with simple substitutions made. I will definitely take away your animal meat and dairy, but I will give you amazing plant-based substitutes instead, and will not touch your black coffee, your dark chocolate, or your sulfite-free organic red wine! Hey, I'm not crazy!

The Whole Earth Diet will help you lose weight, just like any fad diet that is out there. But this is much more than a weightloss diet. When you lose weight on the Whole Earth Diet, it will be the last time you will ever need to lose weight. The new, healthier, slimmer, more beautiful you will be the "new you" for the rest of your life. But why? How is it any different from the Paleo Diet, or the South Beach Diet, or the This Diet, or the That Diet? No matter what diet you are on or how awesome your health coach or how adorable your fitness trainer with the man-bun, guess what? You are doomed to fail. Of those people who lose weight while dieting, 90–95% of them will put it all back on again (8). Why?

A couple reasons really.

First of all, those other diets address your physical health only. They talk about food. They may talk about fitness. But it is all physical health, and you are not just a body, you are also a heart, a mind, and a soul. Unless you make lifestyle changes that promote emotional, mental, and spiritual wellness, along with dietary changes, you are doomed to fail. You will stay on the diet only as long as your weakest link allows you to.

If your mind is not well, you will not stay the course. You will tell yourself it's okay to skip your morning exercise, or mindlessly nibble on salty snacks when bored, or you will let financial stress from overspending disrupt healthy habits.

If your heart is not well, you will not stay the course. You will allow yourself to nibble on sweets whenever your mood is low or you have fought with someone close to you and you are craving emotional support. After all, if you don't love yourself, you will never feel truly worthy of living a healthy, happy life.

If your soul is empty, you will find no reason to carry on because you do not understand the purpose or meaning behind any of it anyway, and the world is going to hell in a handbasket so who cares how much longer you have to live? When your soul is empty you have a deep sorrow, an existential angst, that will never allow you to live a truly happy life.

The Whole Earth Diet sees you as you are, a whole and complete, complex and multifaceted soul having a human experience, and we will work on all parts and pieces of wellness with the ultimate goal, not just a health body, but a happy life ... because at the end of the day, that is really what we want, isn't it? A long and happy life. No other diet promises you happiness. Whole Earth Diet does, and for this reason it will work.

But there is another reason, too, that Whole Earth Diet works. All of those other diets are purely self-serving. You are thinking only about yourself and how you look. And at the end of the day, none of us can ever care enough about how we look to fire up that willpower of steel that we need to "just say no" to the glorious rush of instant gratification that forbidden food offers. What makes this diet different, what makes this the ONLY diet that will work for permanent change, is this diet is about something much, much bigger than you or I. A true shift in how we eat and how we live can come only from a much deeper place than just a superficial concern about how we look. To be successful, we as human beings need to be motivated by something much larger than ourselves.

Once you start eating this way, once you eliminate the meat and the dairy from your plate, you will wake up to the realization that most of the world's evils stem from our ability to turn a blind eye to the evil we have been inflicting for centuries on animals. You will make changes not just to what you eat but to how you live, what you buy, and what companies you support. This diet is about future generations and saving humanity from itself. Until the world wakes up to see how important this is, we—you and I—must shout this knowledge from the rooftops and be living and breathing examples of good health and happiness ourselves because our children, all the animals, and the planet Earth itself depend on what you are about to learn here in this book. So stop all those silly trendy diets now, stop chasing the latest fitness guru with the six-pack abs and the cool yoga outfits, take a deep breath, and start this journey with me and the many others who have awakened to a new way of thinking about nutrition, food, and life in general.

Whole Earth Diet is about creating a healthy body, a happy life, and a peaceful world. No other diet can make this claim. Welcome to the light, my friend. It is only going to get better and better, starting now.

Who is this diet for?

Before we get into the details, let's address the elephant in the room: why on earth should you take this huge leap of faith with me and give any kind of serious thought to giving up your meat and dairy? Before we begin the next chapter where we get into this in detail, let me first talk politics, religion and labels. (As if I haven't gotten myself into enough trouble already!) This diet is intended for everyone, no matter your politics or your religion. Though I hate using labels, for brevity I will use them here. My tribe is conservative and liberal, religious and atheists alike. But I have seen many conservative religious folks read no further than this without giving it a second thought, thinking it's a "liberal thing". But since 78.4 percent of Americans identify as Christian (9), and 40 percent describe themselves as conservative (10), I want to address politics and religion first before I even start talking about meat and dairy. I want everyone to hear what I have to say, not just one side of the aisle. My tribe is all of you, and I'm not leaving anyone behind. I love both elephants and donkeys equally!

I have many religious conservative friends and family who think I am crazy. They believe that farm animals are meant for us to eat; it's just the way it's always been, and it is what God intended for us. They also hate the idea of the government, or anyone, telling them what to eat. They don't want a "nanny state" infringing on their freedom to make their food choices for them. I get it. But though the PR machine *appears* to be promoting fruits and veggies on the surface, the "nanny state" is actually promoting meat and dairy with tax subsidies, so by eating what you please (which is what the advertisers are tricking you into thinking), you are given the illusion of free choice but actually eating *exactly* what the government wants you to. The government spends **billions** of taxpayer dollars on subsidies that support the production of meat and dairy. The USDA is full of people with financial interests in the meat and dairy industries, so while the government may act like they are promoting fruits and veggies, more than 60 percent of agricultural subsidies either directly or indirectly support meat and dairy production, while less than 1 percent benefit fruit and vegetable producers (11). Follow the money, not the talking heads. These are our hard-earned tax dollars at work, keeping us all sick, promoting what they know is bad for us. Don't buy into the illusion. The nanny state wants you to keep eating meat and dairy because an unhealthy population is so much easier to keep under control. And I know you are MUCH smarter than that. I have faith in my conservative friends.

My atheist liberal friends just think I am crazy period because I believe in God and am contributing to overpopulation and global warming by having five children! I live in conservative Orange County, and I am running a for-profit business to make money, which is bad, real bad. I promote a 100 percent plant-based diet, but have recently disassociated from labeling myself as a "vegan". I will still call foods vegan, or restaurants vegan, but I don't think people should call themselves vegan. Products should have labels, but not people. I don't believe in labeling myself or anyone else; labels are automatically divisive. I don't eat any meat or dairy now, I never will again, and I do it for all the same moral reasons that the so-called "ethical vegans" (or "vegan police") do. But I don't want to label myself as different or endorse this diet as being anything different from what we should ALL be eating. This should be the normal way to eat and shouldn't be set aside as weird or different, put into a box with a nice, neat label called vegan, and held at arms length from the rest of the world. I wouldn't mind bringing back the label "canivore" though, and maybe calling those folks out as weird extremists who continue to eat meat and dairy after they read this book! Finally, the current vegan tribe brings to mind an attitude of judgmental and angry confrontation because of the actions of some of my vocal vegan brethren, creating the notion that all vegans are wild and crazy extremists. And the big food/drug/hospital/insurance companies are loving this; they will continue to paint us as liberal whackos because then the majority of the population will continue happily eating meat and dairy without a second thought, not wanting to be one of "them." After all, an unhealthy population equals enormous profits for meat, dairy, food, drug, medical devices, hospitals, and insurance companies.

I believe that what we all have in common is much more than what divides us—the desire for freedom to live our longest, healthiest, happiest life, and the desire to see our loved ones live their longest, healthiest, happiest lives. I wanted to address this first, since our country is so polarized that even health has become political issue. And I wanted to point out that the misguided politics of nutrition ("conservatives eat meat, liberals are vegetarians") is a bunch of horse manure! Aside from most (but not all (12)) Texan cattle ranchers who may conform to this stereotype, there is no reason that all conservatives need to march to the same drummer, especially after you hear what I am about to tell you.

So why should you listen to me after you know what a wishy-washy political centrist I am? Because of my motivation. Always look at motive before you buy anything that anyone is trying to sell you.

What honestly motivates me? Compassion, deep empathy, and an end to unnecessary suffering and early death. A vision where all living creatures, human and animal alike live long, healthy, happy lives, and the earth itself is healthy and well. And there is peace. And happiness. And lots of love. Sure, there is no such thing as perfection, this may be nothing more than a lovely but naïve dream, but there is excellence in the trying.

My motive is not profit. Even if I never make a single penny from this book, I will be fine. Oatman Architects has finally taken off and Homer is doing an awesome job supporting the two of us with his talent designing incredible custom homes. We certainly don't have the income we once did before the crash, but the kids are (mostly) grown, and we've learned to live much more modestly. Our needs are much simpler and we appreciate everything so much more than before. It's not that I would have a problem with making a penny or two; I'm just saying I don't need to do this to pay rent or survive. I am very blessed to be in the position that I am today, with the luxury of being able to write this book without feeling desperate to make money. And I'm not going to sell out if someone offers me money to do an about-face, to say that "well, the vegan diet just didn't work for me," and start to advocate eating animals again. (Yes, this does happen.) You must look at the motive behind all the folks continuing to advocate eating meat, be they ranchers, advertisers, health coaches, government lobbyists, or celebrity chefs. Even so-called spiritual leaders who may or may not be vegetarian themselves, who keep silent on the disconnect between their flocks continuing to eat meat and struggling with their spirituality. Their motive is money. Profit. Pure and simple. Once they take the meat and dairy away from their clientele, their profits are gone. I don't blame these businesses completely; they need to survive. They know what sells today, and they do need money today, but they need to wake up and shift, and soon. The money will follow when they follow their conscience.

My motive is not anarchy. I am not looking to disrupt our economy or put anyone out of work. I don't have a problem with profit, as long as it's not made on the back of anyone else's life, liberty, or pursuit of happiness. I am not looking to disrupt lives, just to save lives. You cannot say the same of some of the animal liberation groups burning down barns and blowing up tractors. That is not the way to change hearts and minds. Their motive is anger and though I understand it, anger can never change people's hearts and minds. Farmers and ranchers and other agricultural businesses will change when demand for meat and dairy goes down; the supply side will change to accommodate whatever the consumer demands. I am now seeing old factory farms and cattle ranches being converted to organic farms, nut orchards, vineyards, animal rescue farms, and organic manure producers. I don't want to see these old farming families suffer at all and in any way; I just want to help open their eyes and let them see there is another way.

My motive is not attention. I am the most reluctant messenger and have always hated to be the center of attention. The first time I ever spoke publicly, in high school, I walked to the podium, stared into the crowd for about thirty very long seconds, dropped the mic, and walked off the stage! I've done a couple speaking gigs since then, and I will continue to, but every time my heart races, my palms sweat, my stomach churns, and I always have a last thought about sneaking out and hiding before it begins! I am quietly spreading my message every way I can, but you won't see my Facebook wall littered with softly-lit selfies with duck lips, pitching my diet. I have recently had some beautiful photos taken just for this book actually, but it was a long, weird photoshoot day for me to be the center of attention all day with a camera pointed at me. My motive is not narcissism;

the last thing I want you to ever feel is envy or jealousy of me. I don't want the attention. I'm content and at peace. This is not about me.

This is about YOU. And so I must come out of my comfort zone and reach out to YOU, my friend, because I can never be truly happy if you are not happy. We are connected, you and I.

My motive is deep compassion. I know there will always be suffering that's beyond our control, but intentional, inexcusable suffering and death that comes far too early in life needs to end. I have always had an intense ability to feel compassion, a physical ability to feel another's pain, for as long as I can remember. When others are in pain, I am in pain. When I was a kid, if I saw someone injure their arm, my arm would hurt. I have always been this way, and I consider it a gift. So when I awoke to the realization that the reason people were suffering—dying of disease, dying of hunger, dying in battle—stemmed from the suffering and deaths of animals ... well, that was it for me. Slam dunk. This has become my life work now, to get meat and dairy off the plate and save the world in the process.

My passion brings tears to my eyes even as I write this. I want to scream and shout, but I know I need to go slowly and gently and not let my passion be misinterpreted as anger. It is such a fine line, and the written word so much more easily misinterpreted in tone than the spoken word. But there is no anger here, no judgement, only deep passion, deep sadness, deep conviction, and deep urgency. This is what I hope to convey to you, and hope I don't drive you away in the process. I hope that you are feeling me reach out to you as you read these words. I have nothing but deep love and compassion for you, and I want to support you, nourish you, encourage you, guide you, educate you, and love you into your best self.

I went into this much detail because I really want you on board, whether you call yourself liberal or conservative, religious or atheist, old or young, married or single, vegan or carnivore. I am putting together a true rainbow coalition tribe of warriors to save this planet, ignoring all labels around diet, religion and politics, and I need every single one of you on board with me. No stragglers. Hurry up, time is wasting!

Where do we begin?

Your first step? Throw the USDA food pyramid out the window, no matter how many times they "revise" it (as they are doing again this year). It's all a bunch of nonsense, tainted by money and politics. I am about to challenge everything you've been told about the traditional concept of a balanced diet. I am going to educate and support you toward thinking differently, eating differently, and acting differently, and I am going to back it all up with the most recent cutting-edge findings from esteemed medical experts that support a plant-based diet. Your healthy new body will be created by eating a meat-free and dairy-free diet that embraces a variety of global dishes from different cultures around the world.

Unlike some diets that are geographically specific (e.g., South Beach Diet, Swiss Diet, Sonoma Diet, Mediterranean Diet, etc.) that work well for people that live in those locales but not for everyone, I have taken traditional "comfort food" recipes from all over the world and modified them to be meat- and dairy-free, and so much healthier! So no matter where you were born, what you grew up eating, Whole Earth Diet will have recipes that you will love in addition to simple ideas for how to eat every day, with or without recipes, to make it simple for you. It is simple, quick, healthy, AND delicious. You will be able to stick to any diet plan if you are eating foods that you love, particularly meals that remind you of your family, your childhood, your home ... and especially if it doesn't feel like a "diet" at all. And the best part is, you can eat—you can eat A LOT—and you will still lose weight.

Beyond the food itself, besides WHAT to eat, Whole Earth Diet will also help you discover when, where, and how to eat by combining ancient wellness wisdom from China, India, Babylonia, and Greece that today are being proven true via modern science. These tidbits of wisdom will provide you with simple eating and lifestyle guidelines to create your whole healthy body.

In addition to learning about food, you will also learn about the equally important side of the equation for physical health—what you DO with your body, otherwise known as exercise! The word "exercise" has struck fear into the hearts of dieters for years, but I am going to give you a brand new way of looking at exercise so that you will not only look forward to it, you will be able to stick with it. It will not be a temporary fling this time, but a permanent, positive lifestyle change! We will explore the four classical elements of your self: exercising your earth element through weight training, exercising your water element through yoga, exercising your fire element with dance or martial arts (or anything that makes you laugh-out-loud happy), and exercising your wind element with cardiovascular exercise, such as walking, hiking, running, and bike riding. Together we will remake your lifestyle to include both variety AND fun in your weekly routine ... things that make you happy AND just happen to burn calories and keep you fit.

After giving you all the simple and straightforward steps you need for the healthy body, I will also gently lead you down the path of complete, integrated, body/mind/heart/soul holistic health because once the body is totally healthy and happy, the mind, heart, and soul just naturally want to tag along!

I have broken this book into three parts. The first section, Healthy Body, is all about nutrition and the plant-based diet, and it is the foundation of everything that follows. The second section, Happy Life, is about holistic wellness—creating a healthy mind, healthy heart, and healthy soul—which is the foundation for living your happiest life. The final section, Peaceful World, steps all the way back to the big-picture view, that when all of these individuals start to live their best, healthiest, happiest life (yourself included) we will begin a ripple effect that will be unstoppable, that will create an Earth that is healthy and happy and peaceful.

To expand on this a little more, in Part One, I am going to help you to rethink nutrition. As part of my training, I have studied hundreds of nutritional theories and read hundreds of diet books. I have done all the homework for you, and I continue to educate myself all day every day while you are doing what you need to do all day. I have distilled it down to the best possible summary for you so that you can benefit—in just a few hours—from everything I have spent years studying. I will make the case for a whole-foods, plant-based vegan diet and give you some real-world advice on foods to avoid, foods to eat in moderation, and foods to eat as much as you want. I will provide you with interfaith holiday ideas to rethink the way we celebrate our food-centered holidays—keeping all the good stuff, getting rid of the bad. I am going to give you some added bonuses from the combined wisdom of modern technology and ancient philosophy—healing herbs and spices and teas. The last chapter in Part One will be a practical, step-by-step, simple guide for you to put this all into practice, to simply eat well.

In Part Two, we will talk a little bit about ancient wellness philosophies from around the world, and how (and why) we can apply these guidelines to twenty-first-century holistic wellness. We will talk about guidelines around mindful food preparation and mindful eating. We will talk about exercise, the health benefits of routines, and mental, emotional, and spiritual wellness. We will think about finding our life purpose, reviving our heart's passions, and remembering how to pray. The last chapter will be a practical, step-by-step simple guide for you to put this all into practice, how to live a passionate, purposeful and prayerful life, and find true happiness and bliss.

In Part Three, we will learn about the connection between what we eat, and why the world has gone mad. In this section, I will illustrate how my Catholic faith supports me not only with this wellness philosophy, but also how it supports me personally. We will talk about interfaith spirituality and the need for all faiths, all cultures, to not only learn "tolerance" for each other, but true love and respect for each other, as well as friendship. The only way we are going to create a peaceful world for our children to enjoy is to recognize the destructive path we are currently on, acknowledge it, and turn this ship around 180 degrees. It is only with God's help that this will be done. Peace begins on your plate, but becomes a reality when you remember to say grace before your plant-based meals.

At the end of the book, I will give you all kinds of great info—recipes, nutritional charts, further resources (i.e., recommended books to read, movies to watch, websites to visit)—and, of course, I will cite all the various studies, research articles, and books that I used as references in writing this book.

Naturally, I will provide lots of ways for you to stay involved with me and with Whole Earth Wellness through the website, the mobile app, global webinars, or for complete immersion in the Whole Earth Wellness lifestyle, coming to one of our amazing international, interfaith wellness retreats. Finally, I am here for you, live, if you need me, to provide support, encouragement, and accountability as you start this amazing journey to health. If you would like to learn more about the programs that I offer, please visit my website, send me a personal message, and I will be there for you. Not too many books will do that for you! I am literally energetically with you at this moment as you read these words. I am here.

What are these changes you speak of?

Change, change, change. Okay, I'm going to change, but how? Change is scary. Is this going to be a good thing? If I give up meat and dairy, if I start following these unfamiliar ancient lifestyle guidelines that sound a little weird, what results am I going to see? What is going to happen? I'm actually a little bit afraid to change, after all. (And, is this really a cult?)

Do any of those questions resonate with you? Do ALL of those questions resonate with you?

First of all, let me assure you that this is not a cult. I don't want to convert anyone to anything; I just want what is best for you. I don't want you to convert to my religion, or move to my country, or become like me, or dress like me, or change your hairstyle, or switch your political party, or make any drastic changes to who you are and what you believe because I believe that the beauty of our global humanity comes from our rainbow of differences. Dark leafy greens are good, but we don't want only green in our salad. We want reds and oranges and purples and yellows and whites and browns to complete the salad.

I want nothing more than for you to be who you are, but to be the very best, healthiest, and happiest version of you— exactly how you are today, but better! The best you.

If you follow the advice I give in this book, I can promise you all the following and more:

Physically, you are going to lose all your unwanted extra weight for the last time. You are going to finally look and feel absolutely amazing! But that is not all. You are going to gain incredible reserves of energy similar to the energy you had as a young child. Have you ever seen someone that just radiates good health? They seem to almost have a supernatural glow, right? Well, that is going to be YOU in just a few months' time.

If you are suffering from a chronic health issue, it may be cured or at least reduced dramatically. If you are on pharmaceutical drugs, you will be able to reduce and potentially eliminate your medicine altogether (under your doc's supervision, of course!). You will actually look years younger than you do today. You will sleep better, and you will be adding years to your life. Even if you are currently obese, even if you are currently suffering from a debilitating and potentially life-threatening disease, the Whole Earth Diet will help you regain health and strength, and potentially make a full recovery. At the very least, it will help eliminate discomfort and add more valuable and happy years to your life no matter how severe your condition. Whatever your condition, whatever your age, this diet cannot help but improve your health and give you the best fighting chance at a long, healthy, and happy life.

And if you are fearing change because you think it will estrange you from everything that is familiar and comfortable—your traditions, your family, your friends who may still be stuck in the past—never fear. This "diet" respects, honors, and wholeheartedly embraces and celebrates all cultural holidays and traditions (even ones that are not are own!), while at the same time moving things forward toward a new and improved future.

As your body becomes healthier, you will also notice changes in your thinking, **in your mind**. The mind-body connection is always very strong, but when you are eating like this, you will notice it all the more. As you become physically healthy, your thoughts will become healthier, more positive and optimistic. You will start to see the glass as half-full again. Your mind will be less distracted, less scattered. You will have a new focus and a newfound mental strength and willpower to "just say no" to temptations. You will see clearly a path forward for yourself—where you are going with your life, with your career—potentially a completely new direction with a clearer vision. If you are out of work, you will find a job. If you are in a job that you hate, you will find a way to leave it. You will start to work toward a new career that you love, that gives your life meaning and purpose. It just happens. Miracles happen. The universe commands it. The world is changing, and you will change with it. And when you have found your true life purpose, you will find it impossible to be unhappy.

As your body and your mind become healthy, **your heart will follow**. As you now have a healthy body and a new career with more meaning, you will naturally find it so much easier to just love, love, love yourself! You will learn how to love yourself without feeling guilty about doing so. You will step into the amazing person that you were meant to be, without holding back. Once you have learned to truly love yourself, you will finally now be able to truly love others. This abundance of love will overflow for all others—your spouse, your family, your friends, mankind, all other species, and the world. No matter what your life circumstance, whether you are old or young, single or married, living alone or in a houseful of people, you will find your life filled with total, overflowing love. And when you are filled with love like this, you will find it impossible to hate.

With your body, mind, and heart now all in harmony and growing together side by side, naturally, that last and most important element of yourself, **your soul**, will be nourished and will flourish. You will notice an inner spiritual awakening, even if you have never ever been a spiritual person before. You may not call it "God", this feeling of pure love growing inside your heart that comes from eating peace, but that love that is growing is God expressing through you. You may choose to remain purely spiritual, or you may find yourself being drawn back to a certain religion, a tribe in which to manifest, as your inner spirituality grows and seeks an outward expression. All the problems with religions today are the result of traditional religions embracing politics and wordly things instead of inner spirituality. I will always encourage you to first develop and work on your inner spirituality, then go back and revisit the faith of your ancestors, or any faith. Our religions need more people filled with real spirituality and lacking in political motivation or ambition, hatred, and divisiveness. This will infuse our tired, old, angry, politicized religions with new life, with true Spirit, and they will finally be able to serve the purpose for which they were intended. Your renewed spirit will be a part of that change, and as a fully developed spiritual being, you will find it impossible to fear anything.

Once all of this happens, you will understand what it truly means to live a full and happy life. Happiness, peace, and bliss will be yours every day, no matter what life throws at you.

Mahatma Gandhi said, "Be the change you wish to see in the world." The changes you see happening in you will start to also happen all around you, like dominoes falling, like ripples in a pond spreading and becoming waves. Just as you have become physically, mentally, emotionally, and spiritually healthy and happy, you'll impact those around you, and you will help to change our world.

And it all begins with food, with step number one— changing what you eat. Ready, set, c'mon Warriors! Now is the time ... jump on your steed! Let's ride!

PART ONE:

HEALTHY BODY ~ THE WHOLE EARTH DIET

"Let food be thy medicine and medicine be thy food"

~Hippocrates, Greek physician (460-370 BC)

Chapter 1

The Big Leap –
Why Plant-Based?

The Big Leap – Why Plant-Based?

"Isn't man an amazing animal? He kills wildlife such as birds, kangaroos, deer, all kinds of cats, coyotes, beavers, groundhogs, mice, foxes and dingoes by the million in order to protect his domestic animals and their feed. Then he kills domestic animals by the billion and eats them. This in turn kills man by the million, because eating all those animals leads to degenerative and fatal health conditions like heart disease, kidney disease, and cancer. So then man tortures and kills millions more animals to look for cures for these diseases. Elsewhere, millions of other human beings are being killed by hunger and malnutrition because food they could eat is being used to fatten domestic animals. Meanwhile, some people are dying of sad laughter at the absurdity of man, who kills so easily and so violently, and once a year, sends out cards praying for 'Peace on Earth.'"
~David Coats, from Old MacDonald's Factory Farm

Let's start with the big leap of faith, giving up your meat and dairy. There are many diets available out there with variations on the same theme—give up processed foods, cut out simple carbs and sugar, eat more fruits and veggies, eat less meat and dairy. All of them bang this same drum, and I agree 100 percent with all the above. However, they all stop short of completely taking away your meat and dairy. Most other diets tiptoe around this, asking that you eat less meat, or only lean meats, or only fish, or only grass-fed meats. We say: No meat, no dairy is best for you, period. This is the foundation of what makes the Whole Earth Diet different, so let's start with this.

If giving up meat and dairy is so good for you, why do so many other diets allow it? Because the kiss of death seems to follow any business that suggests that folks give up their meat and dairy completely. Most people consider a 100 percent plant-based diet just too extreme and completely unsustainable. They want to lose weight and get healthy, but they would rather go to someone who blesses their meat "in moderation," rather than someone who wants to take it away altogether. So diet books, doctors, nutritionists, health coaches, environmental groups, and non-profit groups all stick with what they know sells and keeps the money flowing: allowing people to keep their meat and dairy—albeit in much smaller quantities—even when they know it is bad for health, bad for the environment, and torture for animals. If they ask people to cut out the meat and dairy, they will lose their audience, lose their clients, and lose their cash flow ... or so they think. This diet is different. This one boldly goes where no other diet dares to go. This diet promotes a 100 percent plant-based diet, giving up meat and dairy altogether. This is your huge leap-of-faith chapter!

WHY should you leave meat and dairy off your plate completely? There are three major reasons (any one of which stands alone as reason enough) that I will present to you here in this chapter:

1) for your health
2) for the planet
3) for the animals

Get ready to have your blinders ripped off and a bucket of cold water thrown over your head; ready?

A Plant-Based Diet is Best for Your Health

Let's start with the health reasons. Once you finish this chapter, you are going to have a fresh perspective and hopefully a zeal for sharing this new knowledge with everyone you know. You are going to be amazed—and saddened—that this information has been hidden from you for so many years.

When I became a vegetarian (for the second time), it was after a visit to the fair when my then thirteen-year-old daughter decided to never eat those cute animals again! So I went along for the ride without any real personal conviction, and I continued to eat occasional fish, chicken, eggs, and cheese for years—a vegetarian diet except when inconvenient, or worse, a junk food vegetarian downing processed white flour carbs and loads of cheese and dairy, which is really just as bad for your health as eating meat. It wasn't until I stumbled onto thw book, "Skinny Bitch," and decided to take the plunge to a 100 percent plant-based diet that real physical health changes started happening. Being thin, having great skin and hair, and looking good is great and all that, but it is only the icing on the cake. When you are looking vibrant and beautiful on the outside, it is generally a sign that you are also physically healthy on the inside.

As more studies are done, more research shows that a good diet is our best defense against disease. As Hippocrates said, "Let food be thy medicine and medicine be thy food." So then when you think about it, your health and wellness is completely in your own hands, and it all boils down to choosing the best breakfast, lunch, and dinner you can eat, one meal at a time, one day at a time. And those three meals should contain the best that the plant kingdom has to offer—fruits and vegetables and whole grains and legumes (beans, peas, and lentils)—prepared and served in a delicious variety of ways. You just need to leave the dead animals AND the products that come out of animals' bodies, off your plate. It is really that simple.

But wait … did I just hear you say, *"Simple? But I could never give up my meat! That will NOT be easy!"* Hold on a minute. Hear me out. This is where the rethinking begins. I'll highlight here a few of my favorite arguments with meat eaters. Consider this both education and your handbook for fighting back once you take on your new 100 percent plant-based lifestyle:

"People have been eating animals for years, since caveman days!" Yes, that is true, but the meat today is very different from the meat of yesterday. In the good old days, they were eating meat with plain old unhealthy saturated fats and cholesterol. Today, every time you consume factory-farmed chicken, beef, veal, pork, eggs, or dairy, you are not only eating the naturally-occurring unhealthy saturated fat and cholesterol, but you are also eating the unnatural added hormones, pesticides, steroids, and antibiotics that those animals were fed to fatten them up more quickly for slaughter or to produce more milk (13). Is it any wonder it is fattening us up too?

"But my grandfather has been eating steak every day of his life, and he is 101." Well, he's probably one of those guys that smokes cigars and drinks whiskey too! Don't let yourself get sidetracked by anecdotal stories of this grandpa or that. There are some folks that smoke a pack of cigarettes every day for their entire life and somehow live to be 100, yet no one today disputes the fact that smoking is bad for you and

no one encourage you to smoke for your health. While on the other hand, most people we know eat meat, and they get very sick and die far too young from cancer, heart disease, obesity, and diabetes. Studies show that a vegetarian diet increases your life expectancy by 6 years (14).

"But I heard that our brains grew when we started to eat meat millions of years ago. The meat helped us evolve into the intelligent beings we are today." The most likely cause for the burst in brain growth corresponding with meat eating had to do with the fact that humans needed to hunt animals to survive during the Ice Age, and so through natural selection the smartest and most cunning hunters survived. The meat didn't cause the brain growth. Natural selection favored those with larger brains who were the more skilled hunters. Once, we needed to hunt to survive. Today, we go to the supermarket. Albert Einstein is a little bit closer to us in history than the Neanderthal, and his brain development didn't seem stunted given the fact he was a vegetarian (15). I think I'll follow Einstein's lead, rather than that of a Paleolithic caveman, thank you very much.

"Wait, I didn't get to the top of the food chain just to eat carrots," or *"God gave us dominion over the animals for us to eat."* These two arguments tend to get blended together, all based in the belief that man is superior to every other animal. Yes, we are different from animals in our capacity to think and speak and build things and stuff. Maybe we are superior. But does that mean that we should kill and eat anything that is less intelligent than we are? If we are truly at the top, then we should also be superior enough to know that "dominion" doesn't necessarily translate to "kill and eat." Perhaps it means what the dictionary says: "Dominion: the power or right of governing and controlling." I don't know about you,

but I'm so glad we live in a country where our leaders don't show their dominion over us by eating us—or maybe just eating the folks with the low IQs. Since when did power and authority translate to murder and consumption? If we are truly at the top of the food chain, should we not evolve beyond this primitive way of thinking?

"But I have Type O blood, so I need to eat meat for protein!" No, sorry, I'm not buying that argument either. I am a true Type-A personality, blood-Type-O; an overachieving superwoman. According to those blood-type theories, I am the ideal candidate to be consuming raw moo cows, and yet I am just thriving on a purely plant-based diet. Folks, we are all so obsessed with protein. If a person eats enough calories from a broad range of healthy, whole, plant-based foods, they are going to get enough protein, period. Simple. Where does the rhino, the elephant, the gorilla, or the water buffalo get its protein? None of these animals seem weak and puny, or lacking muscle. A better question to ask yourself is, if you eat a lot of meat, dairy, and eggs, which contain NO FIBER, then where the heck are you getting your fiber? If people were as concerned with getting their daily fiber as they are with getting their daily protein, our health statistics would be reversed from what they are today! It is easy for a plant-based diet to meet recommendations for protein, and protein combining is not necessary (16).

"But we have these sharp canine teeth that make us carnivores; doesn't our anatomy tell us that we are meat eaters?" Well, actually, no it doesn't. Our embarrassing little canine teeth pale in comparison to the true carnivores, the lions and tigers and bears (and sharks!) of the animal kingdom. Have you ever looked inside the mouth of a true carnivore? Now those are some teeth! Humans have molar teeth for chewing and grinding up plant foods; we do not

have the same long, sharp, pointed canines to rip flesh like carnivores do. Also, our saliva contains alpha-amylase, an enzyme meant to digest plants and which is not found in the saliva of carnivores. The concentration of stomach acids of carnivores is twenty times that of humans. We don't have claws to tear and rip flesh; we have hands with opposing thumbs for harvesting fruits, vegetables, and grains. All carnivores pant to cool off; we perspire. Finally, meats putrefy much faster than vegetables, so carnivores have short intestines (maybe three times their body length); humans and herbivores have long intestines, ten to twelve times their body length. All very interesting food for thought, right?. (See Appendix B, Table 1, Comparative Anatomy) (17)

"I could never be a vegan. I like the taste of meat and cheese too much." Okay, this would fly if it didn't involve the moral argument (which comes later), but there is also the health argument. Think of it this way: people hooked on painkillers, narcotics, and illegal drugs may like the way the drug makes them feel (and we've heard amphetamines make you *really* skinny, by the way), but most of us abstain from narcotics no matter what, because we know they're bad for our health. We like the taste of cookies and cupcakes, but we know the fat and sugar are bad for us. Some of us like the taste of cigarette smoke and may have thought once we could never quit smoking, but the overwhelming evidence to stop finally caught up with us, and we did. Why should the saturated-fat, artery-clogging meat be viewed any differently? While it doesn't have an immediate effect on our health like abusing drugs does, think of it more like death by 1,000 cuts. Cheese is actually one of the most addictive food types there is. It is filled with casein and casomorphins, which have an addictive, opioid-like effect intended to bond a nursing baby to its mother (18). It's no wonder you can't give

it up! And why are we not hearing more about this? Because, just like for so many years with cigarettes, there is just too much profit in keeping us all addicted. This truth is being very carefully hidden from us by the powerful meat and dairy industries.

"Hey, vegetables feel pain too! Haven't you seen the study done about plants' feelings?" This is ridiculous. It's just a way for people to justify the fact that they refuse to stop the carnage. If plants could feel pain, they would have developed some kind of a defense mechanism to avoid it—they would have evolved to scream or to run away or at least lean away from death. Any sentient animal with a central nervous system feels pain and struggles and fights for its life. Plants do not have a central nervous system. They have no brain to interpret pain; therefore they cannot feel pain or fear death (19). Put a child into a room with an apple and a bunny. How much do you want to bet that the child eats the apple and plays with the bunny, and not the opposite, understanding intuitively that the apple feels no pain or fear, but the bunny does? We have lost touch with the natural intuition we all had as children.

"But, it's the way things have always been." Native tribes needed to hunt wild game in winter for survival, with snow on the ground and no plant foods available. That is where meat eating began, as a survival mechanism in an emergency situation. Had it not become ingrained in the culture along the way, and had people not become inured to the violence of meat eating, it would have ended long ago. Today, we no longer need to hunt to survive, but we still eat meat and dairy. Once we had small family farms that produced meat and dairy. During the 20th century, however, things changed dramatically in the farming industry in a horrible way, turning farms into soulless factories and animals into

soulless production units. And now, because of the Internet, we know the awful truth. As with all of the past mistakes of mankind throughout history, the most dangerous argument remains the same: "But it's the way things have always been." Just as cannibalism used to be normal, just as slavery used to be normal, just as certain types of people being treated unfairly used to be normal ... now it is time to stop treating animals differently just because a dog looks different from a pig, or a cat looks different from a chicken.

"But farm animals are different; they are meant to be eaten," Before, we had been taught to believe that farm animals were meant to be eaten. That they somehow magically felt no pain, no fear of death. That they all lived happy lives and then gladly gave up their lives to become our food. Now we hear stories that prove that the farm animals we've loved since we were kids, yet have been eating for years, truly do feel all the same emotions—love and fear, jealousy and anger—that our beloved pets do, and that we ourselves do. Farm animals feel pain, have a desire to live, and fear death. They love their babies and cannot bear to be torn away from them, just like we do (20). And the meat and dairy industries have been trying to hide this from us for years.

"But I'm afraid of change. I don't want to lose my family traditions." We need to rethink our obsession with eating meat. Sure, it means shifting some of our family traditions that center around eating some particular type of animal, but it is really only a slight shift in thinking about the "entrée" portion of the meal. All the rest of our traditional holidays— the big meal, all the delicious side dishes and desserts, the gathering of friends and family, the gift-giving, the story-telling, the hot chocolate by the fire, the songs, the laughter, crazy Uncle Frank, all the rest of it—remains the same. It is

only the meat that will be missing, that will be replaced by something else. It is only our fear that holds us back from making that shift, a fear that we are truly entering a new age ... and we are. But there is nothing to fear; we can bring along all the good stuff and just gently let go of all the bad. So the sooner you embrace the change, the better.

I know there are plenty more arguments out there, but let's move on. Let's talk facts—pure and simple. Facts. There are over 100 references in this book, and the vast majority of them are primary sources of information, including hundreds of scientific publications from other researchers that point the way without a doubt to a diet that leads to less cancer, less diabetes, less heart disease, fewer strokes, less obesity, less autoimmune disease, less osteoporosis, less Alzheimer's, less kidney stones, and less blindness. Scientific studies and research and publications that are NOT funded via discreet channels by the meat and dairy industries (which are certainly out there and creating a lot of confusion posing as objective studies), but which are instead funded by non-profit organizations filled with ethical doctors, soulful scientists, and revolutionary nutritionists who have all discovered the diet that will heal the world's current health crisis. That diet is a 100 percent plant-based diet.

Let's take these one health problems one at a time, starting with the "biggie"—obesity!

Obesity is the cause of many killer diseases (21), so if we can wipe out obesity, we can wipe out the root of many problems. And let's face it ... the reason most of you picked up this book was likely because you are struggling with your weight. Even though you may be concerned about your physical appearance, being obese (or even just overweight) is much more a problem because of what you are doing to your health, with the fat that is being stored inside and all around your major organs, and inside your arteries and veins! The fat that is causing cancer, heart disease, and diabetes. The fat that is slowly killing you. The fat we see on the outside is only an indicator that there is much more dangerous fat growing wild on the inside, where it is truly life threatening.

Here's something else to think about: some of you might not even appear fat on the outside, but you are still storing up fat on the inside where it is even more dangerous, like those that lose weight on a high-fat, high-protein diet like the Atkins diet (22). Here are the facts. You will lose weight initially on an Atkins-type diet because you will lose a lot of water weight right off the bat. When your body metabolizes the protein found in animal products, you create toxic nitrogen waste that needs to be eliminated through frequent urination. So, of course, if you are eating a lot of animal protein, you are going to be going to the bathroom a lot! This diuretic effect will look good at first, but it is putting an awful strain on your poor kidneys to keep up with all this toxic ureic acid. Also, though you may start looking better on the outside, on the inside your arteries and veins are still getting clogged up with pockets of plaque, ready to burst and cause a massive heart attack at the first sign of distress. At the end of the day, this diet just ISN'T sustainable and isn't healthy. Eventually you will go back to eating carbs because carbs are our body's fuel. They are an essential nutrient. They are everywhere and much more prevalent in our diet than meat. They are in everything from fruits to veggies to grains to beans to nuts to seeds, all the healthiest, vitamin- and mineral-rich, fiber-rich food you would be omitting, just to eat bacon and butter? Sorry, but the Atkins diet is just crazy, on so many levels. Bad for your health, and completely without any sense of morality for the animals or for the earth.

On average, vegetarians are ten to twenty pounds lighter (23), and this ties in with the fact that they live about six years longer than meat eaters (24).

So how does a plant-based diet help you lose weight???

1) By eliminating growth hormones and steroids. Animal meat and animal products like milk, cheese, and eggs are filled with growth hormones that will cause weight gain as surely as if you were eating these growth hormones directly (25). Eating the toxins that are in the factory-farmed animals' meat or milk will lead to weight gain. Think about it. Factory farming has become an industry that is all about the money. The faster they can grow young calves and piglets and baby chicks into big, fat adults, the less time and money it will take to turn them into meat. They feed them hormones and steroids to speed up the weight-gain process. When you eat these animals, or when you eat their milk products or eggs, you are eating these same chemicals yourself, speeding up your own weight gain. Is that REALLY what you want? Yummy, growth hormones!

2) By increasing the fiber. Diet trends come and go, but one constant is that consuming fiber helps more than any other factor when it comes to losing weight. Focus on fiber from plant foods and you will see your weight drop. This happens for a few reasons: (a) eating fiber makes you feel "full" sooner, so you actually eat less; (b) high-fiber foods require more chewing, which slows down the rate of eating; (c) fiber traps nutrients and slows down the travel time from stomach to intestines, delaying the insulin rush and making your feeling of "fullness" last longer; (d) fiber helps keep your digestive system clean and functioning smoothly for maximum efficiency (26). Oh, and by the way, meat and dairy contain no fiber. Zilch. Nada. None.

3) By trimming the fat. Meats and cheeses are full of saturated animal fat, which clogs up your arteries and veins and puts cellulite on your hips. Animal fats are much harder to digest and absorb, so they are stored as fats and toxins in all your tissues (27). Not all fats are bad though. Polyunsaturated plant-based fats, such as those from avocados, olives, nuts and seeds, are actually very beneficial to the proper functioning of your body. As long as they are eaten in smaller quantities, they will not contribute to any weight gain, but will only give you glowing skin and hair!

When you eat a big plant-based meal, all that low-fat, high-fiber, nutrient-dense, deliciously satisfying food not only fills your belly up to the top in the short term, BUT it also makes you feel full longer, giving you a slow, steady, sustained release of energy from burning those complex carbs for hours, without energy highs and lows, without crashing and craving sugar, sweets, or caffeine. Eating three square plant-based meals a day is the most efficient way to lose weight (28).

So you might be thinking, "Okay, maybe a plant-based diet will help me lose weight. But what is the proof that it is better for my health?" Let's focus first on the big three top killers—diabetes, heart disease, and cancer – then will touch on MRSA and mad cow disease, just for the heck of it.

Diabetes: The big news here is that type 2 diabetes can be prevented and even reversed with a plant-based diet (29). In the U.S., two-thirds of Americans are overweight, and one-third are obese. One out of eight—approximately 24 million Americans—have diabetes, and this number increases daily. Of 1,532 autopsies performed on teenagers in the U.S., 1,532 showed fatty patches in the aorta—100 percent (30). With Western fast-food chains spreading to all corners of the Earth, the rest of the world seems to be falling in line.

This is a man-made crisis of epic proportions. Type 2 diabetes stems from obesity because high levels of body fat lead to insulin resistance and progressively lead to an increased need for more insulin. Losing weight by going to a plant-based diet, as well as exercising, will help control your weight and dramatically reduce or even eliminate the need for insulin dosing. Around the world, the prevalence of diabetes is directly proportional to the consumption of more saturated fat, animal fat, and animal protein. Prevalence decreases with greater intake of fiber and vegetable fat (31). Dietary recommendations for people with diabetes used to focus on minimizing the intake of carbs, which caused the diet to shift toward more animal protein and fat. Today, however, the scientific community is rethinking this advice due to the mounting evidence of the harm caused by high intake of saturated fats and animal protein. Many doctors now are prescribing a whole-foods, plant-based diet, using complex carbs to stabilize blood sugar, as the best diet for diabetes. Residential clinics at Loma Linda University are reversing type 2 diabetes with a 100 percent vegan diet. (32).

Heart disease: Heart disease is the number one cause of death in America (33). In most cases, heart attacks are caused by a narrowing of the coronary arteries that supply the heart with oxygen and nutrients. How do they get narrow? Well, a buildup of disgusting plaque in the arteries—directly related to blood cholesterol levels, directly related to consumption of fat—accumulates over the years. Dr. Caldwell Esselstyn, a seventy-seven-year-old heart surgeon who went from performing surgery to promoting nutrition, calls heart disease "a toothless paper tiger that need never exist ... and when it does exist, it need never progress."

Heart disease is caused by plaque that is a direct result of what you eat, an overconsumption of saturated fats, animal proteins, cholesterol, and highly processed foods, as well as an underconsumption of plants and fiber. Blood cholesterol levels of vegetarians is 35 percent lower than of non-vegetarians, and coronary heart disease is virtually nonexistent in plant-based cultures around the world in places such as Papua New Guinea, some parts of rural China, central Africa, and with the Tarahumara Indians of Mexico.

Dr. Esselstyn says that by following a plant-based diet, you will be "heart attack proof," regardless of your family history. That's a pretty strong statement, but with more research, and the longer we see patients reversing their symptoms of heart disease by switching to a plant-based diet, the more evidence mounts that we are causing our own heart disease by what we are eating. A plant-based diet works by keeping the lining of the blood vessels free of inflammation, blisters, and bubbles, and by keeping the passageways clear of dangerous, disgusting plaque that causes heart attacks (34).

World War II provided a graphic example of how the ravages of heart disease could be totally halted. Norway was one of several western European nations occupied by Nazi Germany during the conflict between 1939 through 1945. The Germans removed all animal livestock from these occupied countries. The native population subsisted on whole grains, legumes, vegetables, and fruit. Almost immediately, death from heart attacks and strokes in Norway plummeted. With the cessation of hostilities in 1945, animal products became available again, and there was an immediate return to the prewar levels of deaths from these illnesses (35). (See Appendix B, Table 2, Mortality from Circulatory Diseases). It is a powerful lesson in public health about the cause and cure of our most common killer—heart disease—but this message was not heeded by the medical profession or the public. Instead, it has been just the reverse. The popularity and success of Western culture has adversely influenced Asian and developing cultures, so they seek to emulate our toxic Western diet. As a result, coronary artery disease is predicated to become the number one global disease burden by 2020 (36).

One other thing: According to a recent study by the Harvard School of Public Health, there is something more than just the saturated fat and cholesterol in meat that is causing heart attacks. Eating meat delivers L-carnitine to bacteria that live in the human gut. These bacteria digest L-carnitine and turn it into a compound called trimethylamine-*N*-oxide (TMAO). In studies in mice, TMAO has been shown to cause atherosclerosis, the disease process that leads to cholesterol-clogged arteries, which can lead to heart attacks (37). So there's that too. So, it comes down to which you would prefer: a long, healthy life with a good, strong ticker, or the taste of BBQ with a heart attack on the side. Or you know what? You can still have your BBQ taste without the heart attack, just make that a veggie burger instead of cow burger, and everyone is happy. Especially your heart!

Cancer: If this still isn't enough to convince you, let's talk cancer. Cancer is the second-leading cause of death in the United States (38), and as complicated as cancer seems with the multitude of different types of cancer, it is really very simple. Cancer is uncontrolled, abnormal cell growth. Every single day our bodies make new cells, even cancer cells. On average, a healthy person produces one cancer cell per day. Why don't all these cancer cells turn into cancer? Because your immune system fights it off. The more acidic your internal environment, the harder it is for your immune system to function properly. If you feed your body with alkalizing fruits and veggies rich in sodium, potassium, magnesium, and calcium, you are creating a perfect environment for your immune system to fight off cancer. If you feed your body with acidic animal proteins that cause inflammation, you are creating a perfect environment for your cancer cells to thrive.

Unfortunately, there is more bad news about acidity and meat consumption. When you eat meat and dairy, which themselves are acidic, you are also typically eating factory-farmed meat and dairy, so you are also eating toxic and carcinogenic tranquilizers, hormones, antibiotics, steroids, pesticides, and preservatives. 70 percent of meat sold in stores is treated with carbon monoxide to keep the rotting meat a deceptively red color. Tasty, right? So if you eat a healthy, whole-foods, plant-based diet and eliminate the meat, dairy, and eggs, you'll greatly reduce your risk of cancer (39). If you have already been diagnosed with cancer, the good news is that most cancers respond extremely well to nutrition therapy, no matter how far along you happen to be with the disease. Almost every type of nutritional therapy today has a raw, 100 percent plant-based diet as its base, often flooding the body with massive doses of green plants through daily green juicing.

To be clear, we're not advocating purely nutritional therapy if you have cancer, particularly cancer in advanced stages. However, there is no doubt that supplementing traditional therapies with nutritional therapy is inexpensive, painless, delicious, and many times just as powerful as medical treatments alone. Work with your doctor to find the best course of treatment for yourself, but always include nutritional therapy. Why would you not if your life is at stake? And if you are one of the lucky ones who is NOT currently dealing with a cancer diagnosis, you most likely will never have to because by the time you are finished reading this book, you will be eating a preventative, healthy, alkaline, whole-foods, organic, plant-based diet.

Antibiotic Resistant Strains of Bacteria: The FDA reports that 80 percent of all antibiotics sold in 2009 were administered to livestock animals and that many of these antibiotics are identical or closely related to drugs used for treating illnesses in humans. Consequently, many of these drugs are losing their effectiveness on humans, and the total health care costs associated with drug-resistant bacterial infections in the United States are between $16.6 billion and $26 billion annually.

Of the samples of ground turkey, pork chops, and ground beef collected from supermarkets for testing by the federal government, more than half contained bacteria resistant to antibiotics, according to a new report highlighting the findings. The data, collected in 2011 by the National Antimicrobial Resistance Monitoring System—a joint program of the Food and Drug Administration, the Agriculture Department, and the Centers for Disease Control and Prevention, show a sizable increase in the amount of meat contaminated with antibiotic-resistant forms of bacteria, known as superbugs, such as salmonella, E. coli, and campylobacter. Pigs have been identified as a big contributor to the rise in MRSA lately. Apparently (but quietly) recognizing the catastrophic potential of all of this, on December 11, 2013, the FDA asked drug makers to "stop marketing antibiotics to farmers" (40). It will take a long time for them to ask them to just plain STOP, but until then, I'm not taking any chances. In the world's worst-case doomsday scenario, a superbug that cannot be killed because people have developed immunity to it by eating antibiotic-filled meat could potentially wipe out everyone on earth except for those of us who don't eat meat. Hopefully this will never come to pass, but it isn't nearly as outrageous as you might think.

Mad Cow Disease: Mad cow disease (bovine spongiform encephalopathy or BSE) is a fatal disease of the central nervous system. The latest case in the U.S. was found in 2014 in a dairy cow in a random USDA test of dead farm animals in California. Alive, the cow showed no signs of BSE. Affected cows often show increased apprehension, poor coordination, difficulties in walking, and weight loss. In this case, it's a wonder that the disease was detected at all. The agency conducts BSE tests on only 0.1 percent of cows, or about 40,000 of the 34 million cattle slaughtered each year, and with budget cuts, the amount of oversight in slaughterhouses has decreased dramatically. When you think about the fact that one hamburger can contain the meat of up to 100 cows, and now the government has ruled that meat producers don't even need to label what country the meat came from, so you really have no idea what you are eating when you eat a single hamburger, and the odds of getting meat that is tainted increases dramatically.

There is evidence that the agent responsible for BSE is the same agent responsible for Variant Creutzfeldt-Jakob Disease (vCJD), the human form of mad cow disease, which is more prevalent than once thought, according to a study published in *The British Medical Journal*. Researchers analyzed 32,441 tissue samples from forty-one British hospitals collected by the Health Protection Agency between 2000 and 2012. Each sample was tested for the proteins associated with vCJD. Results showed the number of people who carry the protein was double that of previous surveys.

By June 2014 in the United Kingdom, there were 183,841 confirmed cases of cattle with mad cow disease, and vCJD had killed 176 people. A British and Irish inquiry determined that the mad cow was caused by feeding cattle the remains of other diseased cattle in the form of meat and bone meal, which caused it to spread like it did. It is notable that there are no cases of vCJD in countries where cattle are grass-fed only, like Uruguay, Argentina and Brazil. (41).

So this highlights yet another problem with eating meat and dairy – the factory farmed cattle and dairy cows, instead of eating grass like nature intended, are being fed commercial grain that not only contains antibiotics, hormones, pesticides, fertilizers but also "protein supplements" in the form of ground and cooked leftovers from the slaughtering process, as well as carcasses of sick and injured animals unfit for human consumption. However, whatever the cattle eats, you eat, when you eat meat. Whatever the cow eats, you eat, when you drink milk or eat cheese. And with industrial factory farming, this is not pretty.

Okay, we talked about diabetes, heart disease, cancer, MRSA and mad cow disease. I could go on and on with a multitude of other chronic and life-threatening diseases that can be both prevented and cured by switching to a whole-foods, plant-based diet: high cholesterol; osteoporosis; all kinds of gastrointestinal illnesses such as gastroesophageal reflux disease, inflammatory bowel disease, irritable bowel syndrome, diverticular disease, and celiac sprue; and all kinds of other disorders such as autoimmune diseases, kidney disease, gout, and even dementia and Alzheimer's. Yes, there are studies showing that a plant-based diet helps to both prevent and in many cases reverse all of these diseases. You can look at my recommended reading list at the back of the book to see where you can get more on this very important subject. For now, just know that the vast majority of illness can be both prevented and cured by eating a diet rich in phytochemicals, fiber, antioxidants, vitamins, and minerals and low in saturated animal fats, cholesterol and artificial crap. An alkaline diet, not an acidic diet. In other words, a whole-foods, plant-based diet.

In case you are still not convinced that an architect doesn't have the credentials to dish out nutritional advice (and I don't blame you if you're not convinced by my ranting yet!), I suggest you start to explore some of this yourself. Here is a short list of some of my well-qualified vegan tribe that has my back when it comes to advocating a plant-based diet for your health:

- **Dr. Caldwell Esselstyn Jr., MD** – The Cleveland Clinic Foundation, Cleveland, Ohio: an American surgeon who conducted a twelve-year trial study on terminal heart-diseased patients with severe atherosclerosis whose diseases were reversed by following a strict low-fat, whole-foods, plant-based diet (no meat, dairy, or oils). His work is documented in the 2011 documentary *Forks Over Knives*. He attributes the success of his trial to low cholesterol and also states that plaque does not develop until the endothelium, or the lining of the arteries, is injured—and it is injured every time people eat meat, dairy, fish, and chicken (42).

- **Dr. Dean Ornish, MD** – physician and founder of Preventative Medicine Research Institute in Sausalito, California: For more than thirty-two years, Ornish has directed clinical research demonstrating that comprehensive diet and lifestyle changes may begin to reverse even severe coronary artery disease without drugs or surgery. He also promotes a whole-foods, low-fat, plant-based diet, and he was the physician consultant to former President Bill Clinton when, in 2010 after the former president's cardiac bypass grafts became clogged, Ornish coached him to reverse the disease by following a plant-based diet (43).

- **Dr. Neal Barnard, MD** – physician, nutrition researcher, author, and president of Physicians Committee for Responsible Medicine in Washington, DC: Dr. Barnard claims there are several significant heart-health gains for people following a 100 percent plant-based diet because there is no animal fat, cholesterol, or fat added to the bloodstream, and the high fiber and vitamin content help people who are overweight to drop the extra pounds and lower their blood pressure (44).

- **Dr. T. Colin Campbell, PhD** – professor at Cornell University, American biochemist who specializes in the effect of nutrition on long-term health, known for his advocacy of a low-fat, whole-foods, plant-based diet: He was one of the lead scientists in the 1980s of the massive China-Oxford-Cornell study on diet and disease known as "The China Study." They examined the diets, lifestyle, and disease characteristics of sixty-five rural Chinese counties, linking the consumption of animal protein (meat and/or dairy) with the development of cancer and heart disease. Like Dr. Esselstyn, he is featured in the documentary *Forks Over Knives* (45).

- **Dr. Joel Fuhrman, MD** – family physician who specializes in plant-based nutrition treatments for obesity and chronic disease: He states that by eating a low-fat, plant-based diet, you can actually make yourself "heart-attack proof." He is the author of six books, including *Eat to Live*, and is featured in the movies *Sacred Duty*, *Simply Raw: Reversing Diabetes in 30 Days*, *Fat, Sick and Nearly Dead*, and *Vegucated* (46).

- **Dr. Michael Greger, MD** – physician, author, general practitioner specializing in clinical nutrition and focused on a whole-foods, plant-based diet: His work can be found at Nutritionfacts.org, which is now a 501c3 non-profit charity (47).

- **Dr. John McDougall, MD** – physician and author whose philosophy is that degenerative disease can be prevented and treated with a low-fat, whole-foods, plant-based diet: At age eighteen, he suffered a massive stroke (which he now attributes to his high animal-product diet). This influenced his decision to become a physician. Some years later when he observed the disease patterns of his patients as a plantation doctor in Hawaii, he began to rethink his approach to medicine. This became the McDougall Program. He has authored many books, including *The McDougall Plan* and his latest, *The Starch Solution* (48).

A Plant-Based Diet is Best for the Earth

Are you still not convinced? Maybe you are young and strong and going to live forever, or maybe you are old and strong, have been eating meat and dairy your whole life, and are healthy as a horse, so none of this health stuff matters to you! Okay, let's pretend there were NO detrimental health effects from eating meat or dairy, that all the above is somehow just not true, and that the motives of the mostly grey-haired gentlemen doctors listed above are extremely suspect. (Think about it, what WOULD their motives be except for truly wanting to help people get healthy, because trust me, this is not getting them rich, famous or very popular!)

So let's say that for whatever reason, you don't trust those guys, you don't buy into the health ramifications of eating meat and dairy, but maybe you are concerned about the environment. You will want to think about eliminating meat and dairy for environmental reasons alone! Let's address the simple and pragmatic concept of a clean, healthy planet right here and now—clean water, clean air, and healthy wildlife.

Let's first talk about current-day water usage. In the U.S. today, 50 percent of our water is used for some phase of livestock production. Yes, 50 percent. That number alone is staggering. The water needed to produce one pound of meat is 2,500 gallons; the water needed to produce one pound of wheat is 25 gallons! Read this again. It takes 100 TIMES the amount of water to produce a pound of beef compared to a pound of wheat. 100 times. This is a HUGE difference, and especially concerning to me as I write this, living in California and undergoing the most severe three-year drought in the last 1,200 years. Current drought trends and declining groundwater with an ever-increasing population point toward severe future water shortages unless we figure out a more sustainable way to eat without using tremendous amounts of water in the food-production process. Growing plants uses a lot less water than growing animals (49).

Next, let's consider the animal-production waste products soiling our water. We all know about the 12 million gallons of oil spilled by the Exxon Valdez, but have you heard about the 25 million gallons of hog excrement that spilled into the Neuse River in North Carolina on June 21, 1995, when a "lagoon" full of hog poop burst? As a result of this, 14 million fish were killed, and 364,000 acres of coastal wetlands closed to fishing, but we never saw much about this in the news. The amount of waste produced by North Carolina's 7 million factory-raised hogs compared to the amount produced by the state's human population is 4:1. Did you know that the relative concentrations of pathogens in hog waste is 10–100 times greater than human sewage, yet it sits out there in open "lagoons" (cesspools really)? North Carolina, it is time to learn how to grow some veggies! (50)

California is not doing so well either with animal waste, even though they try to be so environmentally friendly. The number one milk-producing area in the U.S. is California's central valley, and it is certainly not the beautiful green pastures you see advertised in the "California Happy Cows" cheese commercials or on the sides of milk cartons. Anyone who has ever driven up Interstate 5 from northern to southern California (or vice versa) has driven through this little slice of paradise—and has done so quickly and with their windows rolled up! I know this route all too well, living as I do with family in both southern and northern California and making this drive a couple few times a year. You can see many of these "happy cows" from the freeway, standing there miserably like concentration-camp prisoners, crowded into ankle-deep manure-filled pens; you not only see them, but you are knocked over by the smell of their waste from miles away.

The amount of waste produced by the 1,600 dairies in California's central valley is more than the waste produced by the entire human population of Texas (51). Do you suppose some of that manure is getting into our groundwater and waterways? Do you know how many water quality inspectors monitor the central valley? Four (52). So, who would be affected by contaminated drinking water around there? Los Angeles, San Diego, and all points in between—about 20 million people (65 percent of the state's population). But sure, four inspectors are plenty. No reason to worry, right? Who's afraid of a little pathogen that lives in dairy manure called cryptosporidium anyways? Just forget about the dairy manure cryptosporidium that got into Milwaukee's water supply in 1993 that sickened 400,000 and killed 100 people (53). No reason to worry about that here in So Cal! Wait, what was that about beach closings? The number of beach closings in California due to water pollution in 1998 was 5,285! (54) It would sure be nice to know that our drinking water supply doesn't have any cow manure in it. Is that too much to ask?

So yes, it's time to worry. It's also time to think beyond the borders of my sunny (though somewhat smoggy) backyard here in So Cal. It's time to think about the issue of the globalization of meat eating and factory farming, the bigger issue of the relationship between climate change and cow farts. Maybe this is something you have laughed about in the past, BUT this may sober you up quickly.

The three main contributors to global warming and climate change are carbon dioxide, methane, and nitrous oxide. Although transportation and the burning of fossil fuels have typically been thought of as the chief contributors to climate change, new studies are finding that 51 percent of those three big nasties come from meat eating and the factory-farming process (55). And as the population grows and more countries such as China and India (that previously ate mostly vegetarian) start to adopt the "prestigious" American meat-centric diet, this situation is only going to get worse.

2014 was just noted to be the hottest year on record for the planet, with global temperatures 1.03 degrees Fahrenheit higher than the average temperature from 1961 to 1990. It was also the thirty-eighth consecutive year with abnormally high global temperature (56). Sure, there are a couple scientists claiming that climate change is bogus, scientists paid off by big corporations that benefit from fewer environmental restraints, but the overwhelming majority of scientists state as fact that the climate is changing, the Earth is getting warmer, and the research shows that factory farming is the leading contributor to this (57). You cannot claim to be concerned about the environment and continue to eat cheeseburgers. You just can't.

Adding to the climate change caused by the factory-farming process itself is the problem of climate change due to deforestation. Up to 80 percent of deforestation in the Amazon rainforest in Brazil is due to an increased need to raise more cattle for human consumption. Brazil has become the largest exporter of beef in the world, but they have destroyed millions of acres of pristine rainforest in the process. In fact, today half the world's tropical forests have been cleared or degraded for cattle ranching (58).

Now I'd like you to consider this: all animals breathe in oxygen and breathe out carbon dioxide; plants breathe in carbon dioxide and breathe out oxygen. Forget worrying about carbons and ozone layers and even climate change. Just pause and think about that for a minute. The human population is soaring while the rainforests are being cleared for cattle consumption. You don't have to be an engineer or a scientist to know how this is going to affect our lives when the lungs of our Earth, our rainforests, are cleared to make way for farting cows!

If this argument on air quality doesn't impress you, what about these facts: the number of species of birds in one square mile of the Amazon rainforest is more than exists in all North America (59). The life forms destroyed in the production of each fast-food hamburger made from rainforest beef are as follows: twenty to thirty different plant species, 100 different insect species, and dozens of birds, mammals, and reptiles (60). So you are not only taking the life of a cow when you eat meat, you are also taking multiple lives out of the rainforest.

It would take only three and a half years to clear the Indonesian forests, all 280 million acres of them, to produce enough beef for Indonesians to eat as much beef, per person, as the people of the United States do (61). It would take only a year to completely clear the Costa Rican rainforest to produce enough beef for the people of Costa Rica to eat as much beef, per person, as the people of the United States eat! (62)

These are staggering, irresponsible numbers. Do you know that 25 percent of the world's mammalian species are currently threatened with extinction? (63) Care to guess what the leading threat and/or cause for elimination of species in the tropical rainforests is? Livestock grazing. Or the leading threat and/or cause for elimination of species in the United States (according to the U.S. Congress General Accounting Office)? Livestock grazing (64).

We are wiping out our water supply, our rainforests, our animal species, and quite literally our entire planet with our appetite for meat.

I have one last point I would like to make regarding the feed we are growing for our livestock (beef, pork and chicken). Did you know that 70 percent of the grain grown in the U.S. is fed to livestock? This is such an inefficient use of land because it takes sixteen pounds of grain to yield one pound of beef. If the whole world were vegetarian, there would be enough grain to feed 11 billion people (our current population is 7 billion)—enough grain to feed the entire world and save every child from starvation (65). World hunger would cease to exist.

Which brings me to my final thought on this subject: what are the socioeconomic implications of eating meat and dairy? The consumption of meat is economically unsound and contributes to many problems in societies around the world. If the world was vegetarian, health care costs would drop dramatically, and there would be little to no disease and little to no starvation. There would be more than enough grain and greens to go around to every man, woman, and child. According to the Worldwatch Institute, "Massive reductions in meat consumption in industrial nations will ease the healthcare burden while improving public health; declining livestock herds will take pressure off rangelands and grain lands, allowing the agricultural resource base to rejuvenate. As populations grow, lowering meat consumption worldwide will allow more efficient use of declining per capita land and water resources, while at the same time making grain more affordable to the world's chronically hungry."

Environmental vegetarians call for a reduction of first-world consumption of meat, especially in the U.S. According to the United Nations Population Fund, "Each U.S. citizen consumes an average of 260 lbs. of meat per year, the world's highest rate. That is about 1.5 times the industrial world average, three times the East Asian average, and 40 times the average in Bangladesh." In addition, "The ecological footprint of an average person in a high-income country is about six times bigger than that of someone in a low-income country, and many more times bigger than in the least-developed countries." The World Health Organization calls global malnutrition "the silent emergency," and says it is a factor in at least half the 10.4 million child deaths that occur every year. Stop, listen, and think. We are not making these numbers up! (66)

A 2010 report from the International Panel of Sustainable Resource Management states that a global shift toward a purely plant-based diet is critical for mitigating issues of hunger, poverty, and climate change. The panel declared: "Impacts from agriculture are expected to increase substantially due to population growth and increasing consumption of animal products. Unlike fossil fuels, it is difficult to look for alternatives: people have to eat. A substantial reduction of impacts would only be possible with a substantial worldwide diet change, away from animal products." (67)

Cowspiracy is a great film that just came out last year. If you are at all interested in learning more about this, I beg you to watch this mind-blowing film—and to watch it with your friends and family. We need to spread the word.

There can be no doubt that a global shift toward a plant-based diet would help ease both world hunger and disease, save water and precious farmlands, save both air and water quality ... and save lives. And save our planet.

Still not convinced? Still enjoy the taste of meat too much to change?

Read on...

A Compassionate Diet is Best for the Animals

So if the health reasons didn't sell you, and the environmental reasons weren't compelling enough for you, the third and final (and most compelling reason of all) are the moral and ethical reasons. You can give up eating meat for health reasons or environmental reasons, but once you have made the emotional connection between what we call "food" and what we call "animals," there is just no turning back. You cannot call yourself an animal lover and eat meat. You just can't. Wait, wait, hear me out! Please don't get defensive. Most animal lovers do eat meat, at least right now, today, they do. And I know a lot of you are animal lovers and you don't want to be told that you don't love animals. Of course you adore your cats and dogs and rabbits and hamsters. But somehow you are able to turn off your brain when it comes to the meat you are eating, that your meal was once a life exactly the same as your dog or your cat. And I so totally understand that. I do. I get it. That is how I lived for most of my life, loving animals my entire life, almost more than I liked humans, and still eating meat without giving it a second thought. It now is amazing to me that I was able to live so blindly for so long.

But the following is my personal story, and I hope to provide you with both inspiration and camaraderie as your own story unfolds:

I was always an animal lover, even as a young girl. I had at least one dog and at least one cat in my home for as long as I can remember. Animals have always been my best friends. Even though I grew up in LA and lived nowhere near a farm, my favorite stories growing up were about animals—farm animals particularly, especially horses and cows and sheep and pigs and chickens—from *Charlotte's Web* to *Watership Down* and *Animal Farm*. I always told my mom and dad that one day I would grow up and move to Texas and live on a farm because of all the farm animals. I still lived in that naïve childlike reality where one doesn't make the connection that all of these beloved animals would one day be killed and eaten. I had a storybook mental image. I saw them as if in a fairy tale, living their lives in green pastures and bright red barns with white picket fences; the sun was always shining and the birds were always singing.

I remember one day questioning my mom about food: Is a hot dog really made out of dogs? No, don't worry, of course not! Is a hamburger made out of ham, whatever ham is? No, of course not. Beef was beef, bacon was bacon, sausage was sausage, pork chops were pork chops, and lamb chops were ... oh, who knows, and who really wants to know? It was so confusing that I stopped asking. Food was food and animals were animals; the names had been changed to protect the innocent. It had always been that way. So time went by, and the last thing I thought about was where my food actually came from. These were the days of Space Food Sticks, Koolaid, Otter Pops and Swanson frozen TV dinners with brownies! The connection between food and nature just wasn't there. I just turned off thinking about it. It was so easy to do; everyone ate these same food-like products wrapped in brightly packaged boxes and bags, that really didn't resemble anything from nature, as the food industries back in the sixties and seventies worked on developing food-like products that were further and further removed from nature.

It wasn't until much, much later, as an adult with my own five children visiting the farm animals at the Orange County Fair, that my thirteen-year-old daughter made the connection for me. We were visiting the animal exhibit as we always did, and she asked, "Mom, do we really eat all of these animals?" Looking around at all the doe-eyed calves and the sweet baby lambs and the rows of fat pink piglets nursing on the fat warm sows, something moved in me and reminded me of how I loved these animals when I was a kid. When we got home that day, my daughter announced that she wanted to become a vegetarian and never eat those cute farm animals again, and I decided that day too to join my daughter on her new vegetarian path!

My journey to becoming a vegan was a series of baby steps forward and back. A healthy vegetarian at age 17, then went back to eating meat at age 20 as I adopted all kinds of unhealthy habits to survive the stress of graduate school at UCLA. Became a partial vegetarian again at age 41 when my daughter became one, with my philosophy being that if I couldn't kill the animal with my bare hands (in theory of course) then I didn't deserve to eat it. So I stopped eating all red meat, all mammals, because I felt the most connection with them. They are after all warm-blooded like us, nurse their babies like us, our beloved dogs and cats are mammals, and knew I could never kill any mammal with my bare hands. But I continued to eat small amounts of fish and chicken on occasion, when it was inconvenient to do otherwise. I wasn't firmly committed, still not making the complete connection.

A few years later, at age 49, after reading *Skinny Bitch* and having my bell rung, and giving up ALL animal products for good, I decided to look online for more information on factory farms and slaughterhouses to confirm if what I had read in that book was true. I discovered the horrible truth behind Paul McCartney's words: "If slaughterhouses had glass walls, everyone would be vegetarian." The Internet provided the glass walls that I needed to convince myself that I had been hiding my head in the sand for years. I was being willfully ignorant, but the Internet woke me up. It was a rude awakening, but a necessary one.

Today all slaughterhouses now have glass walls, and the only people that are not vegetarians yet are the ones that still refuse to look. The Internet and the videos that can be found there, especially the undercover slaughterhouse footage shot by our heroes—those brave guys at Mercy for Animals and the brutally persuasive *Earthlings* movie by Shaun Monson—tell the truth. After doing a little Internet surfing to see what the truth really was, I became fully and passionately convinced to never eat meat or animal products again. The fairy tale reality of life on the farm for my beloved farm animals was completely blown away by the stark reality of what I saw with my own eyes. This stuff is really hard to watch, but remember, what they must endure with their bodies, we must endure with our eyes. It is the least we can do to advocate for the more than 150 billion animals who are slaughtered worldwide every year for food.

If you are an animal lover, if you own cats or dogs and know in your heart that they are capable of feeling emotions and pain like we do, if you look into the eyes of your dog and you see a soul, then you must take an honest look at what goes on in slaughterhouses. I used to think that I knew, but I really had no idea. The demand for animal products has increased so much that changes have been made to the meat and dairy industries so that they are unrecognizable from what they were even fifty years ago. The current mass demand for meat cannot be satisfied without a system that completely disregards the welfare of the animals, without a system that thinks of animals as "units" and not living beings, where time is money so their lives are shorter and their death more quick and brutal than ever before.

While they are alive, they are kept in tiny areas because the more animals you can fit into a warehouse, the more "product" you have to sell. And the faster they can grow them up to a size suitable for slaughter, the more money they can make, because time is money. So most of these animals live their entire lives inside tiny cages inside warehouses without ever seeing the light of day or feeling the sun on their bodies except perhaps for a moment, if they are lucky, when being prodded down the chute toward the transport truck that will take them to their slaughter. They are fed genetically modified grains instead of the grass that they should be eating—special grains that are filled with hormones and steroids to plump them up faster, filled with antibiotics to make sure they stay healthy and wounds don't become infected, filled with preservatives to preserve their shelf-life, and filled with pesticides to keep the bugs away (68).

And then, after they have lived their short, unnatural lives, they are taken to the slaughterhouse where again profit takes priority over their welfare. In the U.S., about 10 billion animals are slaughtered for food every year; that is 27 million each day or 19,000 every minute. Worldwide, the slaughter count is staggering. Every second worldwide, 1,680 animals are killed for food, and most animals are killed when they are barely adolescents (69). We are actually killing babies and eating them. Not just veal, not just lamb. All meat comes from youngsters.

If you are a vegetarian eating only eggs and dairy, don't think you are off the hook because you are not eating meat. Your eggs and cheese are causing plenty of death. Think about it. In the egg and dairy industries, the newborn males of the species are never needed - baby male chicks are unable to make eggs and baby male lambs, calves, and goats will never grow up to make milk. They need only a single male, maybe two, for their thousands of profitable female units. Baby males in the egg and dairy industries are worthless.

So, the egg industry suffocates, gases, or grinds up alive 250 million unnecessary, freshly-hatched male chicks each year (70). And the dairy industry is even worse. The 4.5 million calves in Europe and 1 million calves in the U.S. annually destined to become veal are forcibly pulled away from their mothers, the dairy cows, within hours or at most one to two days after birth (71). The milk naturally produced by the mother for her calf is taken for sale to humans while the calf is fed nutritionally deficient formula and his movements severely restricted so that his flesh will be the pale color desired by customers wanting to eat his flesh. In addition, with the rise in popularity of the "healthier" and trendy sheep, goat, and feta cheeses, there is suddenly an increase in "lamb popsicles" and baby goat meat on restaurant menus (72). I dare you to google a lamb or veal slaughterhouse video. No, actually, I like you too much to do that to you. I witnessed it for you. Trust me when I say I had nightmares for weeks after accidentally seeing a slaughterhouse for veal. It was worse than you can even imagine. And this all comes from drinking milk and "not being able to ever give up my cheese!!"

Speaking of the slaughterhouse process itself, no matter the age or the type of animal being killed, no matter if he has lived his short life on a factory farm or a family farm, his final stop is a literal hell on earth. Deep breath here. Slaughtering animals on a large scale—and quickly (remember, time is money)—presents some horrific realities. For cattle, step number one of the killing process is to knock out the animal with an electric shock to the back of the head or a bolt pistol to the front of the head. Pigs are usually rendered unconscious with gas stunning. (Note: these steps are prohibited under kosher or halal methods.) Due to the speed of the slaughterhouse assembly line now, many times the shock to the head, or the bolt through the forehead, or the gas stunning is not applied perfectly or correctly as the animal is struggling and throwing its head around and fighting for its life. Therefore the bolt gun often misses, and the animal goes onto the cold, emotionless, mostly mechanized next few steps ... fully conscious.

They are often fully conscious as they are hung upside down by their hind legs and put into the processing line with all the other animals they had been standing next to moments before. They are often fully conscious as their carotid artery and jugular vein are severed with a knife and as the blood drains from their body. They are often fully conscious as they have their noses and their feet cut off and the skin stripped from their bodies. They are often fully conscious as their digestive tracts are stripped out to avoid fecal contamination. They are often fully conscious as their internal organs are removed and inspected. And they are finally put out of their misery when their heads are removed and they are split in half, quartered, cleaned, and sent on to distribution centers to be turned into nice neat clean packages for the supermarket shelves, packages that have no indication of the sheer horror that hides behind them.

The slaughter process is the almost the same whether it is a cow, a pig, a goat, or a sheep, a baby or an adolescent, humanely raised or factory farmed. By the way, there is no such thing as "humane slaughter," so lose that phrase, please. It doesn't exist. "Humane meat" only means that the young animal may have been raised humanely; for the short time it was alive, it may have lived a good life. But the death, however, is always the same. There are no humane slaughterhouses; there is no humane slaughter. Being killed when you are just a baby can't be pleasant, no matter how pleasant your short life may have been leading up to that day. (73). To determine whether something is "humane", decide whether you would want it done to you, or someone you love.

You may read all of this and still think, "Well, that's okay. That's what these animals were bred and raised for—to be eaten." But if you think this, then you are living in complete disregard for the fact that all animals, even farm animals, have proven through multiple documented examples that they have consciousness and that they exhibit behavior that can only be attributed to very real emotions like fear and love, anger and jealousy. Animals feel pain and fear just the same as humans do; in fact, one could argue that animals feel more deeply than humans do. Human beings live in their minds, cluttered with words. We are intelligent, thinking animals with this constant chatter of conversation going on in our minds. One could argue that this constant chatter in our minds can distance us from experiencing life deeply in the moment. Animals don't have that verbal chatter in their minds. It just may be that animals, free of mental chatter, may be experiencing life more fully, more present, and more in the moment than most humans do, as any yogi does who has learned to live with a quiet mind and in the present moment.

It also is true that animals have stronger sensory perception than we do—a stronger sense of smell, hearing, and taste; in fact, some animals may have senses that humans do not have at all, such as the echolocation in bats and cetaceans, the electroreception in sharks, or the magnetoreception in birds and bees. Just because they do not speak or write novels, just because they do not build cities or write poetry, does not mean that they lack consciousness, intelligence or emotion. It is only a different type of consciousness, a different kind of intelligence, and one could argue that animals may have a more direct interpretation of feelings and emotions based on direct sensory perception, living in the moment without words.

Because they may feel fear and pain and love even more strongly than we do, they are filled at all times with only this great big emotional heart. They have learned to live guided by their heart rather than their mind as we are. If you own a pet, think about how they respond so deeply with sadness when you leave the house, with such happiness when you return or get ready to take them outside, with excitement when they smell something cooking in the kitchen, with obvious joy when they are experiencing sensory comfort—warm sunlight on their bodies, or a human scratch on their belly. They live for these simple sensory comforts. They revel in their senses. They live in their hearts rather than their minds. They are living Buddhas.

And so, if you think about it in these terms, if you accept the premise that maybe, just maybe, animal consciousness is not language but feelings based on sensory perception, imagine now how that dairy cow feels when her newborn calf is taken away from her. Stories abound about how the mamas and the babies scream for days after their separation. About how the highly intelligent, highly emotional pig feels being herded quickly through the chute toward its certain death, hearing the sound of his friends ahead in the line, screaming in pain, smelling the blood and urine and excrement and fear hormones that are being excreted during the slaughters going on up ahead, and finally seeing and fully understanding the horror of the inescapable end that awaits. There are stories in the slaughterhouses of the pigs nuzzling the slaughterhouse workers like puppies, almost as if they are asking for mercy and compassion, and of course they get none.

Guys, we are not making this stuff up. This is happening, right now, every second as you read this book, and the only way it is ever going to change is for YOU to change. YOU can change this because when you change, those around you will change. And slowly but surely the world will change, and this barbaric practice will finally stop.

It is not okay just because it has always been done this way. We are living in a new century and we know that we do not need to eat meat to survive; it is a choice that we make because of a taste that we think we like. We are not cavemen or Neanderthals anymore. I know the Paleo diet is trying to take us all back into the cave, but I encourage you to come out of the cave and into the light. We have a wealth of healthy plant-based food choices in front of us. It is as wrong to kill animals for food as it is to kill humans for food. If we are truly at the top of the food chain, if we are truly the moral superior to the animals, if we are the pinnacle, then shouldn't we behave that way and hold ourselves to a higher standard than that of a predatory carnivorous beast or a prehistoric man?

Everything in the animal agricultural industry is designed to maximize profit at the expense of the animals' welfare. It is true that there are agencies and programs that exist that promote the notion that animals raised for food are treated "humanely." In the U.S., the Humane Slaughter Act of 1958 was enacted that required that all pigs, sheep, cattle, and horses be stunned unconscious prior to being hoisted up on the line. However, we see undercover footage that shows numerous examples where this is not always the case, many animals are fully conscious throughout their brutal slaughter. (74). (By the way, chickens are exempt from this law. I guess because they must not really be real animals!) There simply are not enough USDA inspectors to enforce that animals are unconscious before slaughter and not only that, there are religious restrictions that counter this law as well. The kosher and halal slaughterhouses are probably the most awful videos I have ever seen. There is nothing humane or religious about being trapped inside a huge mechanized steel drum that rolls you upside down, practically decapitates you with a rolling steel blade while fully conscious, blood spurting everywhere, while a hose sprays you down with cold water to make sure your life blood goes down the floor drain. So spiritual, right? Horrible, just unbelievably horrible.

More recently, in the latter part of the twentieth century, the layout and design of most U.S. slaughterhouses were influenced by the work of the autistic Dr. Temple Grandin. She believes that her autism gives her a better understanding of what animals are feeling, so she suggested ways to funnel animals headed to slaughter into single file, curving lines that prevent the animals from seeing what's going on too far ahead. This design "attempts to override the animals' survival instincts and prevent them from reversing direction" (75). Survival instincts? Wait, I thought they couldn't feel fear? Sorry, but there is no "humane" way to kill. Death is death. Killing is killing. It hurts. It's terrifying, and it's permanent. No one has the right to take another life, especially for something as ridiculous as a flavor, a taste, a single meal, or an added layer to a burger. All life is precious.

So, have I made my case for the moral reasons behind a plant-based diet yet? Whether you are concerned about your own personal health, losing weight, or preventing or even curing a disease; whether you are concerned about the environment, global warming, the extinction of species, or social issues like world hunger or global health; whether you care deeply about animals and just cannot ignore the massive, nightmarish scale of pain and suffering anymore, giving up meat and dairy is a win-win-win no matter what angle you look at it from. Which is why I didn't hesitate for a minute after learning all of these facts to give up meat and dairy for good, forever. Period.

I hope I didn't scare you too much with this chapter because it can be scary and difficult to get through, but I am so happy you are still here with me. The overwhelming evidence is that you must transition as soon as possible, as intelligently as possible, and as simply as possible to a whole-foods, plant-based vegan diet, which is every bit as nutritious as what you have always eaten, minus the death and disease. You can go cold turkey or you can take baby steps, whatever suits you. I will never judge you or criticize you for taking baby steps if that is what you need to do. The Whole Earth Diet takes everything into account—your personal physical health, your holistic wellness, AND the big picture health of the whole Earth. You can't be successful if you are on a diet that is focused only on your own waistline and how good you look in your selfies. None of those other diet plans will stick with you like this one will. You need to see this as something much bigger than yourself, because it is. I am so glad you picked up my book because that is exactly what I am going to help you with.

I am going to help make this as easy for you as possible, and I am here to support you and love you and guide you every step of the way. You will quickly find that through our network you will have a permanent new tribe of Rainbow Warriors surrounding you and supporting you as well, if not in person, at least in spirit through the miracle of technology at all times. Let's do this! Let's ride!

Chapter 2

Plant-Based

Nutrition

Plant-Based Nutrition

—•—

"Tell me what you eat and I will tell you what you are" ("You are what you eat")

~Jean Anthelme Brillat-Savarin, French lawyer, politician & gastronome (1755–1826)

In this chapter I will expand the notion of healthy eating from eliminating meat and dairy to also eliminating the other giant stumbling block to health—processed, packaged Frankenfoods! Because you know, it is possible to be a very unhealthy vegan, and I want you to absolutely ROCK this plant-based diet, to become a model example of how this diet makes you glow with health inside and out so that others will follow your path as well. If you look like you're dying of anemia and anorexia, no one is going to follow your example. You can eat a pure junk-food diet of nothing but Twinkies, Oreo cookies, Diet Cokes, Twizzlers, and those other foods you can buy at a 7-Eleven and call yourself a vegan because there are no animal products in there. Well, there are also no plant products either! In fact, there is NOTHING from nature AT ALL (animal, vegetable or mineral) in most of the "food" that you pick up at the corner gas station, or for that matter, from most of the center aisles of the typical supermarket in middle America. I like to call these foods "Frankenfoods," created in a laboratory to offer the perfect trifecta of food addictions—fat, salt, and sugar. They are created with artificial colors, artificial flavors, artificial fats (hydrogenated vegetable oils), artificial sugars (high fructose corn syrup), a long list of ingredients you cannot pronounce, and finally preservatives. All to maximize shelf life, maximize food addictions, and maximize profits. All at the expense of your health.

So what exactly is the Whole Earth Diet? We omit the meat and the dairy, of course, but we also omit the processed foods and sugars. We eat real foods—fruits, veggies, grains and legumes, nuts and seeds—cooked and raw both. We also know that folks cannot be perfect, so we preach the 90/10 rule: eat right 90 percent of the time, and 10 percent of the time you can cheat just a bit! To be clear though, the cheating does NOT apply to the meat and dairy; we must be 100 percent there. The 10 percent cheating rule applies only to the other foods that we know are far from perfect from a health perspective: the vegan cupcakes, the big bowl of pasta with soy-meatballs, the gallon of vegan ice cream! And we do allow black coffee, dark chocolate and organic red wine in moderation, just to make sure that folks don't turn and run away.

We apply the "lesser of two evils" philosophy. If we take away all your fun, you will not even consider this for a moment. But if we promise you a wee bit of vice here and there—a little coffee, a little red wine, a little sweet treat once in a while—we know this will be sustainable. And that is the key word, *sustainable*. This is not a temporary fling. This is a lifetime commitment. This is a marriage, not an affair! And after thirty plus years in my marriage, you know I take these things seriously, and so should you. You are now officially married to Whole Earth Wellness. You are one of my Rainbow Warriors, and there is no backing out now!

So these are the rules: No meat, no dairy, and no processed foods, but there is room for a couple vices here and there! As long as those vices do not impact the pain and suffering of another, which means those cheats do not involve meat or dairy. But an occasional frozen vegan entree thrown into the microwave, a can of plant-based soup heated up over the stove, a little vegan sweet treat now and then, French fries dipped in yellow mustard (that's MY personal weekness), a lovely warm cup of black coffee to greet your day, an indulgent matcha green tea almond milk latte in the middle of the afternoon, and a lovely cool glass of red wine to end it. All okay, now and then; the 90/10 rule applies. A little bit of pain and suffering? Nope. Never. Off the menu, and off your plate. 100 percent. No excuses.

The most amazing thing about Whole Earth Diet is that you can still eat so much of what you are used to eating. If you have family recipes, you can tweak them to eliminate the meat and dairy quite easily. You will eat familiar dishes, familiar comfort foods, but you will have stripped the bad stuff away. The flavors will be slightly different without as much fat, salt, and sugar, but there will be new and different flavors coming through that you may not have noticed before when the recipe was swimming in animal fats—the richness of deeply colored organic vegetables, beans and whole grains; the taste of fresh green herbs and spices; that perfect squeeze of lemon or lime at the end to finish. It's a whole new world of eating.

Remember when you once drank whole milk? You noticed the taste difference when you changed to skim milk, thought you didn't like it at first but grew used to it, then later you tried whole milk again and it tasted way too rich, right? The same will happen once you switch over to plant-based milks, and plant-based everything. The richness and thickness of the saturated fats and cholesterol in the way you were eating with the Standard American Diet will taste overwhelmingly rich and horrible if you ever go back and try them again. But honestly, once you give up meat and dairy, it is almost impossible to go back. Once you make the soul connection between the suffering and the food, once you realize that meat is nothing more than a corpse, and dairy is the product of a baby's suffering, it's impossible to go back to eating that way.

So, the first chapter was the WHY; this chapter is all about the WHAT. What on earth is the Whole Earth Diet? First we will get into a bit of a nutrition lesson, then we will talk more specifically about foods to eat, foods to avoid, and foods to enjoy in "mindful moderation"! In the next chapter we will get into the HOW—how to implement and work this new way of eating. So if you are eager and want to skip right there, please feel free. BUT it really is important for you to educate yourself around this topic because trust me, you will get plenty of challenges from folks trying to tell you that you "need to eat meat" or you're going to "get sick." That you "need your protein." The more you learn, the easier it will be for you to truly rethink nutrition and understand like I did that everything I THOUGHT I knew about nutrition, everything I had always been taught to believe, was DEAD WRONG! So let me try and pass along some of this good info to you so that you are better equipped to really understand this and debate any Paleo diet dinosaur out there!

101 Dietary Theories + Nutrition 101 = Whole Earth Diet

Studying to be a holistic health coach with the Institute of Integrative Nutrition, I spent years immersed in nutrition, studying all 101+ current, competing, compelling, and usually contradictory diets put out there over the last few decades. And my education never really ends. I am in an eternal process of learning, studying, and keeping up with all the latest news, reports, research, studies, and findings on health and nutrition. No matter your country of origin, those of us living in developed nations seem to be obsessed with food, constantly chasing after the latest fad diet promoted by the current pop culture celebrity or television doctor. Every day there is breaking news with regard to the latest and greatest new miracle food for disease prevention, or Dr. So-and-so's new scientifically-proven miracle pill for weight loss. (Can you say "sales gimmick"?)

It's been hard to keep up with all this! Are we supposed to eat "high protein, low carbs," or "low protein, high carbs"? Are there "good carbs" and "bad carbs"? "Good fats" and "bad fats"? And how on earth do those French ladies stay looking so good with all those croissants, red wine, and Brie cheese? Hold on ... probably all those old folks on Okinawa got it right with their macrobiotic diets—all brown rice, veggies, sushi, and seaweed. But wait, folks can't eat that way every day if they grew up and live in South America or Mexico! (Besides, let's be honest—that seaweed really is an acquired taste, right?) Well, perhaps the South Beach Diet with a nice piece of grilled salmon on the BBQ is the way to go? But, that's so "last Tuesday." Aren't all the celebrities doing "Paleo" now?

They all can sound so good when you're listening to a friend brag about their weight loss on a particular diet or reading that inspiring new diet book that gets you all fired up. And these trendy diets may even work for you, for a little while, but most are too specific to their country and culture of origin to apply globally, or too restrictive or incomplete for long-term success. Many rely on portion control and calorie counting, which leads to cravings and unhealthy binge eating. Prepackaged diet plans (where you purchase their packaged entrees) will definitely work for a short while, but sooner or later you have to learn how to feed yourself. At the end of the day, it becomes too difficult to stay the course, and you really don't feel you deserve to be healthy and thin anyways. Many folks will actually self-sabotage their diet, feeling personally unworthy for lacking in willpower. Again, this is why 95 percent of diets fail.

I've studied all of these diets for you, scratched my head over completely contradictory studies, got completely confused by them all, worked through it all again and again, went down this road and that road, tried lots of different things myself, and finally came to a solution that can and does work: the Whole Earth Diet. This is the last "diet book" you will ever need because once you understand the concepts and facts presented here—the overwhelming latest scientific research viewed through a lens of deep and astonishing ancient wisdom, the breathtaking irresponsibility and immorality behind eating any other way—then the light bulb will go off for you, just as it did for me. And though it is called the Whole Earth Diet, it is not truly a "diet." Whole Earth Diet is a new way of life, and the only way to save ourselves and our planet.

Time for our lesson in Nutrition! Ready to be schooled? Here goes:

The Three Macronutrients – Protein, Carbohydrates, and Fat

There are three **major** macronutrients: fats, carbohydrates, and proteins. All the foods you eat are composed of these three macronutrients in varying proportions. Food groups like meat or diary or veggies or fruits are not simply "a protein" OR "a carb" OR "a fat." All food groups are a mix of the three macronutrients, and you need to eat all three to be healthy. You need protein to build tissue, carbs for fuel, and fats to support bodily functions. Think of your body like a car. Proteins are what your car is made of—metal, glass, rubber, plastic. Carbs are the gasoline that runs your car. Fats are the motor oil that keep everything lubricated and running smoothly. Just as a car needs its parts, its fuel, and its oil to function, you need all three macronutrients for your body to function. You cannot omit any of the three just because the latest trend in weightloss tells you that fats or carbs are bad! (76).

What happens if you run out of gas? Your car stops running. It's the same thing if you go on a low-carb or no-carb diet. Your body will run out of gas. You need healthy, complex carbs to fuel everything your body does all day, or you will have zero energy and you will just stop running. Then you will find yourself binging on donuts (unhealthy simple carbs) at two in the morning and quickly putting all that weight back on!

What happens when you forget to put oil in your car? You'll probably fry the engine! It's the same thing as being on a low-fat or no-fat diet. You need healthy plant-based fats for healthy heart and brain function. You may only experience feeling fuzzy or confused at first, but you are heading down the fast lane to Alzheimer's, dementia, or a sudden-death heart attack. Seriously, no joking.

What happens if you get a flat tire? You need to change it with a new fresh tire or you can't drive. It's the same thing as being on a low- or no-protein diet. You need healthy plant-based protein, or your body cannot heal itself when wounded: broken bones won't mend; flesh wounds won't heal. Your hair and nails breaking will be the first sign you're not getting enough protein, NOT feeling a lack of energy. (That would be a lack of carbs or B vitamins, typically.)

Eating a well-balanced diet of fruits, veggies, whole grains, and legumes (beans, peas, lentils) will give you the perfect balance of healthy fats, carbs, and proteins you need for optimum health. You do not need meat or dairy for protein. You will get all the protein you need from a plant-based diet (77).

Drilling down a little deeper, here is more of what you should know about the three macronutrients—proteins, carbohydrates, and fats.

PROTEIN: Proteins are the building blocks for the skeleton and flesh of your body. The flesh in animals and the organic material in plants are made of protein. Protein builds muscles, strengthens tissues, repairs cells, and maintains the structure of your body. Of the twenty different amino acids that your body needs to function, eleven are made by your body, but nine "essential amino acids" must come from food (78).

Animal proteins are called complete proteins because they contain all nine essential amino acids in every bite.

Plant-based proteins are called incomplete proteins because they may be missing one or two of these nine essential amino acids, but each plant is different. Each plant contains a different variety of amino acids, so there is no problem if you are eating a variety of fruits, veggies, beans, and grains every day, as you should anyway. Do you think every bite of food should contain all your daily essential vitamins, minerals, proteins, amino acids, enzymes, carbs, fats, phytonutrients, in perfect proportion and balance, in every bite, from every food source? Of course not, we get a little bit of this from this, and a little bit of that from that. It's the same with the essential amino acids. There is no need to worry about food combining; this will happen naturally.

Most plant-based foods are roughly 10 percent protein, 10 percent fat, and 80 percent carbs, which is exactly the proportion you need in your overall daily caloric intake (79). In addition, the lightweight amino acids found in plant foods are much healthier for you because they're not accompanied by all the unhealthy saturated fats and cholesterol and other toxic junk that meat and dairy contain. Plant proteins are rich in complex carbs for energy and full of healthy fiber for digestive health; meat has no fiber, so it is not easily digested, and it has no carbs for fuel. Meat eaters should be more worried about constipation and colon cancer than about not getting enough protein!

Most people have a tendency to go protein-overboard, thinking they need way more than they do! Watch out for those "high-protein, no-carb" diets that promise quick weight loss. They work at first because (a) excessive protein causes frequent urination, so you'll lose water weight right away, and (b) you will be limiting your calories by restricting a whole class of food from your plate. But at the end of the day, these diets are not only unsustainable, they're unhealthy. Your body can't function for long, nor burn fat efficiently, without carbs. The saturated fats in your high-protein diet are slowly but surely filling your arteries with deadly plaque. Excessive protein also puts added strain on your kidneys, so folks at risk for kidney disease should follow a diet that is very low in protein and eliminate meat completely (80).

Being 100 percent plant-based, the most common question I hear is, *"Where do you get your protein?"* The most common argument against? *"Oh, no, I could never give up my protein!"* And then there is always the restaurant server who, whenever I order a salad, asks if I want any "protein" on that salad. I always reply, *"You know what, this salad has plenty of protein, thanks!"* As if meat equals protein and protein equals meat. This is how brainwashed we all are! ALL FOODS contain protein. Protein is not a food group; protein is not meat. Protein is a macronutrient. By eating a whole-foods, plant-based diet, you are getting more than enough protein. You are not giving up anything except the taste of meat (which, by the way, is so easily imitated now with some amazing plant-based "meats" made from whole grains, peas, nuts, and beans).

There are some instances where people do need to up their protein intake – the young and the elderly, athletes, pregnant women, and people healing from surgery or injury. If you are in one of these categories, I suggest adding non-GMO tofu or tempeh to your daily diet (on your salad or added to just about any cooked entree), as well as an 18-20g green protein powder to your daily morning smoothies.

If your hair and nails start falling out, this is a sure sign you are not getting enough protein. I sure wish some of my hair would fall out so that I wouldn't have to spend so much time trying to get it under control with a blow dryer and flat iron! No one has told my hair that it's not getting enough protein and should be falling out now, and no animal products have passed through these hair bulbs for five years now. If you are new to a plant-based diet and feeling low energy, this does NOT mean you need a steak (as clients have told me that was their first thought). It means you are low on fuel (or B12 or iron, which we will get into later). But first let's talk about fuel—carbohydrates!

CARBOHYDRATES: Carbs are our fuel, our energy source (81), and unfortunately today, when we hear "carbs," we usually think "bad," right? But not all carbs are bad, not all are created equal, and in fact they are absolutely necessary to fuel your body! Most nutritionists recommend that carbs make up 60–80 percent of your daily calories; they are your primary form of energy and a great source of vitamins, minerals, and fiber. Your body uses carbs for immediate energy and also stores energy for later. If you are feeling tired, don't assume you need protein. If you are feeling lethargic, it is probably because you are cutting your carbs to lose weight. You have basically run out of gas!

So let's have a little lesson on carbs. There are three types of carbs: simple, complex, and fiber. **Simple carbs** are really simple sugars (82). They satisfy your sweet tooth, enter your bloodstream quickly, and provide a fast jolt of energy—often followed just as quickly by a drop in energy. Simple carbs are found mostly in processed foods - soft drinks, bottled fruit juices, white bread, white pasta, cakes, cookies, crackers, candy, and sweets. Simple carbs are the culprits behind why carbs have such a bad reputation; overdoing simple carbs really will pack on the pounds!

Simple carbs lead to rapid changes in blood sugar, which lead to mood swings, compulsive eating and snacking, sugar and food cravings, weight gain, and ultimately diabetes. The ONLY good simple carbs are raw organic fruits, which should be eaten daily, two to three servings at least, and best if first thing in the morning on an empty stomach. But, why is fruit okay? Because fruits are perfect natural foods, Mother Nature's sweet, all-natural treat, filled with vitamins, minerals, phytonutrients, enzymes, and fiber in perfect balance, unlike any other simple carb. All the other simple carbs are unnatural, processed foods, mostly made with bleached white flour, and almost always filled with artificial high fructose corn syrup. Feeling low blood sugar between meals and craving something sweet? Have a peach or banana, not a cookie or candy bar!

Complex carbs are the good guys (83); they break apart slowly in your digestive system and release a slow, steady stream of energy into your body for hours. Complex carbs are found in whole grains such as quinoa, rice, and corn, and whole grain breads, cereals, and pasta. These foods all contain both carbs and protein. Eating a meal with whole grains, legumes, vegetables, nuts, and seeds gives you ample protein AND carbs, not to mention tons of vitamins and minerals and fiber, without all the crap that comes with meat and dairy. Ideal healthy complex carbs are the whole grains that are not genetically modified, and that are gluten-free and low in sugar—colorful quinoa, tiny black rice, brown or wild rice, and steel cut oats, for example. Legumes of all kinds are practically the perfect food; they're low fat, high fiber, high protein, complex carb energy, full of vitamins, minerals, and fiber. So what is a legume? Anything that grows in a pod—all manner of beans (red, black, white, kidney, navy, garbanzo);

all peas including English peas, black-eyed peas, snow peas, sugar snap peas, chickpeas, green split peas, and edamame; and lentils and lima beans.

Fiber is also a complex carb (84). Unlike protein, fats, and other carbs, fiber is not exactly a nutrient absorbed by your body, but it is still essential to good health, passing through your body and acting as a companion for all those good nutrients. There are the juicy, soluble fibers (foods that absorb water) found in oatmeal, beans, and lentils that help to slow down your digestive system so that blood sugars are released more slowly into your body. They also delay the emptying of the stomach, which makes you feel full longer and helps you lose weight. Then there are the hard, dry insoluble fibers (foods that don't absorb water and act like a broom) found in whole grain wheat, nuts, and actually most vegetables such as broccoli and cauliflower, that help to speed up the passage of waste through your intestines, keeping you regular, keeping your colon clean, clear, and disease-free. Soluble fiber is a natural remedy for diarrhea; insoluble fiber is a cure for constipation. Eating both keeps your digestive system healthy and regular. In other words, fiber keeps you skinny, healthy, and pooping perfectly! It's no wonder we love fiber!

So, in this era of trendy eliminate-the-carbs-and-go-for-the-meat diets, hear this: healthy **complex** carbs and fiber-rich foods do NOT make you fat! But, overeating processed foods, and in particular, processed **simple** carbs are the real villains here. Many simple carbs are snack-type foods, so by eliminating snacks, even those "healthier" snacks like gluten-free crackers and hummus, or chips and guacamole, you will eliminate the bad simple carbs that make you fat and unhealthy. Eating three square meals a day - breakfast, lunch, and dinner - with organic, natural complex carbs will not make you fat or unhealthy; in fact, the opposite is true. The sustained energy release and filling fiber from complex carbs will help control your portions and keep you feeling full longer. The bottom line is that overeating calories from any food source—whether proteins, fats, or carbs—will make you fat. There is no one macronutrient here to simply eliminate, as so many dietary theories will have you believe. All three macronutrients are essential to good health, but they can all be overdone as well.

FATS: Fats are another one of our three healthy macronutrients that have been singled out as the villain a lot lately (85). It seems that everything in the grocery store is screaming "Low Fat!" or "No Fat!" As with the no-carb, low-carb diets, this implies that if we were just to eliminate all fat from our diet, we would be healthy, happy, and thin! It sounds right, too. Wouldn't fat make you fat? While it's true that eating too much fat leads to weight gain and disease, it is important to know this: healthy fats in moderation play an essential role in brain function and heart health. (Oh, and by the way, healthy fats are primarily responsible for beautiful skin and hair.) Seriously, though, a lack of healthy fat in your diet can cause sudden death heart attacks and severe mental disorders, among other things. Yikes! But how on earth are you supposed to know which fats are good and which fats are bad? Hang on to your love handles, folks. Here we go with our nutrition lesson on fats!

Fats can be divided into three classes: (1) *bad* saturated fats; (2) *simply evil* trans fats; and (3) *healthy & essential* unsaturated fats.

Bad **saturated fats** are fats that are solid at room temperature, and are found in all animal products - meat, butter, bacon grease, and cheese (86). The big problem with animal fats is that they contain cholesterol. You will hear that cholesterol is needed to promote brain, nerve, and hormonal function, and this is true. BUT your own body makes the perfect amount of cholesterol for you. You do not need to ingest any extra cholesterol by eating animals that, just like you, made cholesterol in their bodies for themselves!

When you have excess cholesterol, this lovely semi-solid waxy substance is stored as plaque in your arteries. This leads to blockages in the arteries, coronary heart disease, high blood pressure, and high cholesterol. Do yourself a favor and avoid saturated animal fats altogether. Think about it. If it's solid gunk at room temperature when you eat it, it will probably be solid gunk when it gets inside your veins and arteries. Why would you eat bacon if, when you fry it up, the fat is so bad for your plumbing that you can't pour it down the drain? Why are you pouring this fat into your arteries then? Is your body less important than your kitchen sink?

Avoid all animal products and you will eliminate *almost* all saturated fats. I say *almost* because there are a couple of plant-based sources: palm oil and coconut oil. Palm oil is out of the question, though, as THE leading cause of rainforest and orangutan destruction, so don't buy products with palm oil, ever. Nuff said about that. Coconut oil, however, does have some beneficial uses. Some plant-based folks like to use coconut oil for cooking because it does have a delicious flavor and can handle very high heats for cooking, but it's best to stay away from cooking using any oils if you want to lose weight, lower your cholesterol or blood pressure, or have heart health issues of any kind. For me personally, I prefer to eliminate cooking in oil of any kind, instead cooking with low-sodium veggie broth. Then I use coconut oil as one of nature's best all-natural skin and hair moisturizers! Comb it through your hair the night before you will be shampooing next day, sleep in a shower cap with your coconut oil mask on your hair all night, then see how silky your hair is the next day after shampooing. Rub it onto your skin BEFORE you shower, let it soak in a bit, then shower as usual. You will start to see amazing results—more beautiful, juicy skin and silky hair—right away, while your waistline shrinks from the elimination of those saturated fats and cooking with oils! (Men, this applies to you too! You will never have dry, cracked skin or unhealthy dry hair again!)

So anyways, if saturated fats sound bad for your health, then **super bad trans fats** (87) are downright evil! They are Satan himself! Honestly. Trans fats are a nickname for "partially hydrogenated vegetable oil." They are not found in nature, but are the result of an unholy, artificial process called hydrogenation. See, when corporations realized that butter was causing heart attacks, but the healthier liquid vegetable oils were not as marketable, they developed hydrogenation as a way to turn a liquid oil into a marketable solid by altering its chemical composition. Now partially hydrogenated vegetable oils, or trans fats, or better yet, Frankenfats, are in everything. Margarine was the original resulting product, but now Frankenfats are found everywhere and in everything—in cakes, crackers, cookies, baked goods, fried foods, just about every processed food you find on your grocery store shelves. When you go to the market, look for the words "hydrogenated oils" on those labels, and you will be shocked to find it everywhere.

The bad news is trans fats are even worse than saturated fats. Like saturated fats, they raise your blood cholesterol levels, clog your arteries, and lead to heart disease, but it gets even worse. Your intelligent body doesn't recognize trans fats as food, simply because they are not. Your body can't begin to metabolize artificial trans fats and doesn't know what to do with them. They have no place to go but to be stored away in your fat cells and organs as toxic waste. There are currently studies underway that show that trans fats may be causing Alzheimer's disease, cancer, diabetes, obesity, liver dysfunction, infertility in women, and major depressive disorders. With trans fats in all processed foods and fast foods, is it any wonder we are experiencing an epidemic of all of these illnesses? To be healthy and live a long life, you have no choice but to avoid all trans fats by avoiding margarine, fried foods, and fast foods. You have no choice but to avoid processed foods, period. I know, I know, this sounds hard. But you will thank me later when we are in yoga class together doing tree pose side by side when we are 110 years old.

Good **unsaturated fats** are your good fats, the healthy fats, and there are two kinds—monounsaturated and polyunsaturated. (Don't worry—there's no test. But it's not as complicated as it sounds!)

Monounsaturated fats (88) are found in nuts and high-fat fruits, such as olives and avocados, and current studies support what people living in Mediterranean climates have known for years: a diet rich in monounsaturated fats is a recipe for a healthy heart and a slim body! Research shows that diets rich in monounsaturated fats decrease the risk for breast cancer, reduce cholesterol levels, lower the risk for heart disease and stroke, aid in weight loss, reduce pain and stiffness for sufferers of rheumatoid arthritis, and reduce belly fat. Olive oil and sunflower oil are high in monounsaturated fats, but oil is a processed food with a very condensed high-fat content, so Whole Earth Diet recommends eating your fats as whole foods rather than processed oils. The best way to get your daily dose of healthy monounsaturated fats is simply to eat half an avocado, a few olives, or a handful of raw macadamia nuts, almonds, or pecans every day. By the way, did you know that olive oil has a very low smoke point and should never be used for sautéing anything over the stove? A drizzle of olive oil here and there over cooked or raw food is okay, but use cold and not over a stovetop.

Polyunsaturated fats (89) are the *essential fatty acids* that you hear so much about, and there are two types— omega-6s found in soybean, corn, and safflower oil (which are a big part of the typical Standard American Diet), and omega-3s found in walnuts, flax seeds, fish, algae, and krill (which we typically do NOT get a lot of in our Standard American diet, which is why we all supplement like crazy). While omega-6s are inflammatory, the omega-3s are anti-inflammatory, and most of us, whether meat eaters or vegetarians, just don't get enough healthy omega-3s to balance out all the omega-6s we eat. There is an ideal healthy proportion of 2:1 omega-3s to omega-6s (twice as many omega-3s to omega-6s) that is almost impossible to achieve without supplementation. The omega-3s have been shown to reduce cardiovascular disease, prevent circulatory problems, reduce blood pressure, reduce effects of rheumatoid arthritis, reduce anxiety and depression, reduce risk of stroke, improve brain function, and may help prevent breast, colon, and prostate cancer. Wow! And also, omega-3s are the best-kept beauty secret in the world, nourishing collagen production, the great stuff that supports hair, skin, and nail health.

Without getting too bogged down with info, it is also important to know that there are three types of **omega-3s** (90): "long-chain" EPA and DHA, which are found primarily in marnie-based sources - fatty fish, algae and seaweed; and "short chain" ALA, which is found primarily in plants, such as flaxseeds, hemp seeds, chia seeds, pumpkin seeds, sunflower seeds, leafy green vegetables, and walnuts. Mammals thrive on the EPA and DHA omegas (lending credence to the theory that perhaps our genetic ancestors did come from the sea?), and though we have an ability to convert the short chain plant-based ALAs into the long-chain marine-based EPAs and DHAs, it is somewhat limited and may decrease with age. So it is important to supplement with a long-chain EPA/DHA omega-3 oil. While eating fatty fish or taking a fish-oil supplement may sound like a good idea, since fish is rich in EPA and DHA, fish also contain mercury, PCBs, and other toxins and contaminants, and the over-fishing of our oceans is leading to an environmental crisis of unprecedented proportions.

So what do you do? No worries. There are great algae-oil supplements that will provide you with those same super-healthy fish-oil-style "long chain" DHA/EPA omega-3s that everybody raves about. After all, where do you think those fish got their omega-3s in the first place? From marine algae and phytoplankton (91). So we are just going straight to the primary source by consuming an algae-oil supplement instead of a fish-oil supplement, and we're saying "no thanks" to the mercury and the over-fishing. Whole Earth Diet wholeheartedly recommends—in fact, demands—that you take only two supplements no matter who you are and what the diet; one is B12 (see Vitamins below) and the other is a plant-sourced omega-3 EPA/DHA oil supplement, usually a combination of flaxseed oil and algae oil. Make sure to take at least 600mg of DHA daily. You really should have no other oil in your pantry, either for cooking or for salads, IF you have any concerns about obesity, heart health, high blood pressure, or high cholesterol. Just coconut oil for your bathroom beauty routine!

That was our lesson on macronutrients, folks. You are all now experts on protein, carbs, and fats! Now let's turn our attention to the equally important *micronutrients*. We need them just as much as the macros, but only in lesser quantities.

The 3 Micronutrients – Vitamins, Minerals, and Water

Selling vitamin and mineral supplements has been big business over the last few decades. Most of us pop pills every day, half of which we have no idea what they do or why we are taking them. But do you really need all those pills? The truth is, most of the vitamin and mineral supplements you take are either not absorbed at all or have exceeded your daily requirements, so they are quite literally being flushed down the toilet. But worse than the vitamins and minerals that you are flushing down the toilet are the ones that do not get flushed—the fat-soluble ones that get stuck in your body and become toxic.

Don't misunderstand. You definitely need vitamins and minerals in your diet in order for your body to be healthy. However, vitamins and minerals are called micronutrients for a reason—you need only a small amount of them! That being said, there are more than thirteen vitamins and twenty-two minerals that are essential for healthy body function.

The thirteen **vitamins** fall into two classes—four fat-soluble and nine water-soluble (92). The **four fat-soluble vitamins (A, D, E, and K)** dissolve in fat not water, are stored in your body's fat and liver, can build up in the tissues, and become toxic if the amount you eat is more than you need. But of course the right amounts are essential and necessary for health. **Vitamin A** promotes good vision, healthy skin, and healthy bones. **Vitamin D** plays an important role in building and maintaining strong bones and teeth as it's responsible for your body's ability to absorb calcium. Current research on vitamin D has shown that it goes far beyond bone health to preventing multiple sclerosis, arthritis, psoriasis, diabetes, depression, and may decrease your risk for colon, breast, and prostate cancers! **Vitamin E** is needed for the formation and functioning of your blood cells, muscles, healthy skin and eyes, and protects your essential fatty acids. **Vitamin K** is needed for blood clotting, and fortunately 80 percent of the vitamin K you need is created by the bacteria in your intestines, so if your digestive system is healthy, you've got plenty of K!

Of these 4 fat-soluble vitamins, there is really no need to supplement vitamins A, E or K. There have been more problems with toxicity resulting from taking supplements than there are problems with deficiencies. If you are eating a healthy diet, there is no need to supplement any of the oil-solubles, except for the Vitamin D. Most people are deficient in Vitamin D. If you live in a sunny area, you may get enough Vitamin D simply by sitting outdoors at noon every day for 30-45 mins. But if you are indoors every day or live in areas of very low sunlight, you will probably need to supplement with a vegan D2 supplement (which comes from plant sources; D3 comes from animals). Get your vitamin D blood levels tested. The vitamin D test you're looking for is called 25(OH)D or 25-hydroxyvitamin D. This is the officially recognized marker of overall D status, and is most strongly associated with overall health. You are looking for a blood level of 40-60 ng/ml. The corresponding input of Vitamin D from all sources combined is 5,000 to 6,000 international units daily; not just from supplements per se. We do need supplements, but the 5,000–6,000 IU figure is the total input every day needed to sustain a blood level of 40-60 ng/ml.

Unlike fat-soluble vitamins, the **nine water-soluble vitamins** dissolve in water, so if you take too much, it's not a problem; it will all just be peed out into the toilet later! They won't be stored in your body. On the other hand, it's important that you eat enough of these nine vitamins every day since they are not stored and are flushed out so quickly.

There are **eight Big B vitamins**: thiamin (B1), riboflavin (B2), niacin (B3), pantothenic acid (B5), pyridoxine (B6), biotin (B7), folic acid (B9), and cobalamin (B12). Without going into all the gory detail, basically the B vitamins all work together to support cell metabolism, maintain healthy skin, enhance immune and nervous system function, promote cell growth, and provide stamina and energy. Feeling low energy? Take some **B12**, which brings us to the most important supplement that we suggest everyone take - carnivores, vegetarians and vegans, but especially vegans since B12 is found mostly in animal products. Take a methylcobalamine B12 supplement in a dose of 500mcg per day, dissolved under the tongue. Vegans who don't supplement tend to have low B12 levels, which at the very least means low energy and anemia, but also means elevated homocysteine, which is linked to dementia and brain atrophy, as well as birth defects, stroke, and low bone mineral density. Very serious stuff, solved with a simple cherry-flavored pill!

Next, there is water-soluble **vitamin C**, one of the most important vitamins of all! Vitamin C helps keep your bones, teeth, and blood vessels healthy, helps heal wounds, boosts your resistance to infection, and participates in the formation of collagen. Mega-dosing 1000 mg/hr of vitamin C at the first sign of a cold or flu is almost guaranteed to drive that puppy away! (See Appendix B, Table 3, Vitamins.)

MINERALS, and the Mysterious Acid/Alkaline Balance! Together with vitamins, there are at least **twenty-two minerals** that are needed for your body to function properly (93). And actually, as important as vitamins are, minerals are even more so! Minerals run 95 percent of our body's activities, not vitamins. Microminerals (less than 100mg/day) include copper, iodine, chromium, iron, fluoride, tin, zinc, nickel, vanadium, manganese, silicon, molybdenum, and selenium. Macrominerals (more than 100mg/day) include calcium, magnesium, sodium, potassium, chloride, phosphorus, and sulfur. Minerals are working away in your body right now as you read this, basically running the entire show. To obtain the highest quality and quantity of minerals in your diet, your plant-based foods should all be as wild, as deeply colored, and as organic as possible. However, even if you are eating well and buying only organic, because our soils have been so overworked and all produce is less nutritious than it once was, you may want to consider adding in a raw, whole-foods, vegan mineral supplement just for health insurance purposes. I add minerals to my purified alkaline drinking water just to be sure my body is getting all the healthy minerals it needs (See Appendix B, Table 4, Minerals.)

We have known how important vitamins and minerals are for many years, but the latest research reveals just how critical minerals are to our overall health. Let's talk for a minute about the **acid/alkaline balance**, inflammation, and minerals.

Most nutritionists argue and disagree on just about everything, but the one thing they all agree on is that maintaining a balance of acidity and alkalinity in our bodily tissues is the best way to achieve and maintain good health (94). Your body's pH level will tell you how acidic or how alkaline you are, on a scale from 0.0–14.0, with neutral being 7.0. Below 7.0 is acidic and above 7.0 is alkaline. An acidic body is a breeding ground for unhealthy bacteria, yeast, and fungi while an alkaline environment helps keep things in check. People assume colds and viruses happen when they catch a bug, but many common infections are actually caused by bacteria that are part of the normal flora already present in their systems. When our diet and lifestyle become too acidic, they create fertile ground for the pathogens (not just colds and flus, but inflammation of every sort) to multiply and flourish. This is why when you give up eating acidic meat and dairy, you will notice that you never seem to get colds or flus anymore, which is a good indicator that your alkaline body is kicking some serious pathogen booty! I have not had a cold or flu since I gave up meat and dairy in 2009—not a single day of sickness. Sometimes I feel a cold coming on, but by mega-dosing Vitamin C, it is gone the next day.

An acidic body leads to inflammation which leads to disease. An oxygenated, mineralized, alkaline body will not allow inflammation to grow, will not only kill colds and flus but will also kill serious disease before it begins. Every disease—cancer, heart disease, diabetes, arthritis, Alzheimer's—begins with inflammation; disease cannot exist in an alkaline environment, only an acidic environment. What does all this mean?

Most people eating a Standard American Diet with lots of meats, cheeses, alcohol, caffeine, and sugar become very acidic. Did you know the most acidic food you can eat is ice cream made from cow's milk and the most alkalizing is lemon water? So it is not what your logical brain might think. A diet rich in minerals, with lots of fruits and vegetables, will lead to a more alkaline environment in your body, which will lead to less inflammation, which will lead to less disease. Eating mineral-rich fruits and veggies is like pouring water on the fire of disease, whereas eating acidic foods like meat and dairy is like pouring gasoline on the flames. This helps to make sense of all the scientific studies of late, whether it's a study on prevention of heart disease, cancer, diabetes, osteoporosis, autoimmune disorder, or Alzheimer's. Across the board, all the studies on prevention of any disease say the same thing—eat more fruits and veggies and drink more water. Always. Simple.

The primary determinant of what foods are alkaline and what foods are acidic is their mineral content. Foods rich in alkaline minerals (calcium, magnesium, silicon, iron, sodium, and manganese), which coincidentally are the equivalent of a vegan diet, create alkalinity in your body, which prevents inflammation, which prevents disease, which leads to a longer, healthier life for you. They say that once a cancer tumor is found, oftentimes it has already been growing in your body for around ten years. Why not start eating today to prevent or reverse that cancerous growth that may be floating around in there already? Why wait until it is too late? (See Appendix B, Table 5, Acid/Alkaline Balance.)

This brings us to our last but most important micronutrient of all—**water**—though we think water should be recategorized as a macronutrient because it is so important to health and we need LOTS of it! Water is one of nature's most important gifts to mankind, and it is of major importance to all life (95). Your body is approximately 70 percent water. People have survived without food for weeks or even months, but we can't live without water for more than a few days.

Drinking pure water is one of the simplest but most important things you can do for good health. It is necessary for the digestion and absorption of your food; it helps maintain your muscles; it supplies oxygen and nutrients to all the cells in your body; it helps rid your body of wastes; and it serves as a natural air conditioning system. Health officials emphasize the importance of drinking at least half your body weight in fluid ounces of water each and every day to maintain good health. For example, a 150-pound person should drink 75 ounces of water each day (96).

How important is water? Because water contains no calories, serves as an appetite suppressant, AND helps the body metabolize stored fat, it may possibly be one of the best-kept secrets for weight loss around. If you're reading this book because you are interested in losing weight, you can just set the book down now and walk away with that one tip in your mind. It is so simple. Drink more water—tons of it. Often when we think we are hungry, we're really just dehydrated (or bored). I can't help you with your boredom, but I can tell you that helping yourself to a large glass of water every time you get a stirring of hunger in between meals could be the simplest yet most effective diet secret you have ever heard. So drink lots of water, and do not wait for your body to tell you that you are thirsty; by the time your brain gets the thirsty message, you are already dehydrated. This is the weight-loss secret that should be screamed from every health channel, health publication, TV show and magazine, but you don't hear it talked about too often. Why? Because there is no profit in water, and you could be advertising instead the latest miracle weight-loss pill patented by the pharmaceutical industry!

Beyond weight loss, water may actually be a simple yet powerful key to disease prevention and cure. "You're not sick; you're thirsty. Don't treat thirst with medication," says Dr. Batmanghelidj, author of *Your Body's Many Cries for Water* (97). Dr. Batmanghelidj says that unintentional chronic dehydration (UCD) contributes to many degenerative diseases—asthma, arthritis, hypertension, angina, adult-onset diabetes, lupus, and multiple sclerosis—that can be prevented and treated by merely increasing water intake. The simplest cure for a headache is often just a glass of water. This ties in to all the findings regarding keeping an alkaline environment in the body for disease prevention. Drinking water, especially lemon water, will keep your body alkaline; coffee, sodas, alcohol, and black tea are all acidic beverages and should be mostly avoided. Water also helps you to dilute and flush out all your body's toxins. The only beverages that you should be drinking that are truly healthy and alkalizing are water with lemon, kombucha, green tea, or other naturally caffeine-free herbal teas such as ginger or peppermint. Search today for a source of pure, alkaline water distribution near you.

So what have we learned so far? We now know that a healthy diet consists of a nice balance of all three macronutrients—carbs, protein, and fats (80/10/10)—without omitting any one of the three. We know that all of these macronutrients should be as wild and organic as possible to ingest the highest quality and quantity of micronutrients (vitamins and minerals). We know that we should supplement with vegan DHA/EPA omega-3s, vitamin B12, and most likely vitamin D2 and minerals as well. We know that we should eat plant foods that are more alkaline than acidic to reduce inflammation to avoid or reverse disease. We know that we should drink lots more water. And we know that throughout every recent study on health and nutrition, there seems to be a consistent theme of eating more fruits, veggies, legumes, and whole grains no matter what the health issue or disease. What we eat not only has the potential to cause disease, it also has the potential to reduce, eliminate, and in some cases even reverse and cure disease. Powerful stuff, food. We are just really rethinking this now, here in the 21st C, but it is not a new concept. It all started in ancient times, before we had modern medicine. And we are only now reawakening to this ancient wisdom today. As Hippocrates said so many years ago, and which we seem to have forgotten but are only now remembering, "Let food be thy medicine, and medicine be thy food!"

You can start to eat the perfect diet today by tossing out the USDA Food Pyramind and eating from the PCRM Power Plate instead. Eat from the four healthy food groups - fruits, veggies, grains, and legumes. Forget the meat and dairy. Simply perfect (98). (See Appendix B, Table 6, Power Plate.)

So enough nutrition education. The foundation for good health starts with a healthy body, which starts with our favorite subject—FOOD! We are literally alchemists creating our own physical bodies, for better or worse, with what we put into our mouths. Did you know that every twenty-eight days your skin completely replaces itself? Your liver, every five months? Your bones, every ten years (99)? Your body makes these new cells from the food that you eat. What you eat literally becomes you. Just as Jean Anthelme Brillat-Savarin said, "Tell me what you eat and I will tell you who you are." You are what you eat. It is an art and a science; it is the alchemy of creation. We are what we eat, so why not create for ourselves the most perfect healthy bodies that we can by eating nature's most perfect foods? Living plant foods with life-giving energy, not dead animal foods with life-extinguishing energy.

We are now going to talk food—the foods to avoid, the foods to eat in unlimited quantities, and the foods to eat in moderation—and we will end with some super-cool ancient herbs, teas, and spices to use with our foods that have healing properties.

Foods to Avoid like the Plague!

Animals/Meat: Animal fats, particularly those found in red meat, factory-farmed meat, and processed meat, are not good for your health, no matter what you previously thought; in fact, they are very unhealthy and are the root cause of our declining health. This goes against everything you have learned since you were a child, and your mom probably told you to eat your meat for strength. We have been brainwashed from birth to eat meat, and even as adults it is almost impossible to avoid, as everyone around you eats meat. There is a ton of money going into the promotion of eating meat, so we are deluged with advertisements for it.

But just for a moment, forget all you have learned, and listen to these facts that are being proven in study after study. Meat clogs your veins with cholesterol and plaque, and it clogs your capillaries with fat. Contrary to the popular notion, ancient civilizations very rarely ate red meat except during ceremonial occasions, and when they did eat animal protein, more often it was fish. In fact, the oldest cultures (dare we say "wisest cultures"?)—the Hindus, Buddhists, and Jains—adhere to a purely vegetarian diet. This is the first time in history where most people are eating red meat almost daily, and sometimes two to three times a day! Eating large amounts of animal protein is bad for your heart and arteries and causes stomach and colon cancer and obesity, which can lead to diabetes and heart failure. Is it any wonder we have a health crisis going on?

Red meat is very high in cholesterol and saturated fat, but even worse than red meat is processed meat, such as hot dogs, salami, and lunch meats. These foods not only pack all the fat and cholesterol of red meat, they have the added bonus of cancer-causing nitrates, which are preservatives that increase the shelf life of the meats. (Obviously packaged dead-body parts need a heavy-duty chemical preservative to keep them from rotting in the packages on the shelves, right?) Have you seen the pink slime they use to make hot dogs? This is not food. This is just plain gross. Stay far, far away from both processed meats filled with nitrates, and red meats filled with hormones, antibiotics, and steroids (100).

Factory-farmed anything, whether mammal, bird, or fish, should be avoided. The factory farms feed their animals growth hormones, antibiotics, and pesticide-laced GMO grains you do NOT want in your body. Speaking of birds and fish, don't think you're off the hook if you are only eating chicken and fish." If you are interested in health and longevity, you should know that those who eat chicken have a 55 percent higher risk for colon cancer than vegetarians (101). A recent study shows that bird flu is still very much alive and well in our poultry farms, and much of our poultry is contaminated with salmonella. (In one chicken-processing plant, they found 90 percent of the meat to be contaminated.) (102) On the moral side, chickens are the most abused animal on the planet. Factory-farmed chickens have short miserable lives, and brutal deaths. For some reason, they are exempted from the Humane Slaughter Act, which attempts to make the slaughter of cows and pigs "more humane" by "ensuring" that they are unconscious before the slaughter process begins. Chickens are not protected by this act, so they are always fully conscious when they are shackled upside down and their necks are slit. (103).

From a health perspective, fish isn't much better than chicken. Factory-farmed fish share the same issues of other factory-farmed animals; they contain high levels of pathogens and pesticides. And most wild-caught fish contain mercury, a carcinogen that can alter immune function, raise blood pressure, and even cause irreversible brain damage (104). And while many are now awakening to the negative health effects of red meat, they still believe they need animal protein and have switched to eating a lot more fish. The results of this increased demand are these enormous super-trawler fishing vessels with giant drag nets that are sweeping our oceans dry of fish, scooping up and killing any and all marine life that falls into their broad reach. If we keep this up, our oceans will be completely depleted of all marine life by 2040 (105).

"But what about organic, free-range, grass-fed, 'humanely-raised' farm animals?", you might be wondering. Well, you may be eliminating the hormones, antibiotics, and pesticides, but no matter how you slice it, consider these facts: (1) you are still consuming artery-clogging saturated fat and cholesterol that will slowly but surely give you heart disease; (2) you are still consuming an acidic food with no fiber that will sit in your colon for days putrefying and creating inflammation leading to cancer; and (3) you are still consuming a high-fat food that will cause weight gain and potentially lead to diabetes—even if your meat IS happy and free-range throughout his or her short life.

At the end of the day, if you understand that all food has a certain energy, then you know you are also consuming terror, fear, violence, and death when you eat meat. No living being, no matter how idyllic their life might have been, no matter how humanely they were raised, is killed without feeling terror and fear. The violence of their awful death is released into their bodies through stress hormones of adrenaline and cortisol shortly before they die—"humanely raised" or not. Having your throat slit, no matter how kind the hand or gentle the voice that talks you through it, is still not enjoyable. It's more like the worst terror and pain and fear you can imagine. Consuming terror and fear in the form of slaughtered animals is not good for your physical, mental, emotional, or spiritual health, period.

Animal By-Products/Dairy: So, maybe you tell me you don't eat any meat, but you still enjoy eating eggs and cheese. I used to think this was okay too. I was a vegetarian for years before I recognized why I was still holding on to those thirty extra unwanted pounds of weight. (Can you say, "Baked Brie Cheese"?!) Once I took out the animal products, the weight fell off. Once I took the blinders off to the cruelty still inherent in dairy, the ignorance fell away as well.

There are two categories of animal products: dairy milk products, such as milk, butter, cream, and cheese from mammals (cows, goats, and sheep), and eggs from birds (chickens, ducks, or turkeys). Let's take each separately, starting with the dairy milk products.

When we talk about dairy, cow's milk and cow cheeses are most frequently consumed and are what have become the most commercialized and unhealthy of all. Factory-farmed dairy is now the norm worldwide. Long gone are the days where folks had the family cow in the backyard that they milked. Dairy farming is now big, big agribusiness. Cows are no longer seen as sentient beings; they have become moneymaking milk machines.

From a moral perspective, think about how we obtain milk from cows. Dairy cows are literally kept pregnant or lactating their entire short life, either standing in a crowded, manure-filled pen or lined up at the milking trough connected to a machine that takes the milk from their body—the milk that was intended for their annual newborn calf that gets taken away from them shortly after birth every year. If her calf is female, she is sold to another dairy farm; if he's male, he's put into a veal crate to be eaten later, still just a baby. Anecdotal evidence abounds regarding the emotional trauma experienced by the mama cow and her baby when they are separated after birth, both crying and bellowing for days. Then, once the dairy cows are "spent" and not producing milk any longer, they are sent to the slaughterhouse and killed for lesser-quality hamburger meat, sometimes while they are pregnant. So if you think because you don't eat meat that you are not participating in the killing of animals, you are sadly wrong. Dairy is liquid meat. Just because you like the taste of ice cream, baby male calves are killed and eaten, and mama cows are killed and eaten (106). And even if you cared nothing about animal welfare, there would still be absolutely no reason to consume milk or cheese for health reasons.

Dairy cows are fed antibiotics, pesticides, steroids, and bovine growth hormones because higher production means bigger profits. When you drink milk, you are also drinking these same antibiotics, pesticides, steroids, and growth hormones. Recent studies are linking factory-farmed milk and the consumption of school-cafeteria hamburger meat (which is made from old dairy cows) to the prevalence of premature puberty in young girls today (107). And the prevalence of MRSA, a new antibiotic-resistant bacteria popping up in hospitals, prisons, schools, and nursing homes, is also linked with the consumption of milk and hamburger from dairy farms (108). This is now fortunately being addressed with new governmental regulations asking for antibiotics to be quietly phased out of the dairy industry altogether before we risk a serious health disaster. In addition to all the additives, cow's milk and cheese by itself is mucus-forming and sticky; if you have respiratory conditions, all this of extra mucus is problematic, causing allergies and asthma. (109)

Cow's milk is fattening; its purpose by design is to quickly grow a ninety-pound calf into a 2,000-pound cow. If you too are trying to fatten up quickly, there is no better way than consuming dairy! Milk and cheese are very difficult to digest; being "lactose intolerant" is actually more typical than not, as the human body was never intended to digest milk beyond the age of two! 65 percent of the human population is lactose intolerant, increasing to 90 percent among people of East Asian descent. So all this undigested lactose sits in our intestines causing all sorts of bacterial overgrowth and indigestion, and a much more inflammatory environment for growing a host of diseases (110). We know this, yet we still LOVE our cheese! Why? Because cheese addiction is very real.

The casomorphins found in milk and condensed and compounded in cheese have an opioid effect, producing a mild feeling of euphoria, intended by nature to strengthen bonding between a nursing baby and its mother (111). So of COURSE you are going to have trouble giving up cheese; you are addicted to it. You will break this addiction only by watching videos of baby cows being taken from their mothers so that you can have your cheese and by knowing that, instead of the baby cow that it was intended for, you are going to be the recipient of all that growth instead—in your middle, on your backside, on your hips! Cheese is a drug, and we need to get over our national addiction. There are artisanal plant-based cheese shops opening up everywhere now, so soon there will be no more reason to separate these sweet mamas from their babies ever again.

Cow's milk causes breast and prostate cancer. The China Study, a twenty-year study described by *The New York Times* as "the Grand Prix of epidemiology," was conducted by the Chinese Academy of Preventive Medicine, Cornell University, and the University of Oxford. It looked at mortality rates from cancer and other chronic diseases from 1973–75 in sixty-five counties in China; the data was correlated with dietary surveys and bloodwork from 100 people in each county. The research was conducted in those counties because they had genetically similar populations that tended, over generations, to live and eat in the same way in the same place. The study concluded that counties with a high consumption of animal-based foods were more likely to have higher death rates from "Western" diseases, while the opposite was true for counties that ate more plant foods. In particular, the connection between casein (the protein found in milk) and cancer was so profound that scientists could literally turn cancer growth on and off "like a light switch" simply by altering the level of casein protein in their diets. The same levels of plant-based protein did not promote cancer growth at all (112).

I would also advise you to forget what they say about milk being a good source of minerals such as calcium. You get higher levels of minerals from dark leafy greens and beans than from dairy. A twelve-year Harvard study of 78,000 women demonstrated that those who drink cow's milk are more likely to have osteoporosis and brittle bones than those who don't. The acidity caused in the body from eating dairy products actually causes calcium to be leached from your bones in an effort to balance your internal pH again. The countries that consume the most cow's milk – the United States, England and Sweden - have the highest rates of osteoporosis, while the countries that consume the least milk – China and Japan – have the least (113). So why are we drinking milk again? Oh yah, because advertising tells us that "milk does a body good"!

Well, the good news is that there are great sources of plant-based milks that make it so simple to give up dairy: almond milk, coconut milk, rice milk, barley milk, spelt milk, peanut milk, walnut milk, quinoa milk, sunflower-seed milk, sesame-seed milk, cashew milk, soy milk, oat milk, hazelnut milk, hemp milk ... phew, I'm outta breath! And of course all of these milks make lovely ice creams as well, and sour creams, and cream cheeses, and coffee creamers .... all of which are so much are more healthful, nutritious, and delicious. And no mama cows were harmed and no baby cows were killed in the process. Sweet.

I know what you're thinking: "If dairy were really that bad for us, wouldn't more people know about it? Wouldn't our government put something out to educate and protect us? Isn't this all just the ramblings of a lunatic animal-rights activist who loves her moo cows?" Well, the dairy industry is flush with cash and not only has the money to spend on advertising, they also have powerful interest groups in Washington. I don't mean to villainize farmers either. I love farmers and ranchers. They are hardworking men and women that produce the incredible fruits and vegetables we lobby for in our own diet! My dream for as long as I can remember has been to move to Texas and live on a ranch... now my dream cattle ranch has morphed into a farm animal rescue ranch, but nonetheless, the dream is stll there!

Now what I am about to suggest I know sounds simplistic and naïve, and I know it won't be easy as I am making it sound. But farmers and ranchers need to take a hard look at future trends here, and figure out a way to adjust and transition their business models accordingly. As demand for healthier foods grows, and demand for meat and dairy shrinks, it is time to look at how to transition the land from producing animals to producing plants. It won't happen overnight, and the shift can be gradual, but shift it must. Dairy farmers can slowly transition away from giving land to dairy cows and start to plant almond trees. Cattle ranchers can start an animal sanctuary, plant vineyards and grow wine or apples. More consumers are demanding organic produce, so old-school organic farming can substitute for commercial farming (talking fruits and veggie here obviously, not animals).

Being one of those crazy tree-hugging California girls, I know I don't have the street creds to be giving farmers and ranchers any advice at all, but I do have a couple homies here that do. Like my buddy Howard Lyman, a 77-year-old fourth generation cattle rancher from Montana. He was actively engaged in massive meat production operations on his land until a cancerous tumor set him on the path of a plant-based diet. Now an ex-cattle rancher and an animal rghts activist who promotes plant-based nutrition, he transformed his land into a beautiful organic farm. Like my buddy Harold Brown who grew up on the family cattle farm in MIchigan but, after a health crisis, made the connection between the family tendency of heart disease and the cruelty inherent in their ranching practices. In his own words, "Animals who are destined for an abbreviated life that ends in a violent death now called to my conscience and required me to show up, and where I could, show what little bit of mercy I can. Since I have made this conscious decision to show mercy, my life has been blessed a million, million times over and I have found a deep peace. So no, in my experience, there is no such thing as humane animal products, humane farming practices, humane transport, or humane slaughter." Like my adorable new friend Renee King-Sonnen, founder of Rowdy Girl Sanctuary in Angelton, Texas. Imagine what kind of fast talking she had to do after she had her awakening, to make her cattle rancher husband not only convert to a vegan diet himself but convert their Texas cattle ranch into a farm animal sanctuary! Well, she did it, and their Rowdy Girl Sanctuary is now home to many rescued cows and cattle and fast becoming a haven for vegan awareness events and fundraisers... and the list continues to grow of farmers and ranchers waking up to the fact that farm animals are no different than our pets, and honestly no different than us.

So whether you live in the Midwest or the East Coast or the West Coast, we can all have a say in the future direction of the cattle and dairy operations. The power to be a smart consumer of food is in your hands, and every time you purchase a food product at either a supermarket or a restaurant, you are in effect either voting for disease and cruelty, or voting for health and peace. Every single meal you order, every single visit to the grocery store, every single person makes a difference; don't ever let apathy or feeling like "one person won't make a difference" become your excuse. A lack of demand will start to cut off the need for supply, and so the world will shift. It will need to shift, one dairy farmer, one cattle rancher at a time.

Enough about meat and milk. Now let's dive in to America's favorite morning staple—eggs. Our good old American ranch-style breakfast, as if we were all still working manual labor all day on the ranch instead of sitting at our desks all day! Do you really think you need to fuel up with that many calories, fat, and protein as if you were working the fields all day? In addition, most of the eggs you buy today are from factory farms, not those beautiful, old, family-owned farms, and for many of the same reasons that you should stay away from factory-farmed meats or milks, you should stay away from factory-farmed eggs.

When you eat eggs, you are ingesting all the same hormones, pesticides, chemicals, and steroids, as if you were eating the chicken directly. But what if you are eating eggs from the farmer next door, and you know for a fact that they are "pasture-raised," outdoor, happy hens and that their eggs contain none of those hormones, pesticides, chemicals, and steroids? What if you have your own backyard hens that you treat like pets, and you collect their eggs and eat them? What's wrong with that? A couple things. From a health perspective, eggs are very high in cholesterol; elevated cholesterol leads to plaque building up in the arteries, which leads to heart attacks and strokes (114). Do those eggs really taste THAT good when there are other ways to get your protein? Scrambled tofu with a dash of turmeric is every bit as tasty as scrambled eggs, and so much healthier! Any scrumptious hot brunch dish that you would make with eggs, you can also make using tofu.

From a moral perspective, most of us don't have happy backyard hens. Most of us eat eggs that come from the egg industry, which basically works like this: Newborn chicks are immediately sorted upon hatching—males go down one line, and females go down the other. The female babies are shipped off somewhere to grow up and lay eggs themselves, while the males, the unnecessary by-product of the egg industry, are either ground up, suffocated, or just thrown into the trash bins still alive and left to slowly die. This is the awful reality, so every time you eat an egg, you are condoning this violence to newborn male chicks. And even if you do have happy backyard hens, they were sent to you after hatching in a facility that tossed out the baby males like trash down a garbage disposal (115).

In fact, the entire dairy and egg industry is horrific for young male animals. All dairy and eggs come from the pregnant females of the species—either their milk or their offspring—so the unneeded baby males that are born or hatched are either considered trash (like chicks) or are killed and eaten as quickly as possible (like veal calves and lambs). Unfortunately, with the new, increased demand for goat and sheep milk and cheese, we are noticing a lot more lamb ("lamb popsicles"? really?) and goat on menus and in butcher shops across the U.S. and around the world as these baby male lambs and kids are useless by-products of the ever-more-popular sheep and goat milk industries.

I know how you might be feeling right now. I remember how I felt the first time I learned the truth. This information can be overwhelming, upsetting, and may bring up feelings of guilt. I honestly feel bad to be the one to have to deliver the news, but it's important that you know, so you can start thinking differently about how your food—especially meat and dairy—are sourced and about the subsequent impact on your health. Transforming your life once you transition to a plant-based diet is easy; making yourself think differently about food is the hard part. You can make it right by resolving to make real change in your life and helping to stop this needless violence. Never believe that one person doesn't make a difference. You can, and you do.

Refined Sugar and White flour products: Hopefully, I've talked you into giving up meats and animal products, but we're not done yet! Unfortunately, it is possible to give up the meat and dairy and yet still COMPLETELY blow it from a health perspective! You could call yourself a Vegan and live off nothing but Diet Cokes and Twinkies and Skittles, but this won't make you healthy, and in the end your unhealthy vegan life advertises meat-eating as essential to the uneducated masses! That is why you need the Whole Earth Diet. It is (1) a plant-based vegan, and (2) a WHOLE-FOODS diet, which means, after we give up the animals, we also need to give up the sugars, flours, and processed foods that we all know aren't good for us (herein after referred to as *crap*). There are some pretty bad man-made "foods" out there that may be meat and dairy free, but they are still crappy, junky foods! And since you are now my poster child for a plant-based diet, I want to be sure you are eating the very best and most nutritious diet you can so that you don't come running back to me in a year saying that a plant-based diet "just didn't work out" for you. Because it does work, as long as you are eating right.

So, enemy #1 is refined sugar and white flour products (116). Candy, crackers, sweets, cakes, and sodas—these "foods" destroy our teeth and complexion while adding layers of unwanted fat to our waistlines. We all know that sugar is bad, but do you really know how prevalent it is, that it is in almost every processed food you buy? Read the ingredients on your favorite breakfast cereals, breads, and crackers. Sugar turns up in the most unexpected places. Now, in its purest form, raw cane sugar is just a plant and not too bad for you. In its natural form as fruit, sugar is a good simple carb and satisfies our desire for sweetness. But typically you are getting refined sugar—or even worse, high fructose corn syrup—in almost every kind of processed food.

It is usually used in food that is highly processed, high in fat and calories, and as a way to get you addicted because sugar is a very addictive substance. Food manufacturers learned this years ago, so now they put it in everything to get you coming back for more. The problem is, all this sugar is leading to hypoglycemia, yeast overgrowth, weakened immune systems, hyperactivity, attention deficit disorder, enlargement of the liver and kidneys, increase of uric acid in the blood, mental and emotional disorders, cavities, acne, and an imbalance of neurotransmitters in the brain. And the biggie—according to studies conducted by the American Journal of Clinical Nutrition—obesity and diabetes are directly linked to eating refined sugar and high fructose corn syrup.

Sugar's partner in crime is white flour (117). Where you find sugar, you almost always find white flour; they go hand in hand—cookies, cakes, Twinkies, donuts, pastries, piecrusts. These are the obvious ones. Some of the not-so-obvious ones are croissants, bagels, biscuits, sourdough rolls, even cream-based soups, gravy, pasta, mac and cheese, bread sticks, and stuffing. When used in baking products, white flour creates pleasing dishes. However, with the most nutritious part of the wheat kernel removed and the rest bleached—all to create a longer shelf life—the end product is far, far, from pleasing for your body! This is combined with the degradation of soil quality, mutated strains, and genetic modification to the point where many of us (perhaps as high as 75 percent of the population) have developed some kind of gluten allergy or intolerance, from mild all the way to celiac disease.

So, at the very least, switch from white flour products to dark organic whole-wheat or whole-grain flour products. If you feel bloated, fatigued, or moody, you may in fact be gluten intolerant. Try going gluten-free for a week and see if this changes. If you suspect any kind of gluten intolerance, try switching to a gluten-free flour for a while—flours made from chickpeas, potato starch, arrowroot, tapioca, hazelnut, almonds, amaranth, buckwheat, oats, or even coconut flour. Anything that can be ground into flour can be used as an alternative to white flour, and all of them are superior. There are so many alternatives now, and the "gluten-free vegan" community is active online sharing recipes and tips.

Processed and Artificial Foods: Processed foods are anything that has a label filled with artificial ingredients and additives. Most of these artificial ingredients are toxic, and this accumulation of toxins—though it may not kill you right away—at the very least is going to clog up your bloodstream and your lymphatic system (118). So read the ingredients. The fewer ingredients the better, such as "brown rice." Period. Or "lentils." Period. If it says "monosodium glutimate" or "butylated hydroxytoluene" or "high fructose corn syrup," turn around and run. If you can't pronounce the ingredients (-ates, -ites, -enes, -ame, -ose!), then don't eat it. If it contains artificial flavors or artificial colors, don't eat it.

And though sugar is bad, artificial sweeteners are even worse (119). Do not eat anything with aspartame, such as Nutrasweet or Equal. Aspartame was denied FDA approval eight times before they squeaked it through (after years and years and millions of dollars of legal battles). Aspartame converts to formaldehyde when eaten, which just can't be good for you, and there aren't any safe options for artificial sweeteners. Sweet & Low contains saccharin, a coal-tar compound. Splenda is chlorinated sugar, which has been bleached and its molecular structure changed; it has been transformed into sucralose, which contains heavy metals, arsenic, and methanol. It also can give you diarrhea and is found in many "healthy" protein and power bars on the market. Check for sucralose as an ingredient before you decide to carry a sucralose-laced protein bar in any sort of endurance event like a marathon. It is guaranteed to NOT help your performance when you need an emergency trip to the bathroom halfway through! Finally, artificial sweeteners are very acidic, and an acidic environment in your body leads to inflammation, which leads to disease. Period. So stay away from artificial sweeteners. Good substitutes for refined sugar would be evaporated cane juice, agave, brown rice syrup, raw sugar, Grade B maple syrup, molasses, or natural stevia (a newer sweetener on the market, from a plant found in Paraguay). Xylitol is the only natural sweetener that is so low in sugar that it is safe for diabetics.

Fried Foods and Cooked Oils: Fried foods (and cooking in oils in general) are also major culprits in our deteriorating health (120). Acne is frequently associated with eating cooked oils (margarine, hydrogenated oil, cooked polyunsaturated oil, etc.). Cooked oils and margarine and fried foods are probably the most difficult of all cooked foods to break down and metabolize. They require a significant amount of liver energy. Cooked oils and margarines are often incompletely broken down and end up clumping in the bloodstream and causing hormonal imbalances and acne. Cooked oils are inflammatory to the tissues and accelerate the aging process. Though there are oils that you could use for high-heat cooking, such as coconut oil, I don't recommend cooking in oils at all. It is much healthier to cook using low-sodium veggie broth, coconut water, or plain water.

Most "beverages" except for water: Okay, I'm here to tell you that most beverages should just be eliminated from your grocery cart and from your restaurant meal order except for water. WHAT? How boring is that? Well, if you are interested in losing weight, the biggest waste of calories is in commercial beverages. Those sweetened, bottled iced tea drinks typically have the same amount of sugar as four slices of pie. Those cool energy drinks that everyone is drinking—so full of caffeine as it is—have a sugar content equal to six

Krispy Kreme glazed doughnuts! Bottled coffee drinks are equal to a full meal's worth of calories. Orange sodas have the same amount of sugar as six ice cream sandwiches. Those bottled "juice" drinks, which you may think are healthier because they are "juice," can have the same amount of sugar as two cans of Reddi-wip whipped cream! And I know I shouldn't mention any coffee companies by name, but there is a big one that serves a "peppermint white chocolate mocha with whipped cream" coffee drink that is the sugar equivalent of eight and a half scoops of coffee ice cream (121).

All of these beverages exploit our sugar addictions. Just say, "No, thank you" to any beverage but water. Don't put these items in your grocery carts, and get used to ordering "just water, please," maybe with a squeeze of lemon or lime when you go out to a restaurant. Hot or cold water, it doesn't matter. Try it—it's easy. Just make your mouth say the words! Otherwise, you are wasting so many calories on liquids completely devoid of any nutritional value whatsoever. It truly does go "straight to the hips." This one little change in your diet will help you lose weight right away. I guarantee it.

Okay, so now you're thinking, "What the heck is left? You've taken away everything but water!" Don't worry. There are LOTS of things left! Lots of really good things that you can consume freely, and as much of them as possible.

Foods to Consume Freely!

Now that you have all the foods we are NOT supposed to eat, I will briefly go through some wonderful, real food that you can eat to your heart's content. Pull out a fork. You are about to start salivating for some tasty treats.

Greens, Greens, Greens! What food is unfortunately most often missing in our Standard American Diet, yet probably the best thing you can eat for good health? Green vegetables! And that wilted iceberg lettuce on your veggie burger doesn't count any more than the catsup counts as a tomato! Learning to cook and eat deep dark greens is essential to good health.

The chlorophyll found in plant leaves is what's used for photosynthesis, transforming carbon dioxide and water into glucose and oxygen. Chlorophyll is very similar in chemical composition to human blood, to the "hema" in "hemoglobin." The difference is that chlorophyll contains magnesium and blood contains iron. It's interesting that humans breathe in oxygen and expel carbon dioxide, while plants do the opposite; humans and plants are uniquely dependent upon each other for healthy survival. So it makes sense that the best thing we can eat are green plants. Chlorophyll's similarity to blood makes it easy for the body to use. Chlorophyll has powerful antioxidant, anti-inflammatory, and wound-healing potential. It helps to oxygenate your blood, which helps your body cleanse and heal itself. Chlorophyll binds with toxins like heavy metals so that they can be carried away as waste in the bloodstream. And it has been shown to help build up red blood cells, which benefits people suffering from anemia (122).

Variety is the spice of life, and there are tons of greens to choose from. To find what you like, start with the ones that are familiar to you—spinach and lettuce, perhaps? And then start to be adventurous and try greens that you've never heard of before. Rotate between bok choy, napa cabbage, kale, collards, watercress, mustard greens, broccoli rabe, dandelion, and other leafy greens. Green cabbage is great cooked, raw, or fermented in the form of sauerkraut. Arugula, endive, chicory, lettuce, mesclun, parsley, and wild greens are generally eaten raw, but can be consumed in any creative way you enjoy. Some greens are just great eaten raw as salads; others are better cooked. When cooking greens, try a variety of methods like steaming, boiling, sautéing, roasting, or lightly pickling, as in a pressed salad. Raw salad is also a wonderful way to get your greens. Raw veggies are refreshing, cooling, and supply live enzymes and phytonutrients. And, of course, there is my favorite: "a green smoothie a day" is a sure way to achieve optimum health. Take whatever raw greens you have, and juice 'em up with at least one raw apple or pear for sweetness. Throw in some additional spirulina powder for a super-boost of green energy and protein. Get into the habit of adding these dark, leafy green vegetables to your daily diet. Add a tablespoon of condensed super-greens powder into a beverage at least once a day. Try this out for a month and see for yourself the noticeable changes in your health.

That's some fine water, or "You are what you drink": Here I am with water again! But I cannot make this point enough—good, clean, simple, pure water is the key to good health and longevity. You can and should drink water all day long for maximum health benefits. How important is it to our health? Because water contains no calories and fills you up, it serves as a powerful appetite suppressant AND helps the body metabolize stored fat. Drink a big glass of water every morning when you first wake up and every hour throughout the day.

What kind of water should you be drinking? Ideally, water from a mountain spring—pure with minerals. Unfortunately, not all of us live close to a mountain stream. Just find a way to get pure, alkaline, mineralized water, and lots of it, into your home. By the way, water doesn't have to be boring. You can drink it cool, warm, or hot; you can throw into your glass a wide variety of fruits (lemons, limes, berries, peaches, pineapple), veggies (cucumber, celery), and/or herbs (ginger, mint, basil). There is also a staggering array of herbal teas available on the grocery store shelves now, all with zero calories and many with healing and curative properties. Make tea a part of your daily afternoon routine as a great weight-loss tip.

Fruits: Including fruits in your diet is one sure way to a healthier body. A daily intake of these delicious, all-natural foods can be of great benefit to your body in various ways. As you begin to eat more fruit, you will begin to realize how much better you feel. Fruit contains 80 percent water, so adding fruit to your diet increases your overall water intake. No other food on this planet contains that much water (123).

Digestive problems, such as constipation, diarrhea, or abdominal cramping, can be alleviated by eating fruit. Fruits that contain natural fiber can also help regulate bowel movements. Fruits have also been proven effective when it comes to lowering cholesterol levels, which can help you prevent strokes and heart disease. There have even been studies that say fruits can help stimulate your memory. People who consume fruits daily can retain more information and even recall it quicker versus those who don't eat fruits. There have also been studies that say people who drink fruit juices or eat fruit regularly can lower their risk of contracting

Alzheimer's disease by an incredible 76 percent (124). Wow! All this sounds pretty good, right?

One great tip to help you eat more fruit is to keep fruit out in a place where you can see it, like in the front of the refrigerator or out on the kitchen counter. By doing this, you will be more likely to eat it than if it is kept out of sight. Keep in mind that fruits are the most natural foods on this planet. They are the only kind of food that grows on a tree or a bush that you can pick and eat without any preparation or cooking. Your body has a craving for all natural foods. Fruit is how food was intended to be. Don't let the naysayers tell you that fruit is bad or too high in sugar. Fruit is one of our four recommended food groups on the Power Plate from PCRM, along with vegetables, grains, and legumes. For optimal health, don't go on one of these trendy diets telling you not to eat fruit. People have been successfully eating fruits for thousands of years, long before famous diet doctors came up with their dietary theories.

A Rainbow of Fruits and Veggies: There's no question that eating three to five servings of fruits and vegetables daily will improve your health. But more and more experts are saying healthy eating is not only about how many servings you eat. It's about the variety you pick, too. The more colorful your food on your plate, the healthier you will be! (125) Try and eat a variety of deeply colored fruits and veggies every day. Every color that you see is broadcasting its phytonutrient content. The orange fruits and veggies are packed with carotenoids, which help maintain healthy eyes, reduce the risk of cancer and heart disease, and can improve immune system function. Blue fruits and veggies contain anthocyanins, powerful antioxidants that protect cells from damage and aging. The lycopene in red tomatoes, watermelon, and pink grapefruit may reduce the risk of several types of cancer, especially prostate cancer. White fruits and veggies have allicin, which helps lower cholesterol and blood pressure and may reduce the risk of stomach cancer and heart disease.

So now you know why you must strive for a rainbow on your plate every day. What's the old saying, an apple a day keeps the doctor away? Let's change that to, "A rainbow a day keeps the doctor away!" Every day make at least one meal a day a beautiful raw salad containing every color of the rainbow.

Beans, Beans, the Musical Fruit (lentils, chickpeas, mung beans, fava beans, black beans)! Beans or legumes belong to an extremely large category of vegetables, containing more than 13,000 species, and are second only to grains for supplying calories and protein to the world. However, compared to grains, beans have about the same number of calories, BUT two to four times as much protein! They are the most perfect healthy food group—high in protein and fiber, low in fat and calories. Many beans, especially soybeans, are showing some amazing health benefits. Diets rich in beans are being used to lower cholesterol, improve blood-glucose control for diabetics, reduce the risk of cancers, lower blood pressure, regulate functions of the colon, prevent and cure constipation, and prevent many other bowel and digestive issues. Also, just as with fruits and veggies, richly colored beans are full of phytochemicals that offer a high degree of antioxidant protection. Beans also contain a lot of fiber, which helps digestion and to lower cholesterol. Finally, when beans are being absorbed in the intestines, they are carriers of "protease inhibitors," enzymes that counteract the activation of cancer-causing compounds in the colon, so they may help prevent colon cancer as well (126).

Of course, the ONLY negative with beans is their tendency to produce embarrassing and uncomfortable gas in some people! This is caused by a certain type of fiber found in beans that gets broken down in the intestine and can produce a lot of gas. This can be alleviated by properly soaking them before cooking, cooking for the proper amount of time, or sprouting them before cooking. Add in ginger, cumin seeds, or the Indian spice asaephoetida to your beans to increase their ability to be digested in the body and reduce the tendency to produce gas. Also, very simply learning to slow down and chew your food more thoroughly often heals gas problems overnight, and the more frequently you eat beans, the more your body will learn to digest without any problems. One more tip: the smaller beans like lentils and mung beans are easier to digest and produce less gas that the larger navy beans. These tips should allow you to enjoy these protein-rich musical fruits without too much of the music!

The nice thing about beans is how easily you can incorporate them into any meal. You can pour them into soups or salads. You can blend them up into delicious hummus or tahini for use in sandwiches, with pita bread, or as a dip for raw veggies. You can throw them onto pasta or into casseroles, stews, or really just about any dish you can think of. If you use canned beans, just be sure to buy 100 percent organic, with no added salt or sugar. You can eat them right out of the can, after rinsing and draining and with a dash of pepper, and be happy as a clam. (Shhhh, yes, I have done this!) (See Appendix B, Table 7, Beans.)

Ancient Whole Grains: Whole grains have been a central element of the human diet since early civilization. Humans ceased being hunter-gatherers and settled down into farming communities when they were able to cultivate grain crops. In the Americas, corn was the staple grain. In India and Asia, it was rice. In Africa, people ate sorghum. In the Middle East, they used wheat, making pita bread, tabouli, and couscous. In Europe, corn, millet, wheat, rice, pasta, dark breads, and even beer were considered health-providing foods. In Scotland, oats were a staple food. In Russia, they ate buckwheat or kasha. Very few people were overweight, even while on these "high-carb" diets! The difference is, they were eating these grains as whole foods, cooked or sprouted, not processed into sugary breads or pastas. They were eating whole grains, as close to nature as possible (127).

Some ancient grains have been around, unchanged, for millennia. What we are calling "ancient grains" are actually edible seeds with roots going back thousands of years. These seeds come from true cereal grains or grasses, like **spelt, kamut, teff,** and **millet**, or they are pseudocereals, actually flowering plants, like **quinoa, amaranth,** and **buckwheat**. Current studies show that these ancient grains are packed with protein, omega-3 fatty acids, and antioxidants. Part of the reason these grains are so healthy is that they have not gone through the genetic modifications that our modern wheat, corn, and soy have gone through, and they are all low in GI values, so they are low in sugar as well. I recommend you eat all of these ancient whole grains to your heart's content, with just one cautionary note. All grains do contain gluten in varying degrees. If you have celiac or are highly allergic to gluten, then you should avoid spelt and kamut. The others have only trace elements of gluten, so they should be absolutely fine for most people. (See Appendix B, Table 8, Grains.)

So that, my friends, are the foods you can eat in absolutely unlimited amounts! But don't worry—I still have lots more good food for you. We just need to be a little bit more mindful of the portion sizes.

Foods to Enjoy in Mindful Moderation

Modern Whole Grains: While ancient grains have remained unchanged through the years, by contrast, corn, rice, oats, soybeans, and wheat have been bred selectively over thousands of years to look and taste much different from their ancestors. Modern corn, for example, bears no resemblance to wild corn. Modern wheat has been genetically modified to produce a lighter, fluffier white flour for the white bread that consumers wanted, and a new protein called "gliadin" has been added to stimulate appetite. With all the genetic modifications, selective breeding, and hybridization that has occurred, one wonders what has really gone on with our cereal grains.

Did you know that more than 90 percent of all soybeans grown in the U.S. are genetically modified for herbicide resistance and are sprayed with massive quantities of toxic chemicals? Fully 85 percent of all corn grown in the country is also genetically engineered. So I open this section on foods to be eaten in mindful moderation with a warning: always buy organic grains. Until the day (hopefully soon) that we can require GMOs to be labeled, look for products with labels that proudly state "organic/non-GMO"! Good quality whole grains are an excellent source of nutrition; they contain essential enzymes, iron, dietary fiber, vitamin E, and B-complex vitamins. Since the body absorbs grains slowly, they provide sustained and high-quality energy. Finally, remember that all grains contain gluten in varying degrees, but wheat contains a high amount of gluten. If you have celiac or are highly allergic to gluten, you should avoid wheat and all wheat products. The others have only trace elements of gluten, so they should be absolutely fine for most people. (128)

Whole-Grain Breads and Pastas: I don't want to take all your fun away, so, in mindful moderation, you can eat sprouted, dark, whole-grain breads and pastas! Sprouted breads are made from whole grains that have been allowed to sprout, or germinate. The grains are as varied as the edible seeds described above; wheat is most common, but there are also breads and pastas made from millet, barley, oats, lentils, spelt, amaranth, etc. The sprouted grains have slightly more trace minerals and nutrients than non-sprouted, and whole-grain flour has many more nutrients than white flour. So whether you are selecting a bread or a pasta or a flour, choose sprouted whole grains for maximum nutritional quality, and always choose brown over white. You may want to try some of the gluten-free breads and pastas as well, made from quinoa or brown rice. It's all good.

Meat, Cheese, and Dairy Substitutes: Just because you've stopped eating meat and dairy doesn't mean you can't eat almost all the same foods, and make all your favorite recipes as you always have before! The only food I can think of that doesn't really have a perfect meat-free substitute is a bloody rare steak or raw sashimi fish. There is just no faking a piece of dead animal or fish flesh. But once you have been meat-free for a while, a piece of bloody flesh will honestly be the last thing on Earth you would want on your plate! So let's quickly look at all the other options for substitutions for you plant-based

virgins who still crave the taste of meat.

There are great chicken patty substitutes, veggie burgers, hot dogs, Italian sausages, stuffed turkey breasts, soy-rizo, chicken nuggets, and even spicy buffalo wings. You can make or buy meatloaf made out of nuts, grains, and lentils that is absolutely awesome as a main course with some mushroom gravy drizzled on top. Do you want milk for your cereal or cooking or baking? There is a huge variety now—and it grows every day—of plant-based milks, milk made from almonds, walnuts, rice, hemp, oats, coconut ... your choice! You can make your own almond milk by merely blending almonds with pure water, then straining it. Add a dash of cinnamon or nutmeg, and you have a heavenly beverage full of vitamins and protein. You will have no use for cow's milk ever again! Craving butter? Try using an organic, cold-pressed olive oil as a topping on cooked food or toast instead of butter, but if you want something "spreadable," use Earth Balance. Cheese? Yoghurt? Ice Cream? There are cheeses and yogurts and ice cream now made out of all the plant-based milks I mentioned above— almond cheese, coconut yoghurt, "rice" cream .... The products are only now starting to multiply on the shelves of mostly health-food markets, but with time these products will surpass and take over as the only products available. The amazing secret that the dairy industry has been keeping from us as best it can is that there is no real good use for cow's milk anymore.

There are also great substitutions for eggs, depending on what you want to use the eggs for. If you want to replace your scrambled eggs for breakfast, use extra-firm, plain tofu with a dash of turmeric. Do you want to bake and the recipe calls for eggs? Substitute one banana or ¼ cup applesauce for each egg.

Soy is a food product that has been controversial lately, with some studies touting its benefits and some its risks. The studies that show negative health effects, though, used massive amounts of soy in the research, much more than a normal person would consume in a day (and we also have a suspicion that negative effects are coming not from organic soy but from GMO soy) (129). Also, the funding for the anti-soy studies often has roots in the dairy industry. Just because there was a study done doesn't always mean it is objective science. That being said, soy products belong in the "mindful moderation" category. I don't recommend overeating processed soy milk or cheese or yoghurt or ice cream, especially when there are so many other options for plant-based milk, cheese, yoghurt, and ice cream available. I do recommend the more "traditional" soy products—fermented tofu, miso, or tempeh—eaten for centuries in moderation by the centenarians of Japan and Okinawa, and, of course, you can gobble up that gorgeous edamame. Soy-based meat substitutes are fine once in a while if you are craving meat, provided the soy is non-GMO and there are no nitrates or preservatives. These meat substitutes do much more good than harm, as they help thousands successfully transition their taste buds from a meat-based to a plant-based diet. Once you have been purely plant-based for a few months, though, you will most likely crave these meaty flavors less and less, and finally give them up altogether.

Black Coffee, Red Wine, and Dark Chocolate! With these three delicious vices, a little is okay, but only that—a little! I'm talking a single cup of organic black coffee in the morning or after a meal once in a while, not a whole pot throughout the day; a bite of dark 70–85 percent chocolate in the late afternoon (that's ONE of those cute little squares, not the whole bar!); or one glass of sulfite-free, organic red wine on weekends or with Sunday night dinner (not the whole bottle!). Caffeine and alcohol may have benefits if taken in very small quantities. However, both taken in large quantities on a regular basis have detrimental effects.

In moderation, coffee can improve alertness and mood, increase exercise performance and endurance, reduce muscle pain, and generally stimulate your metabolic processes to work faster and more efficiently (130). However, a bit too much caffeine can cause cardiovascular problems, stress, emotional disturbances, blood-sugar swings, gastrointestinal problems, dehydration, and premature aging. Using a stimulant to create energy you do not naturally have can potentially push your body into an energy deficit, sometimes referred to as adrenal exhaustion. Also, coffee, via its dopamine activation, is a very addictive substance that creates highs and lows in energy. In turn, these highs and lows can affect mood and physiological functioning. But if you love coffee and really enjoy a cup in the morning, go ahead. Just make sure it is black and organic (because anything you take in on a daily basis, even if it's only a small amount of pesticide, will build up in your system).

A little bit of sulfite-free, organic red wine is good for you. It helps to relax you and lowers your cholesterol, and the resveratrol in the red grape skins has been shown to have anti-aging benefits, keeping your memory sharp and your waistline slim (131). However, we have all seen the detrimental effects when someone is addicted to alcohol, and too much of a good thing is actually bad for your heart, your waistline, and your overall health ... not to mention your family relationships.

Organic dark chocolate, at least 70–85 percent cocoa, is actually quite nutritious in low doses. It is a great source of iron, magnesium, copper, and manganese, and is a powerful source of cancer-fighting antioxidants. However, it is still loaded with calories and does contain some sugar (though the darker the chocolate, the lower the sugar), so don't go out and consume a large chocolate bar every day. Just a bite or two after lunch or after dinner will satisfy that sweet tooth in a very healthy way (132).

You can have black coffee, red wine, and dark chocolate—but only in very controlled and mindful moderation. If you have an addictive personality or are out of balance in one of the other areas of self, then you should avoid these altogether.

I always tell my clients, "I may take away your meat and dairy, but never fear, I won't even **think** about taking away your red wine, dark chocolate, or black coffee!" Heck, if I did, I would lose my handful of clients for sure!

HERBS and SPICES: Once you've started adding in more fruits and veggies and eating organic, freshly prepared, simple meals, you can then begin to experiment with cooking as you never have before with herbs and spices. You can add both flavor and nutrients to your healthful plant-based meals with herbs and spices. When you shift away from a Standard American Diet swimming in salt, fat, and sugar to a healthy, whole-foods, plant-based diet, it might take some getting used to. Your taste buds are addicted to and will crave and miss the salt, fat, and sugar, and some of the first meals you experiment with may taste very bland to you, accustomed as you are to eating addictive crap! The perfect solution is to add flavor and taste, as well as more nutrients, by experimenting with and adding lots of flavorful herbs and spices. That spice rack in your kitchen is not just pretty to look at; it has healing powers as well!

Healing herbs—whether dry herbs added to food while cooking or fresh herbs chopped up and added on top of salads and cooked foods or into soups and stews at the last minute—add delicious flavor and nutrients. Oregano soothes coughs, improves digestion, and can lower blood pressure. Rosemary can prevent cataracts and ease asthma. Sage fights infections, alleviates menopause symptoms, and may help boost insulin for folks with diabetes. Thyme contains thymol, which increases blood flow to the skin and speeds up the healing of wounds. Mint has been used for centuries to fight nausea, but it also reduces pain and boosts mental alertness. Basil soothes gas and stomach upsets and can help ease muscle spasms. Parsley is a diuretic and helps prevent kidney and bladder stones, as well as reducing water weight bloating during certain times of the month! Finally, I must mention cilantro, my favorite raw herb to add to just about any cooked meal I make. Cilantro has been found to be effective in toxic metal cleansing. The chemical compounds in cilantro bind to toxic metals and loosen them from the tissue. Many people suffering from mercury exposure report a reduction in the feeling of "mercury disorientation" after consuming large and regular amounts of cilantro over an extended period (133).

Spices do more than make food taste great. Recent research confirms what traditional cultures have been saying for thousands of years: the use of specific spices can promote health, well-being, and anti-aging, and inhibit degenerative disease. The vegetarian diet so often associated with good health and lack of disease relies heavily on the use of spice. Cayenne pepper is one of my favorites, and I add it to EVERYTHING! It adds zest and a spicy quality to your food AND is known to relieve pain and inflammation, increase the appetite, improve digestion, and improve respiratory ailments, such as coughs or phlegm. Ginger root is a flavorful herb excellent for treating upset stomachs, gas, and bloating and can be used in hot dishes, grated over hot cereals, or sliced up and used for hot tea. Cinnamon adds amazing flavor to hot or cold meals, sweet or savory, and has the highest antioxidant value of any spice. Fennel adds a peppery flavor to raw or cooked foods and is high in calcium, vitamin C, fiber, and iron.

Turmeric, one of the main ingredients in curry and used in just about every traditional Indian meal, adds a bright yellow color and a warm spicy flavor to your food, AND it has amazing anti-inflammatory properties. Touted for its medicinal properties for years in Ayurveda, today we are proving with modern science that turmeric does, in fact, provide pain relief, is anti-inflammatory and anti-bacterial, helps digest fats quickly, and is being investigated for treating Alzheimer's, arthritis, and cancer (134). There is just way too much info with regard to healing herbs and spices to put it all into this book; that will have to be the subject of my next book, but hopefully this will at least get you thinking.

Where should you start? Begin experimenting with some turmeric and ginger root in your smoothies or ground up in your oatmeal, or add cinnamon sticks to your tea. These three are the top anti-inflammatories, and since inflammation is at the root of all illness, these three are a good place to start. (See Appendix B, Table 9, Herbs and Spices.)

TEAS: Speaking of tea, in addition to herbs and spices, another powerful ingredient to add to your regular routine is tea. First and foremost, tea has less caffeine than coffee; switching over to tea can make you less anxious and jittery, and it is a great substitute to your morning cup of joe. In addition, the cup of tea you're drinking may be the key to a whole host of health benefits. In the East, drinking tea has been one of the key ingredients to good health and happiness for thousands of years. Today, studies have found that some teas may help with cancer, heart disease, and diabetes; encourage weight loss; lower cholesterol; and bring about mental alertness. Tea also appears to have antimicrobial qualities. Interested in giving it a try? Be sure to invest in a high-quality product obtained from good, natural sources.

In Asia, green tea is the most popular, and its high level of antioxidants act as a protectant against bladder, breast, lung, stomach, pancreatic, and colorectal cancers; prevents clogging of the arteries; burns fat; counteracts oxidative stress on the brain; reduces the risk of neurological disorders, such as Alzheimer's and Parkinson's diseases; reduces the risk of stroke; and improves cholesterol levels.

The best variety of green tea is "matcha," elaborately prepared and drank by the Japanese in their tea ceremonies. Matcha tea benefits are higher because when you drink matcha, you ingest the whole leaf as a green powder dissolved in water, not just the brewed water around a tea bag. Even better, matcha also contains a unique, potent class of antioxidant known as catechins, not found in other foods, and powerful anti-cancer fighters. It is also able to reduce the effects of free radicals, which can lead to cell and DNA damage. A daily matcha regimen can help restore and preserve the body's integral well-being and balance and may add years to your lifespan (135).

Over a thousand years ago, matcha came to Japan as an aid to meditation practice. During long hours of sitting, monks would drink matcha to remain alert yet calm. Modern science has recently confirmed the lessons of centuries of tradition. Matcha is rich in L-Theanine, an amino acid that actually promotes a state of relaxation and well-being. While L-Theanine is common in all tea, matcha may contain up to five times more of this amino acid than common black and green teas. Matcha also contains caffeine, providing the unique experience of "calm alertness." Therefore, a bowl of matcha promotes concentration and clarity of mind without any of the nervous energy found in coffee.

Other popular teas are black tea, ginger tea, and holy basil tea. While black tea has the highest caffeine content, studies have shown that it may protect lungs from damage caused by exposure to cigarette smoke and reduce the risk of stroke. Ginger tea, a great digestive aid, is used to curb nausea, vomiting, or upset stomach due to motion sickness. The best way to enjoy ginger tea is to drink it fresh; just simmer a couple slices of raw ginger root on the stove for ten to fifteen minutes; add fresh lemon juice and agave syrup when you have a cold for a powerful germ-fighting combination. The use of basil leaf tea is recommended in nervous system fatigue, insomnia, and painful menstruation. Chamomile tea has also gained popularity in recent years. A gentle, calming, sedative tea made from flowers, chamomile tea can be helpful for insomnia and as a digestive aid after a meal. And all of this is just the beginning. There are beautiful teas made from flowers, roses, lavender, and many herbal medicinal teas. Dandelion root tea helps cleanse your liver during a detox. Senna tea helps move your bowels. Check out the large display of medicinal teas in your local health-food store, and try them out. You just may find that the remedies for many of your chronic aches, pains, and problems can be more simply, easily, and inexpensively cured with a cup of warm tea. Switch over to sipping tea and the options to explore are endless! (136)

Now that you are equipped with a ton of useful fundamental information, you can begin to experiment with different foods, herbs, spices, and teas based on your individual needs. We gave you the WHY a plant-based diet, and we gave you the WHAT—some useful information for you to think about. But maybe you are still feeling overwhelmed. You still need the HOW. I get it. NO worries. Chapter 3 coming up ... how to put all of this very simply to use for you.

Chapter 3

10 Simple Steps to the Whole Earth Diet

10 Simple Steps to the Whole Earth Diet

---

*"Once there was an Englishman who saw a Scotsman eating oatmeal for breakfast,
and he said, 'Ha, that's what we feed our horses in England!'
The tall Scotsman stood up, looked down at the Brit, and said,
'That's why they have such fine horses in England and such fine men in Scotland.'"*

~ Grandma Betty Barr

So, I hope by now you are at least THINKING about changing your diet—for your health, for the environment, and especially for our fellow earthlings. I have given you some good, solid information based on scientific research that supports my thesis that a whole-foods, plant-based diet is the best diet for your health. I have given you some broad categories of foods that you should never eat, foods that you can eat to your heart's content, and foods to eat in mindful moderation. Now it's time to give you some practical, hands-on advice. Let's actually do this! Let's make this work!

Step #1: Set Your Intentions

Before you begin anything new, it is a good idea to sit down and get crystal clear with your intentions. What health goals do you want to have achieved after six months? For anything to become a permanent lifestyle habit, you need to do it for six months, so give yourself that time for this to work. Write down your goals and be specific.

- How many pounds do you want to lose?
- Which medications do you want to reduce or eliminate altogether (of course, under your doctor's supervision!)?
- What would you like your cholesterol to be?
- What size dress would you like to fit into?
- Are there some skinny jeans in your closet that you want to wear again?
- Do you want to start dancing again, or running marathons—maybe even a triathlon?

Write your own physical goals down.

Then, beyond your physical goals, look at other reasons why this book appealed to you on a holistic level. Do you have goals beyond just feeling and looking good?

- Are you feeling convicted about never wanting to eat animals again?
- Is there something else you want to be doing with your life—volunteer work, a career change?
- Do you need more money?
- Are you unhappy in a relationship?
- Are you lonely and seeking a partner?
- Do you feel empty spiritually and want to find a real relationship with God?

Write ALL of these goals down: physical, mental, emotional, and spiritual.

Did you know that your mind creates your reality? All that is negative in your life—your health issues, your emotional issues, your spiritual issues, your financial issues—your mind creates it all. Your mental chatter constantly reminds you about all that is wrong with you, so you believe it and create that reality. So you need to turn this around and create positive affirmations; you need to start letting your mind tell you all about the *new* you, starting with the goals you just created.

Whatever it is that you desire, write it down in the positive, present tense, as if it were already true:

- "I am at my ideal weight."
- "I love the way I look in my bathing suit."
- "I am 100 percent plant-based and am living an authentic life in alignment with all my principles."
- "I have a partner in life that I adore and he/she adores me."
- "I love the feeling of having a big fat savings account."
- "I feel so great whenever I run a marathon."
- "I love working with special needs children."
- "I feel surrounded by love in my faith community."
- "I love my new pit bull rescue operation."
- "I feel a deeper connection to God now that I am not eating animals."
- "I hear God whispering to me at night when all is quiet and I feel such peace."
- "I truly and deeply love my life."

Take these positive affirmations—you may have one or two, or you may have ten or twelve—and create a beautiful artwork. Write all your affirmations down, and leave room for the last line to read: "For all of these things I am so deeply grateful to God." Decorate your words with whatever makes you happy – drawings, photos, squiggly lines. Make it 100 percent you. Make it fun to look at, frame it when you're done, and hang it where you can see it every day. Read these positive affirmations aloud every day, including the last sentence about being grateful to God. Do this, my friend, and watch the miracles begin to happen.

Step #2: Clear Away Clutter

Creating your positive affirmation artwork was step #1. That was fun, right? Well, step #2 is a big one. We are going to clear out the clutter! It's not nearly as much fun, but look at it like this: you are getting a home renovation for free and burning calories while you do it! We have some heavy lifting to do now. It's important to clean up your physical environment, to toss some things out and get rid of the "old" before you bring in the new. Your new life and the new you need a new, clean, clear, clutter-free space! Start with a thorough "spring cleaning" of your home or apartment, from top to bottom. Have a trash bag in one hand and a donation-to-charity bag in the other and fill them up. Fill up several of them. Clean out your closets and your garage, and look at this as a new beginning. The really cool thing about an intense Spring cleaning (any time of the year) is that, after it is done, your space looks much better than if you had gone out and spent money buying and adding more stuff, which is the mistake we often make when trying to refresh our environment. It is just as satisfying, maybe more so, clearing out the crap.

With this behind you, next you will want to really dig in and get rid of specific toxins in your home—in your bathroom and your kitchen particularly!

Clear Out the Toxins from Your Bathrooms:

Don't worry, I'm not asking you to throw all this stuff out and replace it 100 percent with all natural products immediately! I'm suggesting that you take this book with you when you go shopping to REPLACE your toiletries one by one. Starting in your bathroom cabinet and shower, you want to eventually get rid of anything that you put on your body, skin, face, or hair that contains any of these ingredients: (137)

- **Formaldehyde** – found in deodorants, liquid soaps, nail polish, shampoos; causes lung cancer and damages DNA, eyes, lungs

- **Phthalates** – found in hairsprays, perfumes, and nail varnish; damages the liver, kidneys, lungs, and reproductive organs

- **Parabens** (alkyl parahydroxy benzoates & butyl methyl/ethyl/propyllisobutyl paraben) – found in toothpastes, moisturizers, and deodorants; linked to breast cancer and testicular cancer

- **Sodium lauryl sulphate (SLS)** – found in most shampoos; can cause cataracts and urinary tract infections and can damage eyes

- **Toluene** – found in nail enamels, hair gels, hair spray, and perfumes; can damage the liver, disrupt the endocrine system, and cause asthma

- **Fluoride** – found in toothpastes and mouthwash; has been linked to Alzheimer's, osteoporosis, neurological disorders, and bone cancer

- **Propylene glycol** – found in moisturizers, skin creams, baby wipes, and sunscreens; clogs pores and causes skin to age faster

- **Talc** – found in baby powder; linked to ovarian cancer and general urinary tract disorders

- **Perfume** – can contain up to 100 chemicals, 95 percent of which are synthetics derived from petroleum; linked to allergies and breathing difficulties

- **Xylene** (xytol or dimethylbenzene) – found in nail varnish; can damage your liver and cause skin and respiratory tract irritation

- **Diethanolamine** [also Tri and Mono (**DEA, TEA,** and **MEA**)] – found in shampoos, moisterizers, sunscreens and body wash; absorbed through the skin, reacts with nitrates and forms carcinogenic nitrosamine

- **Aluminum** – found in most antiperspirants; accumulates in the organs and attacks central nervous system, linked to Alzheimer's and Parkinson's

- **Triclosan** [also 5-chloro-2 (2,4-dichlorophenoxyl) phenol] – found in deodorants, toothpastes and mouthwashes; releases cancer-causing dioxins

- **Chlorine dioxide** – found in most women's tampons; can cause reproductive cancers

Clear Out the Toxins from Your Kitchen:

Phew! Now that we've got the bathroom under control, let's move to your kitchen! Man, do we have work to do there!

In the pantry and refrigerator, get rid of any food items that have: (138)

- **Partially hydrogenated vegetable oil:** found in most processed foods; trans fats raise your cholesterol and increase your risk of blood clots, heart disease, breast and colon cancer, and atherosclerosis.

- **Shortening:** In addition to clogging your arteries and causing obesity, shortening increases your risk of metabolic syndrome.

- **White flour, white rice, white pasta, white bread:** Replace white flour with whole-wheat or gluten-free flour; white rice with black, brown, or wild rice; white pasta with quinoa pasta; and white bread with gluten-free breads or whole-wheat breads. If it's white, it ain't right! Get rid of it.

- **High fructose corn syrup:** found in practically EVERYTHING; it increases triglycerides, boosts fat-storing hormones, and drives people to overeat and gain weight. Lose the HFCS immediately!

- **Artificial sweeteners:** aspartame (NutraSweet, Equal), saccharin (Sweet'N Low, SugarTwin), and sucralose (Splenda); these supposedly diet-friendly sweeteners actually cause weight gain as well as other obesity-related diseases. Toss all artificial sweeteners!

- **Sodium benzoate and potassium benzoate**: These preservatives are added to soda to prevent mold from growing, but benzene is a known carcinogen that is linked with serious thyroid damage. Dangerous levels of benzene can build up when plastic bottles of soda are exposed to heat.

- **Butylated hydroxyanisole (BHA and BHT)**: BHA is another cancer-causing preservative. Its job is to help prevent spoilage, but it's a major endocrine disruptor and can seriously mess with your hormones. BHT is in HUNDREDS of foods, also food packaging and cosmetics.

- **Sodium nitrates and sodium nitrites:** These two preservatives are found in processed meats such as bacon, lunch meat, and hot dogs (which of course you won't be eating anyways!) They cause colon cancer and metabolic syndrome, which can lead to diabetes.

- **Artificial colors:** The artificial colors blue 1 and 2, green 3, red 3, and yellow 6 have been linked to thyroid, adrenal, bladder, kidney, and brain cancers, as well as ADHD in kids, and food coloring is in all kinds of processed foods. Throw it out!

- **Monosodium glutamate (MSG)**: Monosodium glutamate is a processed "flavor enhancer." The jury is still out on how harmful MSG may be, but glutamates have been shown to seriously mess with brain chemistry.

- **Olestra (Olean):** Olestra is a calorie-free artificial fat substitute used in those lovely "fat-free" snacks and chips you see. Olestra inhibits the absorption of vitamins and can cause diarrhea and anal leakage! Fun.

- **Genetically modified organisms (GMOs):** In the U.S., the majority of corn, soybean, cotton, and canola crops are genetically modified, and can be found in nearly every processed food. Studies show GMOs may cause organ damage, gastrointestinal and immune system disorders, accelerated aging, and infertility. GMOs have been banned in many countries, but here in the U.S. we're having a hard time getting them labeled. Until we do, buy only corn, soy, cotton, or canola products that are non-GMO and organic.

- **Brominated vegetable oil (BVO):** BVO is used to keep flavored oils in soft drinks in suspension. When consumed, BVO can't be digested or utilized, so it's stored in fat and can lead to reproductive interference and birth defects. It has been banned in 100 countries, but not the U.S.

- **Refined sugar:** Most people in the U.S. are consuming half a cup of sugar a day, and aren't even aware of it. It's a typical ingredient in processed foods, even things like spaghetti sauce and salad dressing. Sugar causes weight gain, bloating, fatigue, arthritis, migraines, lowered immune function, obesity, cavities, and cardiovascular disease. Throw out the refined white cane sugar, along with any processed foods that have sugar as an ingredient.

In the cupboards and on the stove, get rid of any kitchen items that have: (139)

- **Bleached white paper products:** Dioxins, the by-product of paper bleaching, are 300,000 times more carcinogenic than DDT. Play it safe and stick to natural brown napkins, coffee filters, and paper towels.

- **Volatile organic compounds (VOCs):** Emitted by paints, plastics, cleansers, solvents, air fresheners, dryer sheets, dry-cleaned clothing, and cosmetics, VOCs can cause nausea, headaches, drowsiness, sore throat, dizziness, memory impairment, and cancer. Switch to all-natural cleaning products, such as baking soda, white vinegar, or lemon juice.

- **BPA plastics:** BPAs are added to plastics to make them stronger. Found in food containers, baby bottles, and water bottles, they leach out into foods and liquids. Side effects can include breast and prostate cancers, infertility, polycystic ovary syndrome (PCOS), and insulin resistance. Store foods in glass or non-BPA plastic containers, and drink water from glass or stainless steel water bottles. Drinking your water from disposable plastic water bottles is not only a health hazard, but an environmental disaster, creating huge floating plastic garbage islands in our oceans.

- **Nonstick cookware:** Nonstick cookware contains a carcinogenic chemical, perfluorooctanoic acid (PFOA), that you inhale while cooking. At high temperatures, the coating of nonstick cookware will break down into a chemical warfare agent known as PFIB, a chemical analog of the WWII nerve gas phosgene. It takes only five minutes for nonstick cookware to emit at least six toxic gases. Immediately replace your nonstick cookware with stainless-steel or cast-iron cookware.

Anodized aluminum cookware is also considered safe, but stay away from non-anodized aluminum or copper cookware.

Clear Out the Toxins from Your Bedroom and Office Space:

Okay, so your bathroom and your kitchen are now free of toxins, but in addition to chemical toxins, you may want to also clear your bedroom and office of potential allergens and dust collectors. It's always best from both a physical and a mental perspective to reduce the amount of clutter in your life. Knickknacks and tchotchkes look good in magazines, but unless you can afford a full-time maid to dust every day, I suggest you get rid of all the crap everywhere and really go for the "Zen" effect in decorating. It can be expensive to go out and redecorate your home, BUT it is free to get rid of things that you no longer love. A place for everything, and everything in its place. Put some time into your Friday afternoon schedule to clean up your office space as well. A clean, clear desk is the best way to start work on a Monday morning. You will be amazed at how much better you feel in a clean, clutter-free, dust-free space, whether at home or at the office. A cluttered environment leads to a cluttered, stressed-out mind. An environment free of clutter leads to a mind free of clutter as well.

Clear Out the Toxins from Your Body – START WITH A CLEANSE:

Now that you have a clutter-free external environment, it is finally time to turn to your body! Before you begin your new way of eating, you should begin with a cleanse. Let's clear out the clutter inside your body to make way for the new. A cleanse just means that, for one week, you're going to be cleansing your internal organs, especially the liver and blood, by strictly eliminating all toxic foods and drinks (meat, dairy, processed foods, sugar, alcohol, AND caffeine), resting your digestive system by eliminating harder-to-digest foods (beans, larger whole grains), and doing some juicing-only days for even deeper digestive rest. Ideally you will sign up to do a Whole Earth Wellness seasonal cleanse that includes a guidebook, recipes and a meal plan, a list of acceptable foods, and daily recordings to help support you during your cleanse. You may want to further support your cleanse on your own with herbal supplements, colon hydrotherapy, a lymphatic drainage massage, or some hot yoga classes, all good for assisting your body with the cleanse.

Step #3: Transform Your Space

Transform Your Bathroom into a Spa:

Just as we did when clearing out the old, let's start with the bathroom. Here is the list of what you might consider purchasing for your new, healthy bathroom, starting with your shower:

- **Showerhead filter** – Tap water often contains as much, if not more, chlorine than found in swimming pools. More chlorine enters the body through skin absorption and inhalation from showering in tap water than by drinking it. Inhaled chemicals make their way into the bloodstream faster than when ingested, and chlorine is a suspected cause of breast cancer. Women suffering from breast cancer are found to have 50–60 percent more chlorine in their breast tissue than healthy women, so the first thing you want to bring into your healthy home are showerhead filters for every shower in your home!

- **Natural bath products** – You want all-natural, organic soaps, shampoos, conditioners, and bath salts. Head out to your local health-food store with this book, and don't forget your reading glasses! If you shop at a health-food store, you are going to have access to lots of organic products, but you still need to read the labels. There is a whole new world of delicious smells and textures out there; enjoy your multi-sensory shopping experience! You'll never go back to commercial soaps or shampoos again.

- **Natural after-bath products** – You want all-natural, organic oils, deodorants, and toothpastes. For moisturizing your skin, use natural oils on your body instead of commercial lotions or moisturizers, which are typically packed with pore-clogging parabens and preservatives. Coconut oil, olive oil, jojoba oil, and almond oil are great for moisturizing your skin and hair, both before you step into the shower and after you get out, if needed. Argan oil is great for hair. Look for toothpastes that contain no sugar, artificial sweeteners, fluoride, or sodium laurel sulfate (SLS). Find a natural deodorant that is NOT an antiperspirant; most antiperspirants contain aluminum and clog up your lymph glands under your arms with toxic chemicals.

- **Natural makeup and perfume** – Commercial perfumes are filled with artificial chemical odors that most people with allergies or asthma (or even a sensitive nose!) will react to. Choose instead a natural oil whose scent is pleasing to moisturize your skin AND to provide a pleasant odor. If you wear makeup, look for all natural and organic, and no animal testing was done as part of its production. Beauty should come from what you eat anyways, beauty from the inside out, not from your makeup. If you have anything that bothers you when you look in the mirror (dry skin, chapped lips, unhealthy hair or nails, acne, rashes, pale complexion), don't think what kind of product or makeup you should buy to cover it up; think about what type of food you should consume to fix it from the inside out. Sometimes you are missing certain minerals or healthy fats. Most often it's just about simply drinking more water.The beautiful results of hydration and healthy eating take longer, you will need to be patient, but the results will be permanent and far more authentic. No amount of makeup can hide poor health. Eat well, drink water, let your skin breathe, and the skin will take care of itself.

- **Accurate digital scale and measuring tape** – For your bathroom you should purchase an accurate digital scale that shows your weight to one-tenth of a pound. It's important to monitor your weight and be able to see the numbers on the scale going down! A scale and a measuring tape are both important to help mark your progress, because sometimes your weight loss will level off, but you will continue to lose inches (since muscle weighs more than fat).

- **Steam showers, soaking tubs and infrared saunas** – Why not? Since we're talking about converting your bathroom into a spa, if you have the space and the money, every luxurious healthy bathroom should have a steam shower, a good soaking tub and an infrared sauna. I know we're talking real money here, but I would be negligent to you, my dear readers, if I didn't mention these three luxury bathroom fixtures that will truly transform your bathroom into a spa. A steam shower (preferably with aromatherapy) can help improve your circulation, help you recover from exercise, clear up your skin, and help you relax, especially before bed and with a nice lavender aroma. A soaking tub is also a great way to introduce some healing herbs and minerals into your body in a very relaxing way. And an infrared sauna allows infrared light to penetrate your skin cells which in turn produces a whole host of health benefits such as stimulated collagen production, improved circulation, and weight loss.

Transform Your Kitchen Pantry and Refrigerator into a Health-Food Store:

Consider getting a head start by starting to stock up on all the following supplies for your "newly healthified" pantry and refrigerator:

- **Healthy baking supplies**: whole-wheat or gluten-free flour (there are all kinds of flours, such as blue-corn flour or coconut flour!), aluminum-free baking powder, arrowroot powder (in lieu of corn starch)

- **Healthy bulk beans/grains/cereals:** a wide variety of beans, split peas, brown rice, all colors of quinoa, millet, wild rice, steel-cut oats, organic gluten-free granola, black (or Forbidden) rice. Have plenty of canned, organic beans (no salt, no preservatives added) in the cupboard as well for when you don't have time to cook from scratch.

- **Plant-based milks and yogurts:** Try a variety of plant-based milks to find your favorite; coconut milk and almond milk are my favorites, but try rice, hemp, oat, or cashew milk—and I think there are a few others now. Try them all (as long as the source is a plant, and not a mama!). Also, try some plant-based yogurts; coconut milk and almond milk yogurt are delicious and make a great breakfast combined with granola and berries.

- **Healthy pastas/breads**: whole-wheat or gluten-free pastas; the quinoa pasta has a lower glycemic index than the brown-rice pasta if you are looking to lower your sugar intake. I recommend either whole-grain sprouted wheat bread or gluten-free breads for morning toasties.

- **Low-sodium vegetable broth and canned tomatoes**: I always have these on hand to make quick meals—soups and stews—out of whatever veggies and grains and beans I have on hand!

- **Spices**: all-natural and organic spices, Celtic or Himalayan sea salts, cayenne pepper, fresh black pepper grinder

- **Sweeteners**: blackstrap molasses; brown-rice syrup; dark, amber, raw, organic agave nectar; maple syrup (grade B); raw cane sugar; xylitol; stevia; xylitol has the lowest GI and the only sugar acceptable for folks with blood-sugar issues and/or diabetes

- **Condiments:** Bragg liquid aminos, Umeboshi plum vinegar, rice vinegar, apple-cider vinegar, extra-virgin olive oil, organic catsup, whole-seed organic mustard, Vegenaise, nutritional yeast (for cheesy flavor topping), Ener-G egg replacer, sauerkraut, pickled beets, vegan kimchi, low-sodium nama shoyu (organic soy sauce) or low-sodium tamari (organic gluten-free soy sauce)

- **Healthy drinks:** herbal teas, green teas, coconut water, kombucha

- **Healthy butter replacer:** Earth Balance natural buttery spread

- **Nuts and seeds:** raw almonds, walnuts, cashews, macadamias, pistachios; raw sprouted pumpkin and sunflower seeds; raw nut and seed butters

- **Frozen organic fruits/veggies:** It is always good to have some frozen organic fruits for your breakfast smoothies and frozen veggies as backup between trips to the market when you are out of the fresh veggies.

- **Vitamins:** whole-foods multivitamin/mineral supplement; vegan omega-3 oil supplement with DHA/EPA (algae); Methyl B-12; D2/calcium/magnesium/zinc if over fifty

- **Fresh fruits and veggies:** Finally, your last stop should be your local farmers' market for some fresh, local, organic, seasonal fruits and veggies. Always have bananas, apples, kale, and berries for breakfasts, multicolored veggies for lunch and dinner ... and more kale. Always have ginger, garlic, and onion (yellow onion for cooking, red onion for salads). If you find fresh turmeric root, buy it and use it fresh or freeze what you don't use. Experiment with fruits and veggies you have never tried before, such as dragon fruit or those weird-looking mushrooms. It's a whole new world of eating! At the end of the week, all your unused produce is going into your juicer or blender to be consumed in one giant monster smoothie, so there is no waste!

Transform Your Kitchen into a Healthy Spa Cafe:

- **Juicers and Blenders** – Speaking of juicers and blenders, once you start this healthy new lifestyle, you are going to want both of these babies in your kitchen, which is now being transformed into a healthy spa café. What is the difference between a juicer and a blender? A *blender* works by using rotating blades to chop up the produce. The result contains everything that went into the blender—all the fiber, ground-up skin, seeds, flesh, pulp—everything, no waste, a nice thick drink. **A smoothie made in a blender** makes a perfect, higher-calorie meal replacement for breakfast any day of the week, and it can be loaded with lots of superfoods (especially green protein powder) as a great way to start your day! A *juicer* separates the juice from the fibers to produce a lighter, thinner beverage. The benefit of **juice made in a juicer** is that the body doesn't have to spend large amounts of energy to digest the juice since there are no fibers to break down. It also means that the body can quickly and easily absorb the nutrients from a lot more fruits and veggies in a juice. As you can see, there are reasons to want a juice and reasons to want a smoothie, so both a juicer and a blender belong in any true health nut's home—and that is now you!

- **Basket o' superfoods** – You know that bread basket that used to overflow with bread, bagels, and Danish? Well, you are about to repurpose that as a superfoods basket! If you are serious about losing weight and getting healthy, you really need to cut back on the breads and bagels and any baked goods anyways. You will be having a lot more smoothies for breakfast, and next to the blender you will want to have a basket chock-full of superfoods to add as you wish. Green protein powder should definitely be in your basket. Cacao powder and raw cacao nibs are a close second. Then all the rest, to be added as needed, include maca powder, ginger root, turmeric, chia seeds, and hemp seeds. We will get to all of this later in this chapter (Step #7 to be exact), but for now just know that you officially have changed the name of your bread basket to superfoods basket, and let's leave it there for now.

- **Spices and teas rack:** If you have a great big kitchen with lots of storage, then you may not need to think about this, but if your kitchen is small like mine, you may want to do what I did. I cleared out a small corner of the kitchen counter near the stove and dedicated it to my daily spices and teas. I have a rack filled with my everyday breakfast/tea stuff: my breakfast/tea spices (cinnamon, nutmeg, cloves, allspice, vanilla), sweeteners (agave syrup, stevia), teas (green, dandelion root, holy basil, rooibos), as well as ginger and turmeric roots and lemons/limes. I use all of these daily for either my hot morning cereal or my hot afternoon tea, so I never put them away. If you line them up nicely, they look pretty and remind you to drink some tea instead of reaching for a cookie during those late afternoon energy lulls.

- **Strainer** – You may want to buy a good strainer as well. If you have a blender and not a juicer and want to strain out the pulp or products that have not broken down, you can use a strainer almost as effectively as if you had juiced in the first place. You will also need a strainer when you make homemade almond milk in a blender, which you will definitely want to do, trust me!

- **Cast-iron, stainless-steel, or anodized-aluminum cookware** – No matter what type of cookware you use, when it is heated, a small amount will leach itself into the food. This is why it is so important NOT to use Teflon, aluminum, copper, or other toxic materials for cooking. On the other hand, when you use cast-iron cookware, a small amount of iron is leached into the food, and since most people have iron deficiencies, most actually benefit from this effect (though those with excess iron issues should note this as well, as they could suffer negative effects). Stainless-steel and anodized-aluminum cookware are also safe options and those with iron issues can safely use them.

- **Sharp knives and a cutting board** – One thing you will be doing a lot of during this new healthy (permanent) phase of your life is chopping up lots of fresh fruits and veggies. Make this experience as wonderful and soothing and Zen as it can be with some nice, professional-quality cutlery, which will make slicing and dicing a breeze! Cutting up fruits and veggies will become one of your new lifestyle daily routines, so make sure you have the best you can afford. You will have no more worries about cross-contaminating your fruits and veggies with salmonella and E. coli or other raw-meat-borne parasites since you won't be chopping meat anymore!

- **Drinking water source** – A very important decision for you to make will be how and where to get good quality alkaline, mineralized drinking water into your home. You may want to consider buying a "Kangen" style water ionizer/filtration system, which is a coffeemaker sized device that is hooked up to your kitchen sink. The machine filters and then ionizes the water. Kangen drinking water is by far the best option for drinking water at home; it is purified, alkaline, and restructured into perfectly shaped microscopic hexagons, so it deeply hydrates you in ways other water cannot. The only downside is the cost. If you can afford one, it is the way to go! If not, look for a local water brewery that produces pure alkaline mineral water and pick yours up there.

- **Glass water bottle** – Buy yourself a special glass water bottle that you fall in love with. You will want to carry it with you everywhere, so be sure it is large and something that you love, as it will be as much a part of your life as your cell phone now! Take it with you everywhere. Feel naked without it. Of course, I would love it if you order the Whole Earth Wellness blue water bottle off our website. Why a cobalt blue glass water bottle? According to Dr. Ihaleakala Hew Len, blue glass bottles are a Hawaiian cleansing tool. Water that is placed in a blue glass water bottle in sunlight for an hour will allow one to "transmute memories replaying problems in the subconscious mind and help the body to 'let go & let God.'" Well, why not?

- **Other special equipment for raw foods:** Consider these: a "spirooli" that makes pasta noodles out of raw veggies like zucchini; dehydrators for making breads, pasta, and all sorts of entrees that are still "raw"; and sprouting trays for nuts, seeds, grains, and legumes. Even if you choose not to go "100 percent raw", at least two of three meals each day should be raw. Raw foods deliver all of the vitamins, minerals, phytonutrients and healthy enzymes from the plant that cooked foods do not.

That's it for Step #3—creating the healthiest home environment that you can. Now that your bathroom is like a spa and your kitchen is a cross between a health-food store and a spa café, let's get down to business. Let's start making some meals! Don't panic if you are not a cook or don't have a lot of time. Trust me, I get it. I am not a cook, and I am always running around like crazy. This system that I am going to give you in Steps 4–7 is everything you need to do to transition successfully to a healthy whole-foods, plant-based diet without needing a degree in culinary arts or having all day to create visual masterpieces. This is about simple, practical cooking. It works for me, and I hope it will work for you.

Step #4: Let's Make Breakfast

Let's start with the first meal of the day—breakfast! What do we eat for breakfast on a weekday when there is not much time to prep and we just want something fast and easy? These are my five Go-To Busy Breakfast Recipes to use Monday through Friday, or every day! Some weeks I am so busy I will have the same thing every morning all week. Other weeks I try to have something different each day. It just depends. But you absolutely must not skip breakfast. You want to eat three square meals a day without snacking, and breakfast is the cornerstone of a good day.

The common theme among the five is they all have fresh fruit, they all have complex carbs for fuel, and they all have some fiber, protein, and healthy fats to keep you feeling full longer. So get that cutting board out every morning and start chopping up some fresh fruits—for your smoothie, your oatmeal, your cereal, your fruit salad, or your PB&J!

Of my five go-to weekday breakfasts, the two that I use the most often are the Green Smoothie and Oatman's Oats, very simply typically alternating those two. Honesly, once I find something I like, I stick with it. Simple. But just so that you don't die of boredom, I have added three more options for you that I do enjoy on occasion: cold cereal, a fresh fruit salad, or a toastie (PB&J and some variations on the theme)!

1. Superfoods green smoothie: This by far is my most often-used breakfast. The basic formula for the perfect green smoothie for two is: 16 oz liquid, a banana, an apple, a handful of blueberries, 6-8 kale leaves stripped off their stalks, 2 Tbsp of some type of green protein powder, 2 Tbsp of vegan omega-3 DHA oil, an inch of ginger root, an inch of turmeric root, and the juice from a lime. That is the basic formula, but you can try many variations on this theme. For the sixteen ounces of liquid, you can use water, coconut water, or a plant-based milk, depending on how many calories you want; use a plant-based milk for a growing child, pure water for a chubby parent, or coconut water for post-workout mineral and electrolyte replacement! If you are really hungry and/or need extra calories, you can add some rolled oats, half an avocado, or a tablespoon of almond or sunflower seed butter to the blend. You can add other tropical fruits or other types of berries. You can experiment with other greens like spinach or collard greens. You can use frozen bananas or frozen fruits to make it colder and more like a milkshake. Make sure to always include the omega-3 oil in your smoothie (or half an avocado or tablespoon of nut or seed butter) because the oil-soluble vitamins A, D, E, and K in those fruits and veggies need the presence of fat to be digested. Also, make sure to add the lime juice too, because the extra vitamin C is crucial to absorbing the iron from your greens. Look for my Superfoods Green Smoothie recipe in Appendix A.

2. Oatman's Oatmeal: This is my favorite healthy comfort-food breakfast for Winter—steel-cut oatmeal with "the works"! If you tell me that you don't care for oatmeal, I will say you've never had Oatman's Oatmeal! You can't just cook it up and eat it without adding some toppings that will make your taste buds sing. Steel-cut oatmeal can take up to thirty minutes to cook, so if you typically don't have that kind of time, you can get the quick-cooking kind, or you can also substitute fifteen-minute cooked quinoa for oats (or cooked rice or any cooked whole grain for that matter, from rice to barley to whatever you have on hand!). All cooked whole grains actually make great hot breakfast cereals, but the texture and taste and chewiness of steel-cut oats is my favorite.

Anyways, cook whatever you have according to the package directions. Instead of cooking in water, you can cook in coconut water with a splash of organic vanilla for a lovely flavor. Once cooked, pour into bowls and add nuts (chopped walnuts or almonds), fruit (dried cranberries; raisins; diced apples; diced dates; chopped peaches, pears, or cherries), spices/superfoods (cinnamon, nutmeg, fresh-grated ginger, flaked coconut, raw cacao nibs, goji berries), and a bit of plant-based milk around the edges (almond, soy, coconut, hemp, oat, or rice milk). Shave some raw ginger or turmeric root on top, and drizzle with a natural sweetener like agave syrup or maple syrup if needed. If you don't mind Dr. Seuss–green oatmeal, stir a tablespoon of a good quality green superfoods protein powder into the oatmeal in your bowl before adding the toppings. This dish is so, so filling. You will not be hungry until lunchtime. If you have a big appetite, you might want to make this your go-to healthy breakfast! Look for my Oatman's Oatmeal recipe in Appendix A.

3. Forever-a-kid cereal – This is just like what you ate when you were a kid, only forget most of the packaged and processed cereals in the cereal aisle. If it's got a cartoon character on the front of the box, or if the box says "heart-healthy," don't buy it; it's not healthy. Shop for healthy cereal only—granolas and mueslis—cereals that actually look like real grains, not marshmallow pots of gold. Don't pay attention to the health claims made on the front of the box; instead, check the ingredients label on the side. (Don't leave those reading glasses at home, ladies!) Look for brands that have no more than 10 grams of sugar, 3 grams of fat, or 220 mg of sodium per serving, and have at least 5 grams of fiber per serving. If there is anything on that label that you don't recognize as food, run. Ideally, you want no artificial flavor or color, no tripotassium phosphates, BHA, or BHT. Check your typical "commercial" cereal label next time, just for the heck of it. You will most likely not be able to recognize or pronounce half the words on there. If your brain cannot recognize it as food, imagine what your poor digestive system will think about it.

Cold cereal always reminds me of being a kid; it is my go-to for both simplicity and nostalgia ... except instead of Lucky Charms (or even Cheerios), I reach for my healthy, organic granola or muesli, pour a little almond milk on top, or pour it OVER some delicious coconut or almond milk yoghurt. I always add some fresh blueberries and/or banana slices ... sprinkle with cinnamon and/or nutmeg and/or allspice ... and I am happy as a clam. Remember, only one bowl now, folks—not TWO!

4. Amazing fruit salad – Simple, pure, fresh, raw fruit. It doesn't get any better than this for pure vitamins, minerals, phytonutrients, fiber, and enzymes, and if I was a total health nut, I would eat NOTHING but fresh fruit for breakfast every morning! Plus, it just doesn't get any tastier than fresh, organic papaya filled with wild blueberries and spritzed with a squeeze of fresh lime from the backyard. Whatever fruits you have on hand, you can blend up into a smoothie or cut up into a quick fruit salad. Chopped avocado blends deliciously with all kinds of fruit salads, being a fruit itself (as do toasted coconut flakes)! And adding avocado also contributes to making you feel full longer than just the fruit since avocado also gives you a nice dose of healthy fat and protein, keeping you satisfied longer. Sprinkle on some hemp seeds or chia seeds to add even more protein and healthy fats. Eating fruit salad always makes me think I am on a tropical vacation. Are you serious about wanting to lose some unwanted weight? Stick with only the fresh fruit salad for breakfast. Look for my Superfoods Fruit Salad recipe in the appendix.

5. Toasties: And finally, this is a good one if you forgot to set your alarm, or if you set it but hit the snooze button one too many times! I do not advocate eating on the run AT ALL, but sometimes it is a necessity. On those kind of mornings, I will make myself a good old PB&J. I use a sprouted whole-grain wheat toast (or gluten-free as needed, but always toast gluten-free bread or you are going to have a mushy mess). Use a pure peanut butter (peanuts should be the ONLY thing listed on the ingredients label) ... or pure almond butter, or cashew butter, or sunflower-seed butter, or pumpkin-seed butter! Try them all and discover some amazing new taste treats! The nice thing about the seed butters is that, if you have young kids in school, schools will allow "seed butter" sandwiches. (Most do not allow peanut butter or any nut butters anymore because of kids with peanut allergies!)

Make sure the jam or jelly you are using is made only with pure organic fruits, no sugar added—maybe some lemon juice to preserve, but nothing else. Better yet, instead of jam, just use some very thinly sliced fresh fruit, like apple or pear, and/or throw on some blueberries to stick onto the freshly spread nut butter. You can call this a PB&F (peanut butter and fruit) sandwich. Oh, and spinning further off the PB&J idea, some equally simple, delicious, and healthy sandwiches might be sliced avocado and sunflower seeds, the famous surfer's peanut butter and sliced bananas with cinnamon, or really any nut butter with any sliced soft fruit.

Bottom line, on your gluten-free toast, have some fruit (jam, avocado slices, fruit slices) and have some nuts/seeds (peanut butter, nut butter, sunflower seeds, almond butter). Avocados and marcona almond sandwiches may be one of the best-kept, delicious secrets on Earth. You're welcome.

So now you have some good ideas about what to make for quick, easy, healthy breakfasts at home. IMPORTANT: Take your daily supplements with breakfast because a lot of our ability to absorb various vitamins and minerals depends on the presence of certain other vitamins and minerals. Look at your breakfast time as that time to flood your body with all the vitamins and minerals it needs, certain that there will be all the others available at the same time for maximum absorption.

If even this is too much for you, you can always stop by a juice place on your way to work and pick up a smoothie. Order a smoothie that is mostly veggies (cucumbers, celery, carrots, spinach) with a fruit or two like an apple or pear thrown in to sweeten it (or trust me, it will taste like your backyard lawn trimmings), and have some ginger thrown in as well. If you're feeling the need to detox, add a pinch of cayenne. Make sure your smoothie doesn't have any added milk or yoghurt in there, too.

No juice place nearby? I am sure you have one of "those" corporate coffeehouses nearby! They are on every street corner in the world now. Order an oatmeal with the works, just throw out the brown sugar, and enjoy the fruits and nuts on top ... and don't even look at all those tempting but extremely fattening pastries. I am so glad they are putting the calorie count there now so that we can start to make sense of why our hips were expanding before we had our awakening here on the Whole Earth Diet.

What about weekends when you have more time, and perhaps want to cook up something special for the family or friends? In Appendix A, I have included just a sampling of fancier breakfasts and brunch-type dishes for when you have company or just want to treat yourself or your family. There are plenty of tasty breakfasts to indulge in on weekends, just like back in the day when you were a meat eater, only these are all cruelty-free—tofu scrambles, muffins, scones, waffles, pancakes, tempeh rancheros, breakfast burritos, polenta and potato casseroles ... amazing dishes for when you have more time. Start a Google image search for "vegan brunch" and you will see what I mean. But to make this transition easy and simple for you, I want to highlight that most mornings you should be having one of these five above, not only for simplicity, but for health as well. As much as we love vegan pancakes and cinnamon rolls, we cannot eat them every morning or we will look like vegan pancakes and cinnamon rolls! Too much baked flour and sugar and maple syrup is not good for the waistline, with or without the eggs, butter, and milk. Think of the fancy breakfasts as your once-a-week treats.

Oh ... and in case you are wondering, I do indulge in a cup of organic black coffee or two every morning. I typically make it at home from fresh-ground organic beans, and I don't bother with soy or almond creamer or anything like that, though they do make them. I just drink it black and make sure it is an organic blend. So often we care so much about buying organic produce, but we ignore it when it comes to our coffee, and the majority of what we are drinking every day in coffeehouses everywhere is not organic and has been sprayed with pesticides. So if you are drinking the same nonorganic coffee every day, whether you are making it at home or ordering it from your favorite corner coffee place, you are slowly but surely poisoning yourself with these coffee-plant pesticides. AND I will tell you right now, if you are ordering soy lattes, the soy milk being used in large chain coffee houses is GMO soy ... so your daily morning soy latte is your daily dose of pesticides and GMOs! I know. I used to do it too. Now I purchase organic beans from the local coffee house and brew at home. I end up saving both money and caloric intake this way, instead of going for those daily venti lattes.

Step #5: Let's Make Lunch

The frustrating thing about lunch is that it is the most important meal of the day, yet it's timed to fall in the middle of our busy day with no time to cook. Regardless, it is so important to never skip lunch either. Your breakfast is intended to fuel you from breakfast to lunchtime, about four hours. Your lunch, however, needs to fuel you from lunch until dinner, about six hours, so it should be a hearty meal. You cannot be healthy if you skip lunch and are running around like a chicken all day without eating. Ideally, you want to consume about 60 percent of your daily caloric requirement at noon because it will fuel you through the afternoon, and your body will have plenty of time to digest and absorb all the good nutrients that I KNOW you will be eating. If eating makes you sleepy, consider having your cup of coffee with lunch. The coffee is acidic and helps you digest your food, AND it revs up your metabolic processes to help you digest your food and keep you from getting sleepy. Also, if you have a sweet tooth and want to indulge in that bite of raw dark chocolate daily, after lunch is the time to do it. Lunchtime is AWESOME!

So how do we "make lunch" if we are busy working professionals? I am just going to assume that everyone reading this is a busy working person, whether you are working in a cubicle somewhere or working from home as a hardworking entrepreneur or stay-at-home mom. No matter who you are—a student, a mom, a corporate executive—I think, realistically, that only in our dreams will we be home cooking at lunchtime like they do on those cooking shows.

So this is what we do: We do our cooking at night.

If you live alone, you cook in the evenings and set aside your cooked meal to take to work for lunch the next day. You make a salad for dinner.

If you have a family to feed, you will make both a cooked meal and a salad. The kids and the hungrier folks can eat the cooked food AND the salad. You, my dear friend reading this and looking to lose weight, are going to eat **only the salad** at dinnertime, and you will set aside your portion of the cooked food for your main meal—lunch—the next day. Whether you are working and eating lunch at home, or working and eating lunch at Corporate Plaza, you are going to have this amazing, homemade meal lovingly cooked by yourself the night before, stored in a glass or a BPA-free plastic container!

If for some reason you are not able to cook dinner the night before, and you have no leftover deliciousness to take to work the next day, you can skip down to Step #9 – Eating Out, preferably with a friend, so that you can show them how easy and delicious it is to eat a purely plant-based diet (and get those compliments on all the weight you have lost and how good you are looking!). Because lunch is the main meal of the day, you can totally pig out at a vegan restaurant with them and show them how you are able to eat and yet still lose weight, once you omit the evil trifecta of meat, dairy, and processed foods.

Alright, you don't want to do any of this? You are too busy to cook, and you have no friends to go eat with? You can simply make yourself a quick raw salad (be sure to include beans or tempeh or tofu for protein), or a tortilla wrap filled with raw veggies and hummus, or go back to the good old PB&J standby! Or you can head to your local healthy market and get yourself a salad from the salad bar or something healthy and purely plant-based at the deli. Also, there are more and more "fast casual" purely vegan restaurant chains opening that are perfect for lunch, like Veggie Grill and Native Foods, and many others like Subway, Chipotle, Quiznos and Panera are starting to offer plant-based options. Though I don't encourage supporting fast-food chains, I think you can get a good meal in the slightly more upscale "fast casual" restaurant where the ingredients are much more fresh and healthy.

For me, I know lunch is an important meal, but I have no time to spend cooking at midday. But I think I have found the best balance by typically eating homemade leftovers from the night before ... which brings me to the most important step of all: Step #6: Making Dinner!

Step #6: Let's Make Dinner

Dinner should always be very light, very low calorie, and eaten early in the evening, preferably before the sun goes down. Dinner need only fuel you until bedtime, which is only about three hours later. You really want to go to sleep on a fairly empty stomach. Making dinner is something you need to make sure to weave into your evening routine; no matter how late you work, you are going to make chopping veggies your nightly meditation. Get out your lovely bamboo chopping board and a set of sharp knives, and have a glass of organic red wine in hand, a lit candle, and your favorite music playing. Make chopping veggies as perfect an experience as you can so that it is something you actually look forward to all day—a Zen, moving meditation. Because the key to good health is lots of fresh veggies, five nights per week you are going to create dinner using three things: fresh veggies, beans, and grains. (I am giving you Friday and Saturday night off from cooking. Go out and explore some of those great vegan restaurants with your spouse, significant other, or friends on the weekends!)

So just like with breakfast, I am going to give you five simple, go-to weekday "dinner formulas." As with breakfast, you can vary them up quite a bit but within a theme. So your five go-to weeknight meals are bowls, wraps, stews, roasts, and rainbow salads.

1. Rainbow salads: Every time I get asked to bring something to a potluck, people demand that I bring a salad because I know how to make a good one, and now so will you! I'll start with this because you should make this salad every single night—either huge as your entrée or small as a side to your cooked entree. Even if you are cooking something, you always want raw veggies too for that extra boost of vitamins, minerals, phytonutrients, and most importantly, enzymes that help you digest your food. Make your salad as colorful as possible—a "Rainbow Salad"—to expand the range of phytonutrients you are eating. Your base should begin with a very dark, leafy green like kale or collard greens. Then add some reds, blues, browns, yellows, purples, and whites. You also want to make sure you have a variety of tastes and textures—sweet, salty, soft, crunchy, savory, spicy—so that every bite is a new taste treat.

Chopped red or green onions and garlic are always a good addition for both flavor and health. Then add a savory plant-based protein—tofu, tempeh, or cool cooked beans or quinoa. (When someone needs to get more iron into their diet, a "beans and greens" salad is a great way to boost their iron; don't forget the squeeze of lemon for iron absorption.) After the savory add a sweet taste—cranberries, chopped pears, raisins, pomegranate seeds. Then add a crunchy plant-based protein—chopped nuts, sunflower seeds, pumpkin seeds, macadamia nuts. Finally, don't forget the final touch for flavor and health—the avocado and the freshly chopped herbs: cilantro, parsley, rosemary, dill, or mint! The sky is the limit. Experiment with different fresh herbs on your salad and find the flavor you like.

With the last piece, go easy on the salad dressing. Ideally, you want not much more than a squeeze of lemon or lime, sea salt, and black pepper. You can make your own salad dressings with vinegar, mustard, minced garlic, a splash of agave syrup, and a squeeze of lime. Never add oil to your salad dressing. You don't need it. And try to avoid the bottled salad dressings; they are full of oil, gluten, salt, and sometimes sugar. They can take a perfectly healthy salad and turn it into a high-calorie, high-fat disaster. When eating out and ordering salad, always ask for the dressing on the side and some citrus wedges, and use the dressing sparingly (if at all) after you have used the citrus juice, salt, and pepper.

So every night the plan is to make this gorgeous, colorful salad that is practically a work of art. It may take you awhile to cut and slice and dice, but it is so worth it for the flavors you will experience and for the overwhelming health benefits. Plus, the formula for this salad leaves so much room for interpretation. Your salad will never taste the same twice, depending on what veggies you use, what proteins and nuts/seeds you use, and how you do your salad dressing. Every one will be tasty and unique; like snowflakes, they are never the same twice. If there is only one or two of you, if you are both adults with low levels of activity and you want to lose weight, this salad is all you need to make. You don't need to cook anything at all. Most nights, honestly, this is all that Homer and I need. However, if you are a mom or dad who has a family to cook for, you can make this salad AND a cooked dinner. Just remember, folks watching their weight should eat the salad only and put aside their cooked portion for lunch the next day. The key to weight loss (and good health in general) is to eat a light, raw meal at dinnertime. If you are really eager and ready to lose weight, you might even want to just juice your dinner. Juicing is ideal for partial fasting and cleansing or as a dinner substitute for rapid weight loss. See the appendix for the recipes for both rainbow salad and a few good juice recipes as well.

2. Bowls – Every night is a salad night, large or small, but in addition you may want to make a cooked meal for growing or active or skinny folks in your household AND/OR for you to enjoy for lunch tomorrow. (This is what is otherwise known as Warrior Willpower.) One of my go-to dinners is simply a "bowl." I have heard that Mother Teresa lived her entire life eating one meal a day, at noon—a bowl of rice, beans, and veggies—and she never suffered from lack of protein. So what goes into a bowl? Similar to Mother Teresa, whole grains, beans, and veggies. Even though this sounds boring, depending on what kinds of beans, what kinds of grains, what kinds of veggies, and what kinds of herbs and spices you use, you can make a bowl 1,000 different ways with 1,000 different tastes and textures.

For my whole grain, I prefer to keep it quick and simple. I use the quick-cooking, low-GI grains like quinoa (red, yellow, black, or white, it doesn't matter), and tiny black rice (sometimes called "Forbidden rice"). Both take about fifteen to twenty minutes to cook. You can cook them in water, low-sodium veggie broth, or coconut water to vary the flavor, and you can always throw in a dash of red or white wine while cooking.

For my beans, I usually am too lazy or in too much of a hurry to think about soaking my beans the night before, so more often than not I just open up a can of organic, no-sodium beans of any color or type—red, black, white, pinto, garbanzo (chickpeas), canneliini—whatever I have on hand. You can also use lentils, lima beans, or peas—any other kind of legume. I heat them up in a small saucepan alongside the cooking grains.

Then I do the veggies. First, I sauté a little minced garlic and chopped onion in a little water or low-sodium veggie broth or coconut water. Then I add in three or four chopped veggies of various colors—green, brown, yellow, red. The hardest veggies should be thrown in first, then the medium, then the softest that need the least amount of cooking. I add some sea salt, black pepper, and dried herbs/spices with the veggies while they cook. I add more liquid as needed, splash some more wine in there.

Once the grains are done and the veggies are tender, I make the bowls filled one-third with whole grains, one-third with beans or peas, and one-third with sautéed veggies. Garnish with a squeeze of lemon or lime and freshly chopped herbs of your choice (cilantro, parsley, dill, mint, etc.). For the skinny kids and the active athletes, add chopped avocado, tofu or tempeh, chopped olives, nuts and/or seeds, with a drizzle of olive oil to the top of the bowl as well! And don't forget the salad on the side!

3. Wraps – Wraps are very similar to bowls except they may not require as much work. Find a raw, gluten-free wrap, spread it with hummus, and add chopped veggies—cooked or raw or both. It's always nice to add raw sprouts, even if you are using sautéed cooked veggies in your wrap. Depending on whether you are in the mood for Asian, Mexican, or Italian, just vary the ingredients and you can get a completely different taste. For Asian, use a rice-paper wrap, fill it with chunks of tofu and thinly sliced Asian veggies (bok choy, baby corn, shitake mushrooms), season it with coconut or lemongrass, sprinkle it with sesame seeds, add raw sprouts, and use a Nama Shoyu dipping sauce. For Mexican, use a large corn tortilla; fill it with quinoa, black beans, corn, and typical Mexican veggies like squash, tomatoes, onions, red onions, avocado, cilantro, and a squeeze of lime; serve it with salsa and guacamole. For Italian, use a large wholegrain wrap; fill it with cannellini beans, tapenade, chopped heirloom tomatoes, artichoke hearts, mushrooms, zucchini, capers, eggplant; season it with basil, marjoram, oregano, rosemary, thyme. For Indian, use a brown-rice wrap; fill it with basmati rice, mung beans, cauliflower, tomato, spinach, carrots, peas; season it with ginger, curry, cardamom. And on and on ... I think you get the picture! Wraps are easy and fun, and you can even have your family put their own wraps together by themselves to alter and adjust their fillings to taste. A wrap is really just a healthy new spin on the good old sandwich, except we are going for less processed flour and fewer calories by using gluten-free and, in some cases, raw wrapping instead of fluffy white-flour bread. You can even make a good ol' PB&J wrap in a pinch!

4. Soups and stews – Super easy stews are a staple around here, and you don't need a recipe. Start to experiment with all sorts of different types of stews. You simply start with a little low-sodium veggie broth with minced garlic and onion; heat that up and cook it for a couple minutes. Then add one to two cups of low-sodium veggie broth per person, a legume/bean, and lots of chopped-up rainbow veggies. Make sure you've got a couple root veggies in there like carrots, potatoes, or sweet potatoes for substance and texture. Add rice noodles at the very end for an Asian-style soup. Add chopped dark greens at the very end and a squeeze of lemon or lime. Serve over rice or quinoa with some avocado for the hungry skinny ones!

5. Roasts – There are a variety of veggies that are just awesome when roasted in the oven and served alongside rice or quinoa. Crank that oven up to 400 degrees, line your cookie sheet with foil, and experiment with all manner of roasted veggies—sweet potatoes, yams, all manner of squash (my favorite being spaghetti squash). You can combine a variety of root veggies like carrots, small potatoes, beets, and yams. Roasted broccoli, cauliflower, and Brussels sprouts are amazing. All you have to do is drizzle them with olive oil, salt, and pepper, and enjoy them once they are tender. Small veggies take about twenty minutes; large potatoes can take up to an hour, so you will have to get a feel for this based on the size of the veggies. Stuff the large potatoes or sweet potatoes or yams with cooked beans, quinoa, and veggies, or serve the smaller roasted veggies alongside the cooked beans and quinoa. Or you may want to do an amazing spaghetti squash that you can peel out of the shell and serve with a marinara sauce and veggie meatballs. Sprinkle it with nutritional yeast instead of parmesan, and you will swear you are having the most amazing Italian dinner ever—without those extra white-flour simple carbs!

Step #7: Take Your Vitamins

Okay, so now you know what to eat for breakfast, lunch, and dinner. You know that the best way to eat is to stick with the three square meals per day, so I am not going into any kinds of snacks or hors d'oeuvres or any of that. But before I leave the topic of "what to eat," I would be remiss if I didn't mention a couple more things that you should also be putting into your bellies: supplements and superfoods.

SUPPLEMENTS: Even if you are eating 100 percent correctly, eating all plant-based foods as described above, there are two supplements that you MUST take daily: B12 and essential fatty acids.

1. B12 is found almost exclusively in animal products, but it is safer to take a cherry-flavored pill than to eat the animal products filled with all the bad stuff just to get a single micronutrient. B12 is the most chemically complex of all the vitamins; it comes in several forms, and not all forms are equally effective. The most effective is methylcobalamine, even though the most common form is cyanocobalamine because it is easier to manufacture; unfortunately it is difficult for the body to absorb. The best way to get your B12 is to take the methylcobalamine form sublingually—allowing it to dissolve under the tongue. Methylcobalamine protects against neurological deterioration as we age, and it also keeps our homocysteine levels down. High levels of homocysteine in our blood may result in the buildup of plaque and blood clots, leading to heart disease and stroke. So B12 is super important for both the heart and the brain. Take your 500 mcg of sublingual methyl-B12 daily (140).

2. Essential fatty acids (EFA) are healthy fats that cannot be made by our bodies, so they must be consumed through food. They improve skin and hair, and they reduce blood pressure, cholesterol, triglycerides, and the risk of blood-clot formation. Found in high concentrations in the brain, EFAs are needed for normal brain functioning. Omega-3s are better for you than the omega-6s, and though we (typically) consume plenty of omega-6s (found in raw nuts, seeds, legumes, and unsaturated vegetable oils), we should be consuming twice as many omega-3s (found in oily fish, walnuts, and flaxseeds). Since we don't eat fish (which have particularly healthy long-chain omega-3s called DHA and EPA), we should take an omega-3 supplement. Make sure to take at least 600mg of DHA daily in a vegan DHA/EPA omega-3 oil (usually a flaxseed and algae oil combination) (141).

Those two are critical, no matter who you are and how you eat. Then, if you are over fifty, live in a cold-weather climate, are pregnant, or all the above, you will want to also take a **vitamin D/calcium/magnesium/zinc supplement.** If you live in a cold-weather climate and/or are over fifty years old, chances are you are low in vitamin D as well. Vitamin D is required for the absorption of calcium and phosphorus and is especially important for bone health (though the more we learn about vitamin D, the more it seems we need it for many health reasons). It protects against muscle weakness, regulates the heartbeat, prevents breast and colon cancer and osteoporosis, enhances immunity, and is necessary for thyroid function and normal blood clotting. Vitamin D2 (ergocalciferol) is the vegan type of D, coming from plant sources; D3 (cholecalciferol) comes from sheep's wool. Vitamin D ideally comes from sunlight on the skin, but if you are over fifty or live in a colder climate, you will want to supplement with D2. Vitamin D should always be taken in conjunction with a calcium/magnesium/zinc combo so that it can be absorbed. The RDA for vitamin D is now 600IU for all ages up to age seventy, and 800IU for those aged seventy-one years and older. The RDA for calcium is 1,500–2,000mg/day, magnesium is 750–1,000mg/day (half of calcium), and zinc is 30–50mg/day. (142)

"Health Insurance" Even if you are eating right, there is the possibility that you may not be eating perfectly every day, and/or the fruits and veggies that you are eating may not be as chock-full of vitamins and minerals as they should be (depending on what type of soil they were grown in, as well as other factors). If you want that additional "health insurance," find a good multivitamin that advertises itself as a "whole-foods," plant-based, vegan, raw, real food vitamin/mineral supplement. Look at the ingredients and look for real foods, not chemicals. Here are the daily recommended dosages you are looking for: (143)

- Carotenoid complex (vitamin A) – 5,000–25,000IU
- Vitamin B1 (thiamine) – 50–100mg
- Vitamin B2 (riboflavin) – 15–50mg
- Vitamin B3 (Niacin) – 15–50mg

- Niacinamide – 50–100mg
- Vitamin B5 (pantothenic acid) – 50–100mg
- Vitamin B6 (pyridoxine) – 50–100mg
- Vitamin B12 (methylcobalamine) – 500 mcg
- Biotin – 400–800mcg
- Choline – 50–200mg
- Folic acid – 400–800mcg
- Inositol – 50–200mg
- Para-aminobenzoic acid (PABA) – 10–50mg
- Vitamin C (best as Ester-C) – 1,000–3,000mg
- Biolavanoids (mixed) – 200–500mg
- Hesperidin – 50–100mg
- Rutin – 25mg
- Vitamin D2 – 600IU
- Vitamin E – 200IU
- Vitamin K – 100–500mcg
- DHA + EPA omega-3 fatty acids – 500mg combined
- Boron – 3–6mg
- Calcium – 1,500–2,000mg
- Chromium – 150–400mcg
- Copper – 2–3mg
- Iodine (kelp is the best source) – 100–225mcg
- Magnesium – 750–1,000mg
- Manganese – 3–10mg
- Molybdenum – 30–100mcg
- Potassium – 99–500mg
- Selenium – 100–200mcg
- Vanadium – 200mcg–1mg
- Zinc – 30–50mg

***(Never take a multivitamin that has iron; iron supplementation should be done only under a doctor's supervision)

Vitamin supplements should never be taken on an empty stomach. The more we learn about vitamins, the more we realize that they need to be taken in conjunction with one another and in the presence of other nutrients and phytonutrients to be properly digested and absorbed. For example, vitamin D needs to be taken with calcium. Oil-soluble vitamins need to be taken with fats. Iron-rich foods must be eaten with vitamin C to be properly absorbed. Rather than worrying about all of this, just get into the routine of taking your supplements all at once at breakfast on a full stomach.

SUPERFOODS:

If you decide to not take the horse pill described above, you may want to look into "superfoods" as a more natural way to boost your vitamin and mineral intake daily through foods. If you are making a green smoothie every morning, a great way to do this is by adding superfoods. Superfoods are a class of the most potent, super-concentrated, and nutrient-rich foods on the planet. Extremely tasty and satisfying, superfoods have the ability to tremendously increase the vital force and energy of one's body and are the optimum choice for improving overall health, boosting the immune system, elevating serotonin production, enhancing sexuality, cleansing, lowering inflammation, and alkalizing the body. Nourishing us at the deepest level possible, they are the true fuel of today's "superhero."

Top 10 Superfoods and Tonic Herbs: (144)

1. **Cacao (raw chocolate)** – The seed/nut of a fruit of an Amazonian tree, cacao is the highest antioxidant food on the planet, the number-one source of antioxidants, magnesium,

iron, manganese, and chromium, and is also extremely high in PEA, theobromine (cardiovascular support), and anandamide ("bliss chemical"). Raw chocolate improves cardiovascular health, builds strong bones, is a natural aphrodisiac, elevates your mood and energy, and increases longevity. Put a tablespoon of raw cacao into your smoothie and/or add a tablespoon of raw cacao nibs for a tasty, crunchy, healthy treat.

2. **Goji berries (wolfberries)** – Used in traditional Chinese medicine for over 5,000 years, goji berries are regarded as a longevity, strength-building, and potency food of the highest order. This superfood contains eighteen kinds of amino acids, including all eight essential amino acids, up to twenty-one trace minerals, high amounts of antioxidants, iron, polysaccharides, B & E vitamins, and many other nutrients.

3. **Maca** – A staple in the Peruvian Andes for thousands of years, this adaptogenic superfood increases energy, endurance, strength, and libido. Dried maca powder contains more than 10 percent protein and nearly twenty amino acids, including seven essential amino acids. As a root crop, maca contains five times more protein than a potato and four times more fiber. A tablespoon of maca in your morning smoothie gives you a burst of energy to start your day!

4. **Hemp products eaten in their RAW form** – Hemp seeds are packed with 33 percent pure digestible protein and are rich in iron, amino acids, and vitamin E as well as omega-3s and GLA. Hemp is a perfect food for growing children and adults looking to increase protein intake. Hemp seeds are great sprinkled on just about anything and everything.

5. **Spirulina and AFA blue-green algae** – Spirulina is the world's highest source of complete protein (65 percent). Spirulina provides a vast array of minerals, trace elements, phytonutrients, and enzymes. AFA blue-green algae is a wild-grown superfood that is made up of 15 percent blue-pigmented phycocyanin, which, according to Christian Drapeau in his book *Primordial Food*, increases our internal production of stem cells. Both spirulina and blue-green algae are vital superfoods. The best way to get this is through a supergreens powder that combines all sorts of greens, and if you are looking for protein post-workout, find a green protein powder with up to 18–20 grams of green protein per serving!

6. **Camu berry** – This is the highest vitamin C source on planet. Great for rebuilding tissue, purifying blood, and enhancing immunity and energy, camu berry is one of the best antidepressants, immune building, and eye-nourishing superfoods in the world.

6. **Sea vegetables (kelp, dulse, nori, hijiki, bladderwrack)** – Rich in life-giving nutrients drawn from the ocean and sun, sea vegetables help remove heavy metals, detoxify the body of radioactive iodine, provide numerous trace minerals, regulate immunity, and decrease the risk of cancer. Seaweeds benefit the entire body and are especially excellent for the thyroid, immune system, adrenals, and hormone function. Throw a sheet of nori into your stew right before serving to add a nice salty flavor AND healthy iodine.

8. **Medicinal mushrooms (reishi, chaga, cordyceps, maitake, shiitake, lion's mane, etc.)** – High in polysaccharides and super immune-enhancing components, medicinal mushrooms are one of the most intelligent

adaptogenic herb/superfoods on the planet! They have also been proven effective in healing cancer and a variety of other ailments.

Additional powerful superfoods and supplements – MSM, digestive and metabolic enzymes, mangosteen powder, marine phytoplankton, activated liquid zeolite, algae oil. I could go on and on about superfoods and raw foods, but that will have to wait for the next book!

Step #8: Keep Your Traditions

I think one of the most difficult obstacles to overcome when getting people to consider eliminating meat and dairy from their lives is the concern that this will make them an extremist, and they will never be able to be "normal" again. Well, that is all wrong. You can be a conservative Christian, a patriotic American, a devout Muslim, a Tea Party activist or an Orthodox Jew and still give up the meat and dairy! It is not just for extremist hippie atheist loners and anarchists anymore!

I find myself surrounded by Vegans (capital V) who are quite militant in their approach. They refuse to eat in restaurants that serve meat, they refuse to eat in households that serve meat; in extreme cases, they actually cut all ties with family members that eat meat. Their dietary preference has become their religion. And though a plant-based diet is certainly far more than a diet—it is an all-encompassing, compassionate lifestyle that goes far beyond what we eat—it should never become a religion. I believe so fervently in compassionate eating that it does feel as if I have had a religious conversion experience, BUT I am not going to make the mistake of promoting it like a religion by forcing conversion, harassing people, or shoving the message in their face. I am going to show them by example. If you believe in your path, people will follow your lead. Lead with your actions and by example, not by shouting at people.

The Vegans are why many people won't even consider giving up their meat and dairy. They feel that the people eating this way are nuts, they will have to join a "cult" and never be able to eat with their families again. Nonsense. In my world, I have parents who grew up eating meat and potatoes their whole lives. My dad has started to eat a lot less meat (though he probably won't admit that publicly!), but he still loves to order steak when he eats out. My mom has started to eat mostly vegetarian, but she still eats meat on occasion. Should I disown them? Not eat with them? No way. My husband only eats plant-based in our house (naturally, it's all we have in the kitchen and all that I cook), but when we go out he still will order an occasional piece of fish. Should I divorce him? No way. My daughter is the one who introduced me to a vegetarian diet about fifteen years ago when she was just a teen, and though she has been a firmly committed vegetarian ever since then, she still struggles with the temptations of cheese. Of my four adult boys, they change their dietary preferences like they change their T-shirts— one family event they are steak-and-potato eaters, the next they are vegetarian, the next vegan, then back again, then back again and again. They are going through the shifting tides of change that is a sign of our times in so many areas. So I never know who is eating what anymore. But it doesn't really matter to me, because when any of them come to my house to eat, they are eating purely plant-based, delicious meals, and they love it. When I go to other people's homes for parties, I always bring a huge plant-based cooked entrée AND a huge monster salad to share, never judging the meat and cheeses they might be serving in their homes. I will never disown or avoid any friends or family for still eating meat or dairy. That is their choice. Most of us grew up eating meat and dairy. It is ingrained in our culture. This has been a long, gradual shift for each of us individually, and it will be the same way for society, but I have no doubt in my heart that the change will come and that it will eventually be 100 percent. In the meantime, we can only continue to educate and make people aware, and continue to pray for the suffering of the animals and the people who consume them.

The key to making this change permanent for you and widespread to everyone you know is to make it simple and easy, and to show your friends and family just how easy and delicious it is. Don't preach at them. Don't judge them. Show them. Educate them. FEED them! A way to anyone's heart is through their stomach, so that is why this step is so important. You must show friends and family how to eat at home and how to celebrate your traditional family or cultural traditions, just the same as before, but with a simple twist— the elimination of the meat and dairy: swapping out grain-based meats for flesh-based meats, swapping out plant-based milks for cow-based milks. It usually just means that we have to rethink the recipes for the meals that the holidays revolve around (and don't they all seem to revolve around food?!).

Here are some quick ideas of how to maintain the traditions while losing the cruelty:

Super Bowl Sunday: You can still have that Super Bowl party and have fun watching football and hanging out with your most macho cowboy family members. Cover your coffee table with Gardein Buffalo Wings (neither chicken nor buffalo—shhh ... don't tell your guests). Your old favorite combo of chips, salsa, and guacamole are all meat and dairy free, and of course everyone appreciates having a lower-calorie, higher-nutrient veggie platter with some homemade vegenaise-based onion dip. Serve delicious veggie burgers and a Tex-Mex chili at halftime, but by that time, after all the beer that's been consumed, they may never know the difference!

Valentine's Day: What about strawberries dipped into dark chocolate and a nice bottle of organic red wine—all plant-based, all delicious, all perfect for Valentine's Day? Personally, I don't need to eat more than this on Valentine's Day. The red wine and the dark chocolate release those endorphins, those feel-good hormones, and who needs a big, full tummy on V-Day anyways? So, red wine and dark chocolate only for Valentine's Day dinner. Tell your sweetheart it was your health coach's suggestion!

St. Patty's Day: The only thing missing from your St. Patty's day traditional menu will be the corned beef, but you won't even notice it's missing. You can make a nice colcannon with potatoes, cabbage, and onions (even throw in some kale to make it healthier). You can make a shepherd's pie or a nice dark Irish stew minus the meat, biscuits and gravy, or just a simple baked potato stuffed with sautéed veggies. Trust me, you will have plenty of food to soak up all that Irish beer!

The spring holidays of Easter/ Passover/ Holi/ Mother's Day: When I think of the springtime holidays, I think of brunch. I think of sitting outdoors and enjoying the first warmth of spring in the morning hours. And it is so easy to create an amazing 100 percent plant-based brunch—a huge fruit salad, tofu scrambles with spring veggies. You can easily make any and all pancakes, waffles, scones, muffins, and crepes of any variety purely plant-based, using unsweetened soy milk in lieu of cow's milk. You can replace the eggs with ground flaxseeds, tofu, energy-G egg replacer, bananas, applesauce, plant-based yogurts, or canola oil— your choice. If you are serving dinner, focus on all the amazing fresh, locally grown veggies of spring. Spring lamb should not be on the table; they should be in the fields where they belong, nursing at their mama's side. Leg of lamb is exactly that—a baby's leg. Don't allow your mind to disconnect.

Father's Day, Fourth of July, Memorial Day, and Labor Day summer BBQs: Just because you are no longer eating meat doesn't mean you can't have awesome summer BBQs! Experiment with creating veggie kabobs with eggplant, peppers, zucchini, mushrooms, onions, tomatoes; marinate them in a vinaigrette dressing for a couple hours before throwing them on the barbie. Portobello mushrooms or veggie burgers can substitute for dead-cow burgers, and you can make 'em just as loaded and delicious as any other burger, with all the same trimmings. There are all kinds of veggie hot dogs, Italian sausages, and grain-based roasts that can all be thrown onto the grill. Then there is the usual corn on the cob, but you can experiment also with throwing all kinds of different things onto the grill: watermelon lightly marinated in balsamic vinegar or any summer fruit really, peaches, honeydew melon, Asian pears. Have fun enjoying a whole new world of amazing BBQ taste treats that will not only taste great but extend your life by about six years.

Halloween: The great thing about Halloween is there really is no particular food associated with it except for CANDY of course. And whether you are on the Paleo Diet or the Whole Earth Diet, all agree that we need to stay away from all commercial candy. If you are at all interested in your health, those commercial candies are deadly for you and your trick-or-treaters as they are filled with high fructose corn syrup and artificial colors and flavors. If you absolutely must have a sweet treat to give away or to indulge in yourself, go for raw dark (vegan) chocolates.

Thanksgiving: Thanksgiving is the most traditional menu of the year for American families. However creative and outside-the-box we are when we celebrate the bounty of autumn with all other plant-based meals, we still choose to serve something on Thanksgiving that is reminiscent of what our forefathers might have served for dinner almost 400 years ago. For many vegetarians, it is the one day that they often feel sentimental about not having as the centerpiece of their holiday table a beautiful, oven-roasted turkey. However, if you think about it, each and every other beloved traditional side dish on the table—the cranberries, the mashed potatoes and gravy, the stuffing, the green bean casserole, the yams, the biscuits, the pumpkin pie—are all mostly plants. To make the side dishes and desserts 100 percent plant-based takes only some minor tweaking—substituting all the butter with healthy fats, substituting cow milk for plant-based milk in your recipes, making your meal 100 percent plant-based and 100 percent healthier for you. Then you just have to create a new tradition for your main entrée instead of a dead bird: a delicious, homemade cashew nut loaf decorated with fresh sprigs of rosemary, sage, and thyme; individual beautifully stuffed acorn squashes; a fun plant-based "turkey" shaped like a whole roast turkey if you must. So simple. Moms and grandmas, it's time to create new family traditions based on love and compassion, without a hint of death or cruelty. Let's do this!

Christmas/Hanukkah: Every family has different family traditions around these winter holidays, often with a menu similar to Thanksgiving's, with a turkey, or maybe a ham or roast beef as the centerpiece. But why is this? Really think about why it is that we need to have a dead animal in the middle of our table. I think this goes back to our most primal memories, back to our caveman days, and appeals to our most primal of senses, that the hunt was successful, that the animal was killed and eaten. Probably back in the days of early man this was cause for celebration, and we have carried this through in our DNA until today, which means it will not be easy to shake this feeling that, in order to bring importance to the gathering, there should be offered the results of a successful hunt. But I really do believe in evolution. I'm not talking about the book of Genesis evolution; I am talking about recent history evolution.

Mankind has evolved so much over the last couple hundred years. Not so long ago, murder was much more common than it is today, cannibalism was practiced in many parts of the world, and slavery and torture and rape were condoned. Today we are in the midst of a huge spiritual evolutionary shift. I invite you to look inside your souls to see if this is true. So shouldn't we look at our most holy and sacred holidays as cause to celebrate this new consciousness that celebrates life, love, and compassion, rather than the old consciousness of killing as a means for survival? Just as described above for Thanksgiving, so much of our traditional feasts are plant-based and need few if any tweaks. It is time to leave the dead animal off the center of the table. It is time to step into the new age of enlightenment, and it begins with your traditional table for the holidays.

Family dinners, neighborhood potlucks, and dinner parties, oh my: The best way to spread the word that plant-based eating is both nutritious and delicious is by sharing. Make a tradition of having family dinners on Sunday nights, or if the kids are grown (or there are no kids), have a plant-based potluck at home on Sundays. Find a way to have *Forks Over Knives* or some other documentary playing in the background, or have dinner and then invite everyone to sit to watch a movie. If you have been invited to a dinner party, bring an amazing plant-based dish to share.

Step #9: Eating Out Is Easy

People ask me all the time, "Isn't it difficult eating out when you're a vegan?" Actually, no, it's not hard at all; in fact, I encourage you to eat out as much as possible because it spreads the message to dining establishments that there are more and more folks out there wanting meat and dairy free options, and they will start to offer more ... AND it is working! You are starting to see more plant-based options popping up on restaurant menus everywhere. I love that Yardhouse offers Gardein options with just about all their entrees. Z Pizza has a vegan pizza with a gluten-free option. I was recently surprised to find that 21 Oceanfront, one of our classic old restaurants here outfitted with red booths and staffed by tuxedoed waiters that serves mostly steaks, has a "vegan" section on their menu now! Why? Because people like me refuse to stay in their vegan-only restaurants; we get out into the real world and ask for plant-based choices everywhere. The more people that ask, the more chefs take notice and make changes to their menu accordingly.

So, here are my top ten tips for dining out:

1) Download the Happy Cow app: First things first, download the Happy Cow app to your smart phone! Check out Happycow.net, a free online vegetarian restaurant guide sorted by country and region that provides vegetarian and vegan restaurant dining and health-food store locations.

2) Choose Japanese: Asian restaurants in general have many vegetarian options because of the large percentage of Buddhist vegetarians in their populations. In Japanese restaurants, you can order miso soup, seaweed salad, and a vegetarian sushi roll. If you live near LA, there is an amazing vegan Japanese restaurant in a funky little strip mall in Little Tokyo called Shojin that is to die for!

3) Choose Indian: India has around 500 million vegetarians, almost half their population, because of the many Jains, Hindus, and Buddhists who abstain from eating meat. So any Indian restaurant has multiple vegetarian options. Just ask your waiter which entrées have no milk or cheese, but rest assured there are plenty. Chana masala (garbanzo beans and potatoes) is one of my favorites. Try to order a couple entrées to share, and make sure and get some beans and some greens in there!

4) Choose Thai: Of the entire Thai population, 95 percent practices Theravada Buddhism, so again we have lots of options in those Thai restaurants! The typical and delicious Thai coconut soup is made with vegetable broth and coconut milk (for the creamy texture). Try a little coconut soup, some spring rolls, and maybe a tofu/noodle soup. Most of the noodles in Asian restaurants are naturally gluten-free, made of rice instead of wheat!

5) Choose Mexican: When you think of vegetarian Mexican food, you may think of beans and enchiladas filled with lard and covered with melted cheese, but don't go there! You can order veggie tacos, burritos, or a tostada and enjoy yourself as much as the person next to you loading his arteries with plaque via carnitas. Order anything off the menu, really; just say "no meat, no cheese, no sour cream," ask for plain black beans instead of refried beans, and you're good. You can also nibble on the chips and guacamole, but only a nibble (watch the fat content in those avocadoes!) The original food of the Native Americans was referred to as the "Three Sisters"—corn, beans, and squash. If only all Mexican restaurants could go back to their healthy indigenous roots and serve up a lot more of those three sisters and a lot less of the three devils—salt, sugar, and animal fats!

6) Ask the waiter: When you didn't get to choose the spot and you find yourself at a traditional restaurant without single plant-based entrée to be found, what do you do? Well, I will never walk out, so I look at it as an opportunity. When the waiter comes to take the order, quietly tell him you don't eat meat or dairy, and ask the chef come up with something really good for you! You will be amazed at what comes out—delicious platters filled with colorful grilled veggies, quinoa, polentas, salsas, great stuff! The chef is usually happy to comply, and your friends will look with envy at your colorful plate and wonder why they didn't order THAT!

7) Don't be ridiculous: Don't call attention to yourself when you're ordering. We don't want to present ourselves as being dogmatic extremists because then NO ONE will ever want to be like us when they grow up. Make your restaurant experience simple and easygoing. Everything may not be organic or locally sourced, but that's okay. A wee bit of feta may have slipped onto your salad. Unless it's covered in feta, don't send it back; just take your fork and a make a pile on the side. Don't be rigid. As long as we are living in these times of transition and we are still only 2.5 percent of the population, it is unavoidable unless you crawl into a cave somewhere. We don't want to separate ourselves from the rest of humanity, or we will never change the world. One day, animal products will no longer be on the menu at all, and we won't have to worry.

8) Order side dishes: What happens if you find yourself at a traditional American-style restaurant, and they are CLUELESS when it comes to offering plant-based choices? Often they have a veggie soup on the menu. (Even if you think it is veggie, you will need to ask about the broth used. Did you know onion soup is made with beef broth? Lots of "vegetable soups" use chicken broth ... ugh.) There are always salads; just ask to omit the meat and the cheese, and they are every bit as tasty. If you want something hearty and warm, though, look at the side dishes! Order two to three sides and ask them to bring them on a single plate—whatever veggies they have, as well as something starchy like a potato or rice—and you will be 100 percent satisfied. I promise!

9) Leave a love note: Whenever I dine in a "normal" restaurant, after doing all of the above, I always leave a little note in the tip tray at the end of the meal. It reads something along the lines of this: "Thank you so much for a lovely dining experience here at _____ (restaurant name). _____ (Server name) was kind enough to assist me with ordering the perfect plant-based entrée even though it was not on the menu. It would be great to see more meat and dairy free items on the menu here the next time I visit, and I will! Peace begins on your plate. X, Laura"

10) Help vegan restaurants succeed! I encourage folks to get out there and eat in any and every restaurant they can to help spread the word. Fast food, fine dining, and everything in between. Get out there and into the world of the other 97.5 percent and demand change by simply being the change. That being said, however, I eat 90 percent of my meals out in a vegan-only dining establishment. I love to support any and all vegan restaurants, like Native Foods or Veggie Grill, but especially the small mom-and-pop vegan restaurants around town because I am rooting for their success. If you go back to your Happy Cow app, I just know you can find someplace close by to take all your friends and family and let them experience how delicious vegan food can be. Every dollar spent there is like a vote for a cruelty-free world and, in the end, a vote for world peace.

One other last thought about eating out: We don't always eat in nice restaurants when we go out. Oftentimes, we go out to these networking events or conferences or weddings or bar mitzvahs. Anytime you find yourself in a big hotel ballroom with options to eat yet another piece of rubber chicken OR the vegan entrée, always, always, always choose the vegan option, EVEN IF you are "not a Vegan". The meat they serve in those large banquet-room situations is guaranteed to be factory-farmed, containing not only the saturated fats and cholesterol inherent in eating flesh, but it will also contain the growth hormones, pesticides, parasites and antibiotics that are found in the flesh of factory-farmed animals. Warn your tablemates too. You don't have to "be a Vegan" to ask for a plant-based entrée in a situation where the meat will certainly be factory-farmed and contaminated with a toxic brew of slow-acting poisons. Let's lose the label, lose the need to always eat meat at every meal unless you are "one of them", and just choose the best option, which in this instance, whether you are a dedicated meat-eater or a vegan, is always the plant-based menu item.

Step #10: Keep Learning About Nutrition

Never stop learning about health and nutrition. Every week there is a new study out about health and wellness. Always look to see where the study is coming from. Look for reputable sources like Harvard Medical School and Physicians Committee for Responsible Medicine. I will continue to learn and grow alongside you. If I were to write this book in five years' time, I'm sure I would make changes and add more to it than I already have. But we must start somewhere.

So to continue to be your healthiest self, I would encourage you to not stop with just this book. Keep learning about nutrition and in particular the plant-based diet. Go to **Appendix C: Resources for Readers** where I have a LONG list of books for you to read, including cookbooks and websites to visit. Most importantly, go there and order some documentary movies to watch, especially in the company of family and friends. The best way to make this new diet and lifestyle sustainable for you is to spread the knowledge and get that ripple effect working for you. You will be amazed how quickly others in your circle will start to get this, even those that you think would NEVER give up their meat and dairy. Never give up on anyone, and always encourage the smallest steps forward. Don't become an extremist. Keep encouraging small, bite-sized changes in everyone you know, and sooner or later, step by step, year by year, those small steps will become bigger steps, and soon we will have a cruelty-free world, and we won't have to call it vegan or plant-based or anything special! It will just be the normal way to eat. So continue to educate yourself, and educate the others around you so that your support group expands and your permanent, new, compassionate way of eating becomes the norm.

PART TWO:

HAPPY LIFE ~ THE WHOLE EARTH LIFESTYLE

*"Happiness is when what you think, what you say,
and what you do are in harmony"*

~Mahatma Gandhi

Chapter 4

Ancient Guidelines for Wellness

Ancient Guidelines for Wellness

---●---

"Health is a state of complete harmony of the body, mind and spirit.
When one is free from physical disabilities and mental distractions,
the gates of the soul open."

~B.K.S. Iyengar

Most diet books would end right here. In Part One we focused on a healthy body, talked a lot about food and nutrition, and hopefully gave you some simple guidelines to follow in order to take this knowledge and put it to work for you so that you can make a simple, easy transition to the Whole Earth Diet—real whole foods, no meat, no dairy. The reasons for shifting to a whole-foods, plant-based diet are many, but what differentiates this diet from any other weight-loss plan is this: it's really the only moral choice when it comes to deciding which dietary theory or philosophy to follow.

Though the foundation of the lifestyle is the food, Whole Earth Diet is much more than healthy eating. By its very nature, it causes you to think past your physical issues, to your deeper mental, emotional, and spiritual issues. By its very nature, Whole Earth Diet cannot stop at the boundary of the physical body; it expands into all other areas of health, not just of the body, but of the mind, of the heart, and of the soul.

Holistic wellness means all aspects of a person must be taken into account when staying healthy and preventing disease. Body, mind, heart, and soul are all distinct but integrated parts of self, and they are all equally important. In Part Two: Happy Life, we are going to move way beyond nutrition and on to the meaning of life, which is really about living a happy life. The goal is to live a long, healthy, HAPPY life because that is what is important—more important even than health and longevity.

So here in Part Two, we are expanding beyond the idea of physical health to include happiness as a goal. All parts of self—mind, body, heart, and soul—must be healthy and well in order to find true happiness, peace, and joy. If any of these pieces are unwell—body, mind, heart, or soul—the other pieces will be dragged down and held back, and you will never be truly healthy or happy. It's only when you start to nurture the health of each of these areas that your health and happiness will become an "upward spiral" (the opposite, perhaps, of the downward spiral you may have experienced before). This is the ultimate journey towards joy.

Interpreting Modern Wellness through an Ancient Lens

The modern holistic philosophy of Whole Earth Wellness was born out of studying holistic wellness philosophies from the ancient world, from ancient Babylonia, to ancient Greece, Egypt, India, China, and Japan. I found a very compelling theme that ran through so much of the ancient world, that resonated deep within my bones: the notion that everything in the universe, including human beings, is composed of four classical elements—earth, water, fire, and air. This idea just stuck with me. Maybe it's the multisensory imagery that comes to mind when you think of earth, wind, fire, and air, or maybe it was because it made so much sense at some very primal level to me. So I adopted it and made it the structure upon which the Whole Earth Wellness philosophy is framed. The plant-based diet is the foundation; the classical elements are the structure. (Can't let go of that architect inside me!). The Whole Earth Wellness philosophy is not true to any one ancient philosophy, but it is a modern blending of many. The basic idea is that our physical bodies are our earth element, our minds are the element of water, our hearts are fire, and our souls are air. Some ancient cultures refer to a fifth element, ether, which we understand to be God/Spirit/Universal Life Force that is the same inside every one of us, that makes us all one.

The earliest record we have of the classical elements is from Babylonia from the eighteenth century BC, and they appear again throughout history in Greek and medieval alchemy, in Indian Ayurveda, and in traditional Chinese medicine. Today, the four elements are still alive and well; they are just renamed "states of matter": solid, liquid, gas, and plasma (145). Earth, water, fire, and air really resonated for me when I was looking to clearly define and crystallize my holistic philosophy of wellness for the individual. The fifth element, the ether, suddenly made sense as the driving force behind my desire to take this message from beyond helping individuals to helping the whole earth. I just felt at my core it was right and the world was hungry for it.

So here in a nutshell is the Whole Earth Wellness theory of holistic wellness as defined by the four elements:

Your **earth** element is your foundation, and it is your phyiscal **body**. A healthy body is created by a combination of the feminine yin and and the masculine yang—what you put in, what you put out. You put in whole, plant-based foods (yin); you put out fitness—exercising your earth element with strength training, your water element with yoga, your fire element with dance, and your air element with cardio (yang). The goal is not superficially to be skinny, but to create a strong, healthy, **powerful body** to achieve the longest life possible without fear or physical limitations.

Your **water** element is your **mind**. A healthy mind is created by a combination of (yin) what you feed your mind with education and continuous lifelong learning, and (yang) what you put out, your career or life work, your assignment, your purpose. A healthy, flexible mind and a purpose-driven life are created by a healthy balance of career or life work and education. The goal is to live a **purposeful** life, to know at the end of your life that you made a difference, that the world was a better place because you were here.

Your **fire** element is your **heart**. A healthy heart is created by a combination of what you feed it with self-love (yin), and what you put out with love for others (yang). A healthy heart is created by a healthy balance of love for self and love for others. The goal is to live a **passionate life**, waking up each day excited about what that day will bring, because your day is ruled by love, because your day is all about adding warmth and love out into the universe, not hatred or divisiveness,

Your **air** element is your **soul**. A healthy soul is created by a combination of what you put in with deepening inner spirituality (yin), and what you put out with your beautiful, cultural, religious traditions, your outward prayer and faith (yang). The goal is to live a **prayerful life**, in a real relationship with God, who you speak to in your prayers, who you listen to in your silence, and for whom your life itself has been dedicated to embody living prayer.

The **ether** element is **God.** The fifth element called "akasha" in Hinduism represents that which is beyond the physical world, the universal spirit that connects all of us. For simplicity, we will call this God, and hopefully this will offend no one even the Athiests. God transcends all boundaries of different cultures, faiths, or religions; He resides in all of us regardless of our faith or complete lack thereof; He transcends our individuality; He is all of us. This fifth element is what gives me the confidence to believe that one person can indeed change the world because each of us has the divine inside us, and anything is possible with God. It's what gives ME the courage to get on my soapbox and proclaim that world peace is possible, and it begins with what YOU put on your plate. The power of the individual is limitless because every individual has inside He who is limitless.

Which brings me to this mathematical equation for happiness and world peace!

Individual Power + Individual Purpose + Individual Passion + Individual Prayer = World Peace. Once all individuals start to wake up to this reality, taking full responsibility for their own individual power and purpose and passion and prayer, one by one, like ripples in a pond, we will eventually have healthy, happy individuals, which will lead to world peace. And though the going is slow right now, once we reach a tipping point, this will bust wide open. When less than 10 percent of a population holds a certain belief, it will go nowhere. However, once that number grows above 10 percent, the idea spreads like flame (146).

So, let's check where we are now. In 2008, a Harris Interactive poll found 3.2 percent of Americans identified as vegetarian and 0.5 percent identified as vegan. By 2011, a poll done by the Vegetarian Resource Group found that 5 percent of Americans identified as vegetarian and 2.5 percent as vegan. Vegetarians almost doubled, but vegans quadrupled, in only four years! (147) At this rate we will reach the 10 percent tipping point very soon, and all the rest will follow. Yep, I am just crazy enough to believe this and will spend the rest of my life making sure the world wakes up and hears me until we are all 100 percent plant-based. World peace begins and ends with what you eat, with what you put on your plate.

Alright, so we get the philosophy. The earth, wind, fire, and air sound really cool and everything, but what does this all mean? How do we apply this to our personal well-being and pursuit of happiness?

Believe it or not, it all starts with rituals and routines: (1) ancient rituals and routines around eating, and (2) ancient rituals and routines around lifestyle habits. Why ancient? Why do I have this fascination with ancient lifestyles? Well, if you think about it, in ancient times, they didn't have any of the benefits we have today with modern medicine or modern surgery. Their lives did not have modern Western medicine to support them if they were eating poorly or living unhealthy lifestyles. Their lives depended on intimately knowing what and how to eat, and what things they could do on a daily basis to promote health and longevity. They didn't want to get ill because often there would be no cure, so prevention of disease was much more important then than today, where we rely on doctors and medicine to heal us from everything!

In this modern age, we have amazing doctors and medicines to cure some diseases that were incurable before, and we have emergency medicine for traumatic stress and accidental injuries that are really almost miraculous. That being said, too many of us now rely on modern medicine to the point where it has become a lifestyle crutch. We don't worry about what we eat or how we live because no matter what happens, there is a pill or a surgery that will probably fix it. We have gone from thinking of modern medicine as a backup plan, something to use when all else fails or when we have an accident, to the primary plan for health and wellness ... for dealing with all our everyday aches and pains, and all of the chronic issues that really could be simply prevented altogether or overcome if we would only switch to a healthy diet and lifestyle.

And now we are learning with modern research and studies that many of the ancient lifestyle guidelines really did improve life, health, and longevity. Many of you are familiar with yoga and meditation—two ancient lifestyle techniques that have made it into the modern Western world with great success and are practiced by millions of people around the world to this day. So of course we enthusiastically embrace yoga and meditation as practices that go hand in hand with our wellness philosophy, but those are only two areas of ancient holistic wellness. There are literally hundreds more, so now we are going to introduce you to some holistic guidelines for living that come from ancient times and whose health benefits are being proven with science today.

In the last chapter we talked about WHAT we are supposed to be eating for good health. But there is more to food that just WHAT to eat. There is also the WHEN, WHERE, WHY, and HOW we eat. Because no matter how good and nutritious the food, if we are mindlessly bolting down massive quantities; if we are eating without gratitude, without chewing, without serenity; if we are snacking all day or eating in the car while running errands, it doesn't matter what you are eating, the HOW is going to mess you up. So let's dive down into some ancient wisdom around the rituals and routines and guidelines when it comes to mealtime.

Ancient Rituals around Eating

In ancient times, the act of eating was truly regarded as sacred, and somewhere along the way we have completely lost this. If you think about it, every bite that you eat becomes you. You are what you eat. How miraculous is that? Mindful eating comes from Buddhism and can be defined as the sacred process of eating. When followed, digestion improves, so perfect weight is better maintained, and perfect health follows. The process of sacred eating begins with mindful food preparation and follows through with eating.

Mindful Shopping: Mindful food preparation begins when you shop for your food. Healthy eating includes a wide variety of fruits and vegetables in different colors and seasons. Often we eat the same things again and again, but here is where you want to explore and try new fruits and vegetables. You also want to buy as much organic or locally, seasonally grown food as possible and explore a local farmers' market near you. When you buy fresh produce from a farmers' market, you can be assured that you are getting fresh, organic, seasonal, locally grown food. According to ancient wellness theories, it is always best to eat seasonally and locally, just as any animal would do in the wild. Deer eat the leafy greens that sprout out of the snow in the spring, and this is exactly what their bodies need in spring—the light energy of sprouting baby greens. They also nibble on roots in the fall before winter comes, foods with a little more starch and sugar to put on some weight before the snow begins to fall. Animals eat locally and seasonally because they have to. We don't have to, so we don't ... but we suffer for it. Follow the lead of the animals in nature if you are ever looking for a health guru; they won't lead you astray! (148)

Mindful Food Preparation: Once you are back from the farmers' market, you want to prepare your meals with the freshest ingredients possible. Start with items that are perishable first—dark greens, vegetables, and fruits—and leave others—potatoes, grains, and beans—for later in the week. Wash your produce thoroughly before storage, but wait to cut them shortly before you are going to prepare the meal. The cooking process can be as relaxing and enjoyable as eating if you plan ahead and are prepared. Enjoy the process of cooking and chopping vegetables, and try to prepare your food with love in your heart for the farmers who grew the produce, for the laborers who picked the crops with their hands, for the truck drivers who drove the truck from field to market, for the people that sold you the food, and for the people (including yourself) that are about to enjoy your labor of love. This love and gratitude will translate into the energy of the food. This may be the most powerful reason to stop eating meat and dairy. It is impossible for a slaughterhouse worker to be kind and loving as he slaughters an animal, or a dairy farmer as he separates the mother cow from her baby, or the egg farmer as he kills the unwanted baby male chicks. All of this violence and horror enters the food. A plant-based diet is the only truly sacred diet (149).

Eat in a Calm Environment: Once the food is prepared, it is time to eat. The environment in which you eat is almost as important as the meal itself because your environment will affect your stress level and thus your digestion. The environment should be quiet and serene. Outside is always best, with the sounds of nature as your background music as you soak up some of that vitamin-D-rich sunshine. In today's world, we often find ourselves eating fast, bolting our food down while in our cars, or standing up at the kitchen counter mindlessly snacking. This results in digestive disorders that result finally in weight gain and health problems. Eating mindfully and slowly while sitting in a serene environment is so important (150).

Say Grace: Before you begin to eat, say grace. This may be something you learned from your mother as a child, or something you did in grammar school before the class ate lunch. Or maybe it's something you see "those people" doing in a restaurant before they eat, but they must be weird or something! Actually, saying grace before a meal may be something as simple as just sitting quietly for even a moment before you start to eat, just to reflect quietly and with gratitude for what you are about to eat. I remember my grandmother from Scotland always saying the Robert Burns poem before meals in her lovely Scottish brogue: *"Some hae meat and cannae eat, and some would eat but want it. But we hae meat and we can eat, Sae let the Lord be thankit."* (Of course, I am working on my own version once I find the perfect rhyming word for kale, instead of meat!) Even if you're not actually eating meat, it is still a good grace before meals! Any grace is good; even a simple, silent "thank you" before you begin will change everything in the way that you eat (151).

Eat Mindfully: Mindful eating is a process that uses all our senses. Allow your eyes to feast over what you are about to eat, let your nose smell the wonderful smells, let your tongue savor the first mouthful of food, which is ALWAYS the best bite of the entire meal. Eat some part of the meal with your hands, breaking bread or picking up a piece of food, allowing your hands to feel the texture of the food. Pause between bites, put your fork down, enjoy smaller portions as part of a longer course. Eating with chopsticks is a great way to focus on mindful eating as well and to pause between bites. It's easier to eat smaller portions this way. Go for quality not quantity. By choosing smaller amounts of the best food you can afford, you will not only enjoy it more, you're far more likely to be satisfied without having to overeat (152).

Chew Thoroughly: Chew each bite thoroughly until the food is liquefied, allowing the digestive juices to fully mix with the food and begin the proper digestion process. By the time you swallow your food, it should be the consistency of baby food, pureed in your mouth and mixed with your digestive saliva. Many digestive and intestinal issues start because your stomach cannot properly digest or absorb solid chunks of food. Also, particles of improperly chewed, solid food can get stuck in pockets all along your digestive tract, from the back of your throat all the way through your intestines to your colon, causing inflammation that leads to disease. This was true 5,000 years ago, and it is still true today! (153)

Eat Slowly: Since it often takes twenty minutes or so for our stomach to send signals to our brain when we are full, slowing down the eating process allows this communication to happen properly. Be aware of how full your stomach feels, and when you are tipping to the point of overeating. The idea of mindful eating is to create awareness of how hungry or full we are, and it can also allow us to be mindful of unnecessary snacking and eating out of boredom, sadness, or worry. Ideally, we want to eat three meals a day without snacking—a big breakfast to fuel us through lunchtime, a very large and well-balanced lunch to fuel us through dinnertime, and a very small dinner to fuel us through bedtime. Snacks throw our digestive rhythms off and cause weight gain and digestive problems (154).

Don't Drink Water While Eating: In ancient times, they avoided taking too much liquid with meals because it would reduce the "internal digestive fire" ... like putting water on a fire. Today, we are learning that the body releases exactly the correct amino acids, digestive juices, and enzymes (fire) needed specifically for whatever food is eaten, and when we dilute this perfect acidic brew for digestion with water or other liquids, it severely limits our ability to properly digest. Best practice is to drink a large glass of water about thirty to sixty minutes before your meal. Then eat your meal without much liquid at all, maybe just a small amount of tea, coffee, or wine (which are acidic and helpful to support digestion). Wait for an hour, then begin to drink lots and lots of water until you are about thirty to sixty minutes away from your next meal! (155)

Don't Stuff Yourself: Ancient cultures emphasized we should eat when hungry, stop when full, and leave a little bit of space in the stomach at each meal. Okinawans, some of the longest-living people on the planet, coined the phrase "Hara Hachi Bu," which literally translated means to eat to 75 percent full. Because, as mentioned previously, it takes about twenty minutes for signals from our stomach to reach our brains, stopping at 75 percent full prevents us from overeating. Modern science today is proving the ancient wisdom behind these guidelines. As early as the 1930s, researchers at Cornell University discovered that lab rats fed a calorie-restricted diet lived twice as long as other rats. Since then, similar findings on the age-defying benefits of calorie restriction have also been shown in insects and mice. In recent times, several studies show that caloric restriction improves the body's ability to fight chronic illness, slows down the aging process, improves serious conditions such as Alzheimer's and cancer, and extends longevity. Reducing food intake from 30 percent to 70 percent can increase the lifespan of various creatures by up to 40 percent. So just start eating LESS. So simple. It's probably my least popular advice, but perhaps it's the wisest advice of all (156).

Rest after Eating: Ancient societies, and even some modern European cultures today, would rest for at least an hour after eating. They say this allows for the first stage of digestion to complete before you move on to your next activity. You may be thinking, "Rest after meals? Not with my busy schedule!" If an hour is just not possible for you, any amount of time is better than no time. Strong exercise and strong emotion should be avoided, but gentle exercise like a slow walk or reading a book is ideal to allow the body to do its work. At the very, very least, sit quietly for just a few minutes after your meal is complete, and do some slow, deep breathing with eyes closed before you push yourself away from the table and get back to work. Today we have learned that, after a meal, blood rushes to the stomach to aid in digestion, and most of the body's caloric energy consumption is diverted to this process. Why force your body to compete its digestive energy against other activities? It is best to rest. (157)

Three Meals a Day and No Snacking: Eating three meals a day without snacks in between is the most efficient way for your body to maintain good digestive health. A healthy body digests food completely anywhere from twelve to seventy-two hours after a meal. Most foods take twenty-four hours to fully pass through the entire digestive system, from mouth to bowels. Raw fruits and vegetables take twelve hours while heavier, dense foods such as meat and cheese can take up to seventy-two hours to fully pass through the digestive system. (Of course, you don't need to worry about those colon-clogging meats and cheeses anymore, right?)

Smaller, frequent meals and constant snacking have become popular in recent times. We seem to have developed a fear of feeling hunger! So we snack and overeat all day. Overeating or eating too frequently causes the body to be in a constant state of digestion. The stomach is not designed to be working continuously all day. Like other organs in the body, it needs rest. In addition, food stays in our stomach for five to six hours until it passes to the next stage of digestion. If we eat too soon—if we don't wait at least three hours after each meal—food stays undigested and causes gas, bloating, and discomfort. It then ferments and releases toxins into your system. Repeat this process day after day for weeks, months, and years and the body eventually goes into toxic overload resulting in illness.

Instead of eating and snacking, we should eat three meals with slow-burning, complex-carb-loaded foods with some healthy fats so that we don't feel hungry soon. Remember, you should eat a breakfast that can last you until lunch and a lunch that can last you until dinnertime. Dinner should be light and eaten early in the evening. Replacing dinner with a fresh veggie juice is the best way to lose weight. Never eating after dark is another great way to lose weight. This is the key to weight loss and maintaining a healthy weight: eating a light dinner and never eating after dark (158).

This completes our deep dive into ancient rituals and routines around eating. Now let's expand out to ancient routines and rituals around a holistically healthy lifestyle that is still amazingly appropriate for today.

Ancient Rituals around Body Care

Now that you are eating all the right kinds of foods, eating mindfully, putting only the best and most nutritious food INTO your body through your digestive system, isn't it just as important that you think about what you put ONTO your body as well? Isn't it just as important to take good care of your physical body in other ways, too?

If you had a car that you loved, you would probably not only fill it with the best premium gasoline and oil whenever it was empty, but you would probably also take it to the car wash once a week to make it shine, schedule routine oil changes every 3,000 miles, and also schedule a major tune-up and service every 10,000 miles. If you had a newborn baby at home, you would not only feed her, you would bathe her, clothe her, and take her to the pediatrician for regularly scheduled visits. But how many of us have a body care and maintenance routine that is well thought-out and that we follow for our own selves? Maybe we have a vague idea, but few of us actually have an actual schedule that we follow. This section will help you do just that—to treat your own precious earthly body as well as, if not better than, your favorite car! Imagine that! This chapter will teach you—no, better yet, give you permission—to treat yourself as if you were your own very best and most loving mother on Earth.

The key to making this happen, and to making it simple, is to establish a routine. Ancient holistic wellness emphasizes the importance of routine for health and longevity. Healing cannot completely occur until you remake your lifestyle in a way that has a familiar, comfortable rhythm. This is not to say that you must become like a robot and do everything each day exactly the same without any difference from one day to the next. There is always room for variation. Just as I have the 90/10 rule for eating the right foods, I have a 90/10 rule here for routine. As long as you are sticking to a routine 90 percent of the time, 10 percent of the time you have some wiggle room! Here are some guidelines for establishing a daily, weekly, monthly, seasonal, and annual routine that will contribute to your physical health in so many ways—by reducing stress and anxiety and by ensuring that your body gets the sleep it needs and the care it deserves!

Daily Body Care

MORNINGS:

Meditation: Every morning might begin with sunrise meditation. Sit facing east, preferably outdoors and surrounded by the sights and sounds of nature, preferably with a view of the pending sunrise. Whether you have five minutes or fifty minutes doesn't matter. Obviously the longer you can meditate in the morning, the better. What is important is to just take some time to start your day with quieting the mind. You may want to include time to enjoy your cup of morning coffee or tea as an end to the meditation, as much a part of the morning ritual as the meditation, savoring the taste and feel of the warmth and energy entering your stomach.

Exercise: Start off every day with exercise. If you exercise in the morning as opposed to the afternoon, it sets up your whole day for success. Morning exercise increases your metabolic rate so that you burn calories more efficiently all day. It gives you more energy during your day, it makes you think twice about snacking after working out so hard that morning, and "gets it over with" before your mind has time to wake up and argue with you about it (big one for me!). We will get into this in detail in the next chapter, but I wanted to mention it here as a part of your daily morning body-care routine.

Morning Bathing and Cleansing Ritual: Don't think of your morning shower as just a "shower." Instead, think of it as a sacred time of washing away all that is old and useless to you, and starting each day fresh and clean. Before you step into the shower, you might want to try a ritual that is done throughout India called "abhyanga," which is a daily self-massage done just before bathing (159). You can use sesame oil, coconut oil, olive oil—really any organic herbalized massage oil. Giving yourself a morning self-massage has tremendous benefits: it increases circulation, tones the muscles, calms the nerves, improves the elimination of impurities and toxins from the body, and promotes the health of the skin. Focus on the dry areas of your body, such as your elbows, knees, and hair, and the hardworking areas, such as your hands and the bottoms of your feet. Your skin is actually the largest organ of the body, and it absorbs whatever it is that you put onto it. When you apply oil in the morning before bathing, while the skin is still dry, it will more readily absorb the oil than if it is applied after the shower when your skin has already been saturated with shower water. If you suffer from dry skin at all, doing daily abhyanga might just be the miracle cure you've been looking for!

After abhyanga, step into the shower. Check with your local water company to find out what types of toxic chemicals are in your municipal water supply, and be sure to buy a showerhead filter that filters out whatever those toxins are—arsenic, chlorine, fluoride, and a host of other unhealthy toxins. Using a shower filter will not only prevent your skin from absorbing all of these toxins, it will also prevent your lungs from inhaling all the toxic steam that is created. A showerhead filter may be one of the best investments in your health that you can make.

Use only natural, organic soaps without any synthetic or artificial ingredients, which most commercial soaps contain. Your soap should be biodegradable, all plant-based, certified fair trade and organic, with no animal-tested products and no palm oil.

Use only organic shampoos and conditioners. Be sure to read the labels carefully. Some products claim to be natural or organic but still have some pretty bad stuff in there. Refer back to Chapter 3 to make sure you are slowly but surely replacing all the commercial-grade soaps and shampoos with naturals and organics. In true organic shampoos and conditioners, you will see ingredients like "certified organic tea tree oil," and things that sound like they grew on a plant or a tree or a kelp bed. If the ingredient names are unpronounceable and unrecognizable, just like with processed food, stay away! Anything that you put on your body should actually be safe enough to eat as well. (You may not WANT to eat your soaps and shampoos, but the concept is true,)

After your shower, use a natural organic oil on your skin instead of a commercial body lotion. The truth is, the best things for your body are not fancy man-made products but purely natural oils. Your deodorant should be all natural and should NOT be an antiperspirant, all of which contain cancer-causing aluminum compounds. You are the best, and you want only the best for your body!

Your Environment – Leaving for Work:

Before you leave for work, make it a habit to spend an extra few minutes making sure that your environment is in order so that when you return after a long day, you will return to a clean, serene atmosphere. The three biggies that can really pile up are trash, dishes, and laundry. If you just want to make sure that when you come home the house feels comfortable, just sweep through and make sure all the trash cans are emptied and out to the trash, that all the dishes are cleaned and put away, and that the laundry is either in process or all collected into hampers ready to be processed. Do NOT leave dirty laundry, dirty dishes, or trash out. It will create an unhealthy and unclean energy in the house. And never, ever forget to make your bed. The little things make a huge difference.

Of course, this is the bare minimum. For some of you, it is not nearly enough. Maybe you need to have your entire house in impeccable order before you leave, and that is wonderful if you can spare the time. We are speaking here to the vast majority of people that are pressed for time before they leave for work. It will make a world of difference to your stress and anxiety levels if you make sure that the home you come to at the end of the day, no matter how humble or grand, makes you sigh a deep breath when you walk in the door and think, "It's so good to be home." Simple things that help to decrease your stress and increase your happiness and satisfaction will have tremendous health benefits.

EVENINGS:

Your Environment – Returning Home From Work:

After your long day at work, realize that you have about four hours before you go to sleep, so use this time wisely and well. Sitting in front of the television is not necessarily the best option! Ideally you will spend about an hour preparing dinner, an hour at mealtime, and then two hours of rest and relaxation. When you arrive home, don't go straight to turning on the news. Try instead to turn on some quiet, relaxing music to listen to while you prepare your dinner. Instead of reaching automatically for a glass of wine, try instead to make a cup of herbal tea while you chop your veggies.

The one thing other diet plans have all over us is the five minutes it takes to pop their dinner entrées into the microwave, and dinner is ready. We would love to be able to tell you it will take you less than an hour to prepare and cook dinner, but everything of value takes time. Everything—

including your food. So relax ... there's no rush. You may want to change your clothes or at least your shoes, and put on something comfortable and relaxing so that you don't feel uncomfortable standing and chopping your veggies. With the Whole Earth Diet, there is a lot of chopping of veggies, and there is no getting around that (although you can always do a little food preparation for the day before and knock out the plan/prep/clean-up time)! After your meal is prepared, remember to eat mindfully, and follow the fifteen eating guidelines. Remember that your food preparation and your food itself are sacred. Don't forget your grace.

After your meal, clean up the kitchen right away. Put dishes away and wipe down the counters. Get yourself a large glass of water and leave the kitchen, turning out the light behind you. Brush your teeth right away, long before bed, because once you rid your mouth of any and all food flavors and particles, your stomach and brain get the clue, and all salivary systems shut off and your cravings to eat more will also go away. If you are looking to lose weight, the worst habit you can fall into is mindlessly eating and snacking after dinner. The calories you eat after dark will stay with you a lot longer than you want them to! If the kitchen is clean and dark, there is less likelihood that you will go back in there looking for snacks after dinner is finished. This is the golden key to staying slim and trim. Give yourself at least three hours between your last bite of food at night and bedtime.

Preparing for Sleep:

After dinner is cleaned up, you may have only a couple hours left before bedtime. Use it wisely. Try and use this free time for activities that promote mental wellness instead of anxiety. Your bedroom should be a haven for peace and calm. Before bed, you may read, or knit, or listen to music and write in your journal... Some people prefer not to have a televsion in their bedroom, but if you do enjoy watching TV, avoid those confrontational news programs that put you into an anxious and negative mood before bed. Look for programs with soothing content, such as comedies, classic old movies, travel shows, nature programs, shows that bring you peace and happiness, bring back good memories, or make you laugh. The few free hours that you have during your workweek should be all about reducing stress, not adding to it.

Sleep:

With all the good eating that you are doing and all the other great things you are doing for yourself, it will all be for naught if you are not getting enough rest. Sleep is essential for optimal health and happiness. The quality of your sleep directly affects the quality of your waking life, including your mental sharpness, productivity, emotional balance, creativity, physical vitality, and even your weight. No other activity delivers so many benefits with so little effort!

However, your body and brain don't exactly shut off when you sleep. While you rest, your brain stays busy, overseeing a wide variety of biological maintenance that keeps your body running in top condition, preparing you for the day ahead. Without enough hours of restorative sleep, you won't be able to work, learn, create, and communicate at a level even close to your true potential. You are literally recharging your battery. Regularly skimp on "service" and you're headed for a major mental and physical breakdown.

How much sleep do you need? It depends on your age. Babies will sleep from twelve to eighteen hours a day. Toddlers should sleep eleven to fourteen hours. Kids ages five through twelve need about ten to eleven hours, and kids ages twelve through eighteen need between eight and ten hours. If you have kids, please look carefully at these numbers. So many kids today are not getting enough sleep and are then being diagnosed with all sorts of disorders that perhaps would disappear if the poor kid just got enough rest! Between school and homework and after-school activities, most kids today are running on empty, and it is up to you parents to figure out what time the kids need to wake up; then back up to what time they need to get to bed with lights out, and stick to it. If parents would just step up to this responsibility, getting their kids to bed on time, the world would take a dramatic turn for the better! So, what about you? Sleep requirements vary from person to person, but only slightly. Most healthy adults need between seven and a half and nine hours per night to function at their best. You may think that you need less, you may say that you need less, but the reality is, if you are sleep-deprived, your health may be suffering in ways that are not immediately apparent. Sleep deprivation takes a gradual toll on your mind, body, and overall health in many ways that may surprise you (160).

Research shows that chronic lack of sleep is linked not only to increased colds and flus, but also to diabetes, heart disease, mental health problems, and obesity. Yes, that's right, obesity. When you are sleeping, the cells of your body are hard at work repairing what was broken down or damaged during the day. Your hormones and your immune system behave very differently during sleep. When you are sleep-deprived your body is more vulnerable to infection and disease because your immune system is not able to function properly. Also, you are more likely to become obese because lack of sleep has been linked to lower levels of the hormone leptin, which reduces hunger cravings. The good news is that most of this can be reversed by just getting your eight hours of sleep per night. So, so simple. Why isn't this being shouted from the rooftops? Because there is simply no money to be made by asking people to just sleep. No pharmaceutical company is going to make a profit; no doctors are going to get rich. So we are telling you here and now. Get your eight hours of sleep, and watch your entire life improve dramatically.

Weekly and Monthly Body Care

In addition to your daily routine, you should work out a weekly and monthly routine. Your weekly schedule should incorporate your daily exercise routines, with a variety of different fitness activities across the week. We will get into this more in the next chapter devoted to fitness, so we will leave it at that for now.

Here we will focus on those activities that you might want to add in monthly, and one day a week should be reserved for those monthly activities, maybe Saturday or Sunday afternoon, whatever works for you. Reserve an hour or two each week devoted to four things that you do once a month for self-care to pamper the glorious and wonderful "You." These activities can just as easily be free of charge if budget is a concern. Maybe you will decide that on Sunday afternoons you are going to alternate between going to the park, to the beach, to the mountains, and to the library for an hour, all of which are free. Or, if you really want to indulge yourself (as you should), consider trying some of these self-care activities that will assist you on your journey to more complete and perfect health:

Acupuncture, an alternative treatment, originated in China and has been practiced there for thousands of years. Although there are records of acupuncture being used hundreds of years ago in Europe, it was during the second half of the twentieth century that it began to spread rapidly in Western Europe, the United States, and Canada. Acupuncture involves the insertion of very thin needles through your skin at specific points on the body, and the needles are inserted to various depths. (I know, sounds really awful, doesn't it? But never fear. It is completely painless.) It is thought that these needles send tiny electromagnetic messages to our brains. Although results vary from person to person, acupuncture is well regarded as effective in pain relief and the symptoms of chemotherapy. For those squeamish about the use of tiny needles, acupressure is an alternative that stimulates the same points on the body using pressure. Traditional Chinese medicine, of which acupuncture/acupressure is one part, believes that the root cause of illnesses, not their symptoms, must be treated. Acupuncture has been used successfully in a range of women's fertility issues as well. A monthly visit to an acupuncture clinic is a great way to stay on top of keeping your body working optimally, preventing little things from becoming big things, and staying out of the Western medical doctor's office altogether by preventing disease rather than going back later to try and heal disease (161).

Chiropractic care: Chiropractors use hands-on spinal manipulation and other alternative treatments, the theory being that proper alignment of the body's musculoskeletal structure, particularly the spine, enables the body to heal itself without surgery or medication. Manipulation is used to restore mobility to joints restricted by tissue injury caused by a traumatic event, such as falling, or repetitive stress, such as sitting without proper back support. Chiropractic is primarily used as a pain-relief alternative for muscles, joints, bones, and connective tissue, such as cartilage, ligaments, and tendons.

Spinal manipulation and chiropractic care are generally considered safe, effective treatment for acute low back pain, the type of sudden injury that results from moving furniture or getting tackled. Acute back pain, which is more common than chronic pain, lasts no more than six weeks and typically gets better on its own.

Research has also shown chiropractic to be helpful in treating neck pain and headaches. In addition, osteoarthritis and fibromyalgia may respond to the moderate pressure used by both chiropractors and practitioners of deep-tissue massage. At a deeper level, however, if the body is in alignment, if it is in "balance" and the nerves that connect the brain to the rest of the body are allowed to conduct their messages back and forth, it stands to reason that all parts of the body will be able to heal more readily. Maintaining a healthy and well-adjusted spine enhances the body's ability to heal itself and to stay well. A monthly visit to your chiropractor is part of a healthy lifestyle (162).

Facials: Facials are one of the most popular beauty treatments, but did you know they are more than just an extravagance that make you feel and look good? (And guys, they are not just for women anymore!) Facials also have health benefits. Facials can increase circulation with the warm steam that is applied to the face during a facial. This warm steam not only helps open pores, but it can also open blood vessels and increase circulation. Increasing circulation to the face helps bring beneficial nutrients and oxygen to the skin, which encourages new cell growth. In addition to the steam, the light massage also increases circulation to the face and neck.

Facials may also help reduce blood pressure caused by stress. According to the Mayo Clinic, stress can temporarily raise your blood pressure to unhealthy levels. The hormones that the body releases under stress can cause an increase in heart rate and a narrowing of the blood vessels. Reducing stress, anxiety, and tension can help lower the risk of temporary spikes in blood pressure. The calming atmosphere of the spa room, a soothing facial treatment, and just taking a few minutes to relax may help reduce the risk of short-term high blood pressure due to anxiety and stress.

Facials can also increase lymphatic drainage, which helps stimulate your immune system. The lymphatic system is made up of a network of lymph nodes or glands located throughout the body, including many in the neck and chest. These glands are an integral part of the immune system and also work to drain excess fluid from parts of the body. During a facial, as the esthetician rubs the products into the skin around the neck and chest, the lymphatic system is stimulated. By "awakening" these lymph nodes, the body increases drainage and helps reduce any fluid retention in the face and upper body; this helps one receiving a facial feel and look less "puffy." So go ahead and book those monthly facials without guilt, knowing that you are doing this for your good health. (Oh, and it does feel wonderful to be pampered as well ... which is just as important!) (163).

Manicure and/or Pedicure: Getting a manicure and a pedicure could be a nice way to relax and pamper yourself monthly, or even weekly, but know that there are some risks to going to the local inexpensive nail salon, so you should weigh the benefits against the risks. The benefits of getting a nice manicure and pedicure are mostly obvious: your hands and feet look nice and well groomed. Also, there are health benefits to having someone help you care for your finger and toenails. Having a professional manicurist can help prevent nail damage, hangnails, and overgrown cuticles. Also, the manicure and pedicure typically involves massaging the hands and feet that are typically overworked and ignored, so it is a real treat to have someone massage our hands and feet for overall stress reduction and a greater sense of well-being. Increased circulation, stress relief, and increased movement and flexibility for those that suffer from arthritis are some of the benefits to expect.

That being said, there are some health risks. Some nail salons do not use the best techniques for cleaning and sterilizing their instruments, and the risk of getting infections from less-than-sanitary equipment is present. Also, most nail polishes and nail polish removers are filled with toxic ingredients, including formaldehyde. The nail-drying lamps might actually increase the risk of skin cancer since they emit UV rays. And whatever you do, do NOT get those artificial nails, whether acrylics or silks or gels or whatever the latest rage might be. No matter what the nail industry tells you, artificial nails are going to weaken and damage your natural nails underneath, the chemicals they use to apply and remove the nails are toxic and even flammable, and the risk of infection is greatly increased. The moist, dark space between your natural nail and the artificial nail is a perfect breeding ground for fungus and bacteria. Gross!

So what is the answer here? Do the benefits outweigh the risks? It's up to you entirely, of course. Our solution is to go once a month to a nice, reputable spa and ask only for a "buff" manicure and pedicure. You get all the nice pampering—the nail care, the massage, the nice lotions and oils—and then just a pure, clean buffing of the natural nail that leaves your fingers and toes looking healthy and natural. If you have been wearing polish or artificial nails for years, it will take some time to get your nails healthy again, but start now. The more you do a natural buff manicure, the better and healthier your natural nails will be. Be patient; it may take a few months, but it's well worth it in the end. With all the healthy eating you will be doing, you will have beautiful, healthy, long, strong natural nails in no time (164).

Massage: While there may be a bit of controversy around a manicure or pedicure, there is no controversy around the health benefits of a good massage. Massage has been used in healing for thousands of years in many cultures. Today, the only problem is trying to figure out which one is for you! Oftentimes, the number of choices on a spa menu can be completely overwhelming since there are over eighty different types of massage therapy modalities today.

Swedish massage is the most common type of massage and involves soft, long, kneading strokes on the uppermost layer of muscles, combined with movement of joints. Swedish massage can be both relaxing and energizing. Deep-tissue massage is best for treating painful, stiff "trouble spots" as the therapist focuses pressure more deeply into your spots of pain, eventually relieving chronic patterns of tension. Sports massage helps athletes in training, before, during, and after their sporting event; it promotes flexibility and helps prevent injuries. Shiatsu is a Japanese style of massage; the word "shiatsu" means "finger pressure," and the therapist focuses on applying pressure to precise points of the body, the "acupressure" points of the body, to allow the flow of the body's vital energy, or chi. In Thai massage, the therapist actually uses his or her body to move the client into a variety of positions, utilizing compressions of muscles, mobilization of joints, and acupressure (165).

Extended environment (weekly housecleaning):

Well, we honestly wish there was some way to make this sound like fun, but there's just no way around it. You must find a block of time weekly, whether it's one hour or six hours each week, to cleanse your home environment. Whether you live in a castle or a small apartment, whether you have maids or not, at the end of the day, you are the king of you own castle, no matter how big or small. And if you are taking good care of yourself, eating right, pampering yourself, this same level of care must extend to your extended environment. If you live in a dirty, cluttered mess, your health will suffer. Physically, dirt, dust, mold, and clutter can lead to allergies, asthma, and other physical disorders.

But perhaps more important than that, a cluttered life will lead to a cluttered mind. If your mind is cluttered, you will be stressed. The acts of cleaning and maintaining a clean house can help relieve and prevent unnecessary stress. A clean house makes maneuvering and finding things much easier, and thus reduces stress. Also, a clean and organized kitchen will encourage you to cook more often at home since your kitchen will be a pleasant environment. A clean and organized kitchen pantry and refrigerator will further inspire you to get in there and cook up some healthy meals.

And finally, housecleaning is a great way to burn calories! Doing general housework burns somewhere between 200 and 250 calories per hour, while vacuuming or cleaning out the garage burns even more! So if you look at it all this way, cleaning your house might not be a bad thing to do weekly after all. Maybe "cleaning" becomes your daily fitness activity one day of the week! (Okay, I know I'm stretching here.) But schedule a consistent time every week, get your favorite music going, and dance your way through your housework! Need incentive to clean? Invite guests over for a delicious, home-cooked, plant-based meal!

Seasonal Body Care

In addition to your weekly and monthly routine appointments and schedules, there are certain activities that you may want to plug into your calendar at the start of each new year that will happen at the beginning of each season, four times each year.

Seasonal Cleanses are the perfect way to start every season. Cleanses may seem like the latest trend, but actually seasonal cleanses have been done for thousands of years. Pancha Karma cleansing was originally developed for royalty in India to prolong life and health by removing physical impurities, bringing awareness to destructive thoughts and behaviors, and releasing old patterns. Cleanses were done four times a year, both for disease prevention and for emotional and spiritual growth.

Traditionally a cleanse would be phased like this: Two to three weeks before the actual cleansing phase, you would eliminate all processed foods, sweets, stimulants such as coffee, and most dairy products from your diet. One week before the cleansing phase, the diet would be further modified, becoming predominantly vegetables and whole grains. These foods, especially the vegetables, create a more alkaline (vs. acid) environment in the body, which supports the cleansing and detox process. During this preparation phase, a person's activity shifts to become more internally focused. This means letting go of some day-to-day activities and spending time meditating and taking walks in nature. Deep breathing, focused on the exhalation phase, helps to rid the body of old ideas, emotions, and blockages.

During the cleansing phase itself, we shift into a pure juice fast, or a very light, clean diet of fruits, vegetables, and only a couple types of nuts, seeds, and grains. Foods eaten are mostly raw or lightly steamed, without cooking in any oils. During this part of the cleanse, your digestive system is given a complete break so that the body's energy can go toward healing and detoxifying. Often, supplemental herbal formulas are given that assist with the body's ability to heal, purify, and rid itself of toxins. The cleansing phase can last anywhere from five to ten days.

At the end of the cleanse, we shift into the rejuvenation phase, returning to the simple diet of the preparation phase. It is important to do this gradually, by slowly introducing solid foods, such as legumes and a wider range of grains, nuts and seeds. Many people find that the most profound healing occurs during the rejuvenation phase. Physical, emotional, and spiritual changes may be experienced in the days and weeks to come. Sometimes issues that have been suppressed for long periods of time will surface. The rejuvenation phase can last from twenty-one to twenty-eight days, or even longer. It can and possibly should become a normal way of life, and the normal way of eating (166).

Cleanses are a good way to introduce people to eating whole, real, plant-based foods in a "safe, temporary" way when the reality is that the "rejuvenation phase" should become their normal reality. Sometimes it takes several cleanses to get this, but eventually it happens. So whether you do the Whole Earth Wellness seasonal cleanses, or another cleanse/detox program, it is important to do cleanses as part of your regular routine. Cleanses are an important part of a regular health routine and help the body to detoxify and rejuvenate, giving the overall system a rest and the ability to maintain health and balance in the body.

Hair

Perhaps being a relatively hairless mammal with hair found only on top of our heads is what makes our hair such an object of both admiration and scrutiny. For many people, their hair is their identity. It doesn't matter if you are male or female, if you show your hair to the world or only to your family and mostly wear a hijab, everyone takes pride in this mop of stuff that grows on top of their head. So while the seasonal cleanse will lead you toward better physical, mental, emotional, and spiritual health, equally important are those more "trivial" seasonal activities that you do just because they make you feel good about yourself.

There is no reason to feel that wanting to look good is vain and superficial. This is all part of self-love, of wanting and needing to take care of yourself and pamper yourself without guilt. Going in to the hairdresser or barber at the beginning of every season is a great way to start each season feeling fresh and renewed, and oftentimes I will make a point of seeing my hairdresser at the close of every seasonal cleanse—kind of the icing on the cake ... and just as important. There may be other "superficial" vanity-type things you all would like to do at least four times a year, and there is nothing wrong with wanting to look and feel your best. Schedule these activities to coincide with the Whole Earth Wellness Cleanses across the year, and we will all be looking good and feeling great on this journey to becoming the very best, healthiest, happiest version of ourselves!

Extended environment (seasonal housecleaning)

Well, we've been able to spin just about everything in this chapter to sound like fun, even weekly housecleaning (okay, at least we tried), but seasonal deep housecleaning is a lot more work, and it takes some imagination to make it sound like fun! We're talking about those longer three-day weekends where you roll up your sleeves and tackle a major housecleaning effort. We're talking about cleaning out the garage; cleaning out your bedroom closet and giving away half your unwanted items to charity; completely reorganizing your kitchen cupboards, pantry, and refrigerator; getting into those adult children's bedrooms; giving away those "fat clothes" that you no longer need (because of your new, trim figure, of course!); putting away some of the toys and trinkets. We are talking about those BIG projects that you postpone and put off and procrastinate doing! Put them onto your calendar and act as if they are immovable and inarguable events that MUST occur as if they were important appointments. Then rev yourself up for the actual occurrence. Keep your eyes on the prize. Imagine what your space will look like with this new, clean, uncluttered organized garage, kitchen, closets, and bedrooms. Take "before" and "after" photos to give yourself a tangible reward for your work. Put on some loud and motivating music so that you can dance your way to a clean and organized house! Remember that intensive seasonal housecleaning like this burns lots of calories, gives you a feeling of peace and accomplishment afterwards, and costs you absolutely nothing.

ANNUAL BODY CARE

Just as I encourage you to create your own daily, weekly, monthly, and seasonal schedules, I also encourage you to select one month each year to be your "annual doctors' appointments" month. Most of us have annual exams that we need to schedule, and they always seem to be an intrusion into our normal routine, so why not schedule them all at once and then go light on your workload that month? It also helps you to remember which exams you have scheduled and which you haven't. It's much more convenient to just get them all over with at once. In the end, it will help you live a healthier, longer life if you are on a good annual wellness exam routine, and your doctors can screen for and find early any little things that may be going out of balance before they become big issues.

Now it may get overwhelming at times to follow a diligent set of principles that others in your friends and family may not agree with or may not share with you. At these times, just smile at the world at large and know that you have a happy, healthy body and a clear, tranquil mind in the making, which is the foundation for allowing you to achieve all you want in this lifetime. Lead by example, show the way, and let the results—your glowing skin, pounds shed without much effort, calmer state of mind—speak for themselves much louder than your words.

Chapter 5

Classical Elements
of Exercise

Classical Elements of Exercise

---•●•---

"You are a child of the light, born with the grounding strength of the earth, the patient flexibility of water, the transformative passion of fire, and the forceful energy of the wind. Remember who you are, where you came from, and why you are here."

~Laura Robinson Oatman

The Whole Earth Diet philosophy is to support you to rethink your nutrition, remake your lifestyle, and renew your spirit by transitioning to a plant-based diet. This process is aided by the development of all the other aspects of yourself—your body, mind, heart, and soul.

So far, we have talked almost exclusively about your physical health, focused primarily on food, and offered guidelines for eating and for body care and maintenance. And before we leave our bodies and start to talk about mind, heart, and soul, there is one more important piece of the equation when it comes to physical health—the other side of the coin! The yang of fitness. Aside from the food that you eat, there is nothing else that you can do to improve your health and happiness that is more important than daily physical activity. Today, the folks that live in areas of the world where physical activity is a regular part of their routine will live much longer than those who live a sedentary life. Exercise is critical to good health!

Most long-living communities around the world still use their bodies for chores and activities and have a regular system of physical exercise. There have been studies done on global communities that have the largest number of living centenarians, a person who lives to or beyond the age of 100 years. They have called these areas the "blue zones" to help identify and quantify these particular geographic areas. This concept grew out of work done by Gianni Pes and Michel Poulain who first identified the Italian island of Sardinia as the region with the highest concentration of male centenarians in the world. They further identified other longevity hotspots in Okinawa, Japan; Nicoya, Costa Rica; Icaria, Greece; and the Seventh Day Adventist community in Loma Linda, California. They found common characteristics among all five of these areas: they put family ahead of all else; they didn't smoke; they ate mostly vegetarian (except for the Sardinian diet, all the others are almost 100 percent plant-based); they are all very socially active and integrated into their communities even in old age; they all eat lots of legumes ... and constant, moderate physical activity is an inseparable part of life. Constant, moderate, inseparable (167).

The benefits of getting some physical activity every day are enormous, and these "blue zone" communities are living examples of this: losing weight, having more energy, feeling physically fit and hence mentally more alert, sleeping more soundly, combating major illness, and living longer. The list goes on and on and on.

So think about ways that you can get at least one hour of physical activity every single day. When we were children, we would play outdoors a few hours every day, and it was not something that we did because we "had to"; it was something we wanted to do naturally. We called it "playing." Think about returning to the notion of physical activity as "play," and you will go do it with a different attitude. It will become less of a chore and more fun! So now is the time to think through a few of your favorite physical activities and how you plan to incorporate these into your daily life.

I know I've told you this before but it's worth repeating. Think about your new lifestyle as one that incorporates one hour of "play" each day, preferably first thing in the morning before you shower and get ready for your day. When you exercise first thing in the morning, not only does it get your metabolism up and running on high first thing in the morning (which transmits messages to your body that you are going to have an active day and to burn calories quickly and efficiently all day), but it also gives you a feel-good high that lasts the entire day. When you have taken the initiative to get up early to exercise, you are less likely to sabotage your day with binging or caving in to cravings. By accomplishing something that you have set as a personal goal, you feel confident and motivated to accomplish other things. No matter what your current health situation, if you are sick or fatigued or overworked or bored or suffering from cancer or diabetes or migraines—whatever shape you are in today, you can benefit from some form of exercise. You could start out with a simple twenty-minute walk every day through your neighborhood. Get yourself a dog. There is no better walking buddy, no one who will get more excited about taking a walk with you, than a four-legged companion!

The idea is to get yourself started on the way to forming a new habit. Research states that it takes a person on average twenty-one days of repeating an activity every day to form a new habit (168). So set your goal that for the next twenty-one days you will do an hour of activity, without complaint, imperfectly, to the best of your ability, of your own volition, every single day. I promise, soon it will move from feeling like a chore to something you look forward to! Once you have made up your mind in this direction, say it out loud, "I will exercise every day!"

Creating a daily exercise routine that you will be able to stick with requires participation in a variety of things. Doing the same thing every day will eventually, or quickly, turn BORING! So, following along the idea that we are all created from the four elements of earth, water, fire, and air, our physical fitness should nurture the needs of each of these classical elements inside ourselves. Your body's earth element needs to be fed with strength training; your body's water element needs to be nourished through yoga; your fire element through dance or other creative, adrenaline-charged, physical self-expression; and your body's air element through cardiovascular exercise.

Earth (body) fitness:

Strength Training = Physical Strength = Mental/Emotional/Spiritual Strength

To establish a healthy body, our "earth element" exercise is weight training or strength training. To start on the path to physical fitness, this is the most basic thing you can do and the foundation for all physical wellness. When we talk about weight training or strength training, we are talking about any activity that increases muscles and core strength—weight lifting, or boot camp, or some kind of a "power sculpt" class at your gym where hand weights and barbells are used. You can even just use your own body and do push-ups, leg lifts, planks, and sit-ups. Muscle mass naturally diminishes with age, so we need to do what we can to fight this. There are multiple health benefits to strength training. Besides the obvious visual appeal of having a toned and muscular body, strength training also creates strong ligaments and tendons, which serve to support our joints and decrease the likelihood of injury from other activities. Bone density increases dramatically, reducing our risk of osteoporosis. Strength training enhances quality of life as it enables us to better perform daily activities that require lifting, pushing, and pulling (169). The physical and spiritual benefits of strength training are myriad, and when realized, the goal no longer becomes a "hard body," but the confidence and control that strength training teaches us. Do you have a gym membership? Do they have any good classes you can join? If not, can you buy a DVD and some simple weights to try this at home? There are so many good fitness and exercise programs available now on DVD, so you really have no more excuses. Think this through now and try to make a decision on how you can incorporate strength training into your health regimen.

Water (mind) fitness:

Yoga = Physical Flexibility = Mental/Emotional/Spiritual Flexibility

To establish a healthy mind, our "water element" exercise is associated with yoga, an ancient discipline that increases flexibility/fluidity for the body, which in turn creates mental clarity and calm for the mind and spiritual insight for the soul. The Sanskrit word "yoga" literally means "yoke," meaning "to control," or "to unite." Its purpose is to unite mind, body, and spirit as the purification of the physical body leads to purification of the mind and spirit.

What is the relationship between water and yoga? For those of you that have ever taken a yoga class, you may notice that right after the class you feel as if you have just had a tune-up and an oil change! In fact, while yoga doesn't change any fluids, it does a wonderful job of moving fluids around in your body. Your blood circulates in your arteries and veins, and your lymph flows through the spaces around all your cells; both fluids can be cleansed of metabolic by-products, and your blood replenished with oxygen and nutrients. Yoga also helps circulate the synovial fluid inside your joints, which facilitates smooth, painless movement between bones and delivers nutrients to the muscle cartilage, which doesn't have its own blood supply. As the body ages, we tend to dry up and lose water, and this results in less synovial fluid in our joints, which causes the classic stiffness of old age. Drinking lots of fresh, clean water and practicing yoga at least two to three times a week is essential to keeping the body youthful and flexible, and by keeping the body flexible we also allow the mind to remain flexible as well. Other proven health benefits of yoga include building strength, improving posture and breathing, detoxifying the body, reducing pain, curing insomnia, reducing stress, and promoting deep relaxation (170).

If you want to get started, many yoga studios offer free introductory classes to get you to try it out, and some gyms offer yoga classes along with membership. You may want to shop around and try different yoga teachers as well as different styles of yoga because there are so many variations. Don't go to just one class and decide you don't like it; try a couple and find the right fit for you. Start with some basic **Iyengar yoga** classes. Iyengar yoga, named after founder B.K.S. Iyengar, is really good for learning the fundamentals of yoga, teaching simple but extremely precise alignment; it's a great style for patient perfectionists and detail-oriented folks, but also a good one to start with before exploring out into other styles, to learn the correct way to do poses.

Once you've got the basics, you can start exploring other styles if you wish. There is **Ashtanga yoga**, which is a more intense, rapid-flow yoga taking you from pose to pose without much pause in between, a fairly serious cardio workout that is great for Type-A personalities who want to do yoga for athletic fitness. There is **Bikram yoga**, named after creator Bikram Choudhury, which is a set series of twenty-six poses done in a sauna-like hot room (105 degrees with 40 percent humidity). This is the opposite of Ashtanga flow yoga; in Bikram you move very slowly and deliberately from pose to pose, and in that kind of heat you'll be glad for that. There is nothing quite like Bikram though to get your body both toned AND flexible, if you can stand the heat.

Other great muscle-building, weight-loss focused yoga classes are Anasura yoga (like Ashtanga flow but a little less intense) and Power yoga (like Ashtanga flow but a little MORE intense). Kundalini is a constantly moving flow yoga class as well, but with a bit more spiritual awareness, focused on the kundalini (serpent) energy in your body that sleeps at the base of your spine. Kundalini classes are intended to move the serpent up from the base of your spine through all seven chakras of the body, with a big focus on breathing and energy; it will definitely leave you feeling buzzed.

If you are looking for a more deeply spiritual style, Jivamukti is heavily rooted in the traditions of yogic scripture including yoga philosophy. Expect Sanskrit chanting, references to ancient scripture, and different themes for each class based on the five tenets: scripture, bhakti (devotion to God), ahimsa (nonviolence), nada yoga (yoga of sound), and meditation. This is best for someone looking for the most authentic, traditional, holistic style of yoga being regularly practiced here in the Western world.

These types of yoga are exactly what some folks are looking for, but I personally have two favorite types—Yin Yoga and Restorative Yoga. I look to yoga to be the time when I can relax and stretch and connect my mind with my body in a peaceful way. I like a good flow yoga, but after thirty downward dogs I start looking for the quickest escape route. Bikram was awesome for me for a while, but I had a problem with doing the same exact twenty-six poses over and over. It just got boring.

So I always look first for the yin or Restorative classes at my local yoga studio. Yin (female) is a quiet, meditative yoga style, also called taoist yoga. It is meant to complement muscle-building "yang" (masculine) yoga styles like Anasura, Ashtanga, and Iyengar. The more passive yin poses focus on lengthening and stretching connective tissues, relaxing muscles, and letting gravity work to help stretch out those areas that are tight or bound. The poses are held for a long time, and the classes are extremely relaxing. Yin yoga classes today are still a bit unknown, but once more people start to try them out, I am sure there will be a yin yoga boom.

The other type of class I always look for is a Restorative yoga class. Restorative yoga is best for alleviating stress and for dealing with injuries. There are only about four or five simple poses that are held for up to twenty minutes each and that are intended to direct blood flow to injured areas without straining any muscles. Restorative yoga will leave you feeling completely relaxed and buzzing with good energy.

I encourage you to get out there and try them all. No two yoga classes and no two teachers are alike, so find your favorite and make it a part of your weekly routine. Yoga will increase the fluidity and flexibility of your body and your mind and improve the connection between the two.

Fire (heart) fitness:

Dance/Martial Arts = Physical Passion = Mental/Emotional/Spiritual Passion

The next type of fitness, to establish a healthy heart, is your "fire element." This could be any activity that gets your adrenaline or endorphins (your "feel good" hormones) rocking and rolling, something that makes you happy and excited while burning calories; this might be dance (and there are many types of dance), or martial arts, or rock climbing, or even jumping out of an airplane—whatever turns you on that will both burn calories and keep your emotional heart happy and healthy!

For many of us, particularly women, dance seems to be just the ticket, and this might be something you want to add to your weekly routine. Of course, there are also some who are mortified at the thought of dancing, so no worries! Other forms of fire exercise might be practicing martial arts, karate, kung fu, kickboxing or fencing—something that creates a rise in adrenaline, something that not only makes you smile but makes you laugh out loud, something that, if it is on your calendar, you look forward to with great anticipation and excitement. (This may or may not be true for your "earth" boot camp classes or your "air" cardio sessions on the treadmill.) Fire fitness needs to be something that makes you move and that makes you extremely happy while doing so.

So let's just take dance, as an example (since this is my favorite form of fire fitness!). There are so many types of dance and ways to dance: from square dancing and folk dancing to belly dancing, zumba, and even pole dancing! Dance activity is not only good for your body fitness, but it's also good for your heart fitness. It can be a way to increase your libido and your feelings about your significant other in a very mutually beneficial way, so is not only good for you, but good for your relationships as well.

If dancing is simply not what you enjoy, then you can think of bowling or tennis or anything that is fun, exciting, and you really would enjoy. Think back to when you were a kid. What did you just LOVE to do? You are never too old to do that again, whatever it is. Did you love bike riding, or swimming in the ocean, or maybe even hang gliding or rock climbing? What puts a smile on your face? What would get you really excited and happy about doing again? THAT is exactly what you need to weave back into your life. Get your calendar out, right now. Pick a date, get on the Internet, and make an appointment in your calendar now to do that thing that makes your heart sing. And set it as a recurring appointment weekly, monthly, or quarterly if it's something that you cannot possibly do all the time for practical reasons (an activity that involves travel or money). Ideally though, you might want to look for something you can do regularly (weekly), like a zumba class or a ballroom dancing class. (171)

And then, of course, there is one other thing you can do for your heart health, aside from happy physical activity, and that is LAUGHTER! Perhaps one night a week you can go out and see a funny movie or go to a comedy club. Laughter and dance release very similar beneficial hormones, so if you don't have time to dance, or you don't have the time or money to go skydiving every week, at least find time to laugh! Laugh every day to increase those heart-healthy happy hormones. (172)

Air (soul) fitness:

Cardiovascular = Physical Endurance = Mental/Emotional/Spiritual Endurance

Finally, to establish a healthy soul, our "wind element" exercise is a combination of cardiovascular exercise, deep breathing, and meditation, all involving the breath. Did you know that in many different languages the word for "breath" is the same as the word for "soul" or "life"? The focus here is on your breath, your "prana," or your life force. Something as simple as getting in touch with your breath—whether in exertion, such as on a run, or while sitting quietly and meditating—will get you further and further in touch with your soul, and with the divine life force that lives inside you.

Start with some regular aerobic activity or cardiovascular exercise (otherwise known as "cardio"). Cardio, such as walking, bicycling, or swimming, can help you live longer and healthier and is the best and quickest way to burn calories and lose unwanted weight (if it is weight loss you are after) (173). Need further motivation? See how aerobic exercise affects your heart, lungs, lymph, and blood flow. Then get moving and start reaping the rewards.

During aerobic activity, you are quickly moving the large muscles in your arms, legs, and hips. You'll notice that your body will respond quickly to this. You'll breathe faster and more deeply. This maximizes the amount of oxygen in your blood. Your heart will beat faster, which increases blood flow to your muscles and back to your lungs. Your capillaries will widen to deliver more oxygen to your muscles and carry away waste products, such as carbon dioxide and lactic acid. Your body will even release endorphins, natural painkillers that promote an increased sense of well-being. I do need to insert a warning: sometimes, for the first five minutes, cardio feels like hell on Earth. It is awful when your body first realizes what you are doing to it, and it initially reacts and says, "Oh no, not this again," and you may feel like quitting five minutes in.

But if you just override your brain and keep going, you will slip into a much more relaxed yet energetic state. You will get through your thirty minutes or hour, and afterwards you will be SO glad you did. Get your headphones on and get some good music going, and let the music help you find your rhythm and help the time go faster. So what exactly does aerobic exercise do for your health?

Aerobic activity can help you keep away excess pounds. Combined with a healthy diet, aerobic exercise is the best way to help you lose weight. There are no shortcuts here. You must do cardio if you want to lose weight. Check out the fittest folks in the gym (but don't be obvious); they are the ones who start every workout with thirty to sixty minutes on those darn cardio machines—the stairs, the ellipticals, running on those treadmills. They are burning calories like crazy. Research shows that during the first thirty minutes of cardio, you are burning off the glucose from the food you have eaten in the last twenty-four hours, but after thirty minutes you are starting to actually use the glucose stored in your fat, so it is important to go for at least forty-five minutes. Remember, sweat is your fat crying! And remember to replace all the water lost through sweat with lots of water during and afterwards.

Aerobic exercise may make you tired in the short term, but over the long term, you'll enjoy increased stamina and reduced fatigue. It can help ward off viral illnesses as aerobic exercise activates your immune system by helping the lymph system function properly. This leaves you less susceptible to minor viral illnesses, such as colds and flu. Aerobic exercise reduces the risk of many conditions, including obesity, heart disease, high blood pressure, type 2 diabetes, stroke, and certain types of cancer. It is an effective way to manage chronic conditions. Aerobic exercise helps lower high blood pressure and control blood sugar. If you've had a heart attack, aerobic exercise helps prevent subsequent attacks because it strengthens your heart. A stronger heart doesn't need to beat as fast. A stronger heart also pumps blood more efficiently, which improves blood flow to all parts of your body. It keeps your arteries clear, boosts your HDL "good" cholesterol, and lowers your LDL "bad" cholesterol. The result? Less buildup of plaque in your arteries.

Perhaps one of the best benefits is that it acts as a mood booster! Aerobic exercise can ease the gloominess of depression, reduce the tension associated with anxiety, and promote relaxation. It will help you sleep better at night too, which helps your mood and energy during the day. Aerobic exercise also keeps your muscles strong, which can help you maintain mobility as you get older. It keeps your mind sharp. For whatever reason, studies have shown that at least thirty minutes of aerobic exercise three days a week seems to reduce cognitive decline in older adults. Finally, studies show that people who participate in regular aerobic exercise live longer than those who don't exercise regularly. (173)

Now you know the health benefits of cardiovascular exercise, but how does it relate to spirituality? A couple ways actually, and both have to do with breathing. Breathing exercises are about creating awareness in your body, to know at what exertion level you can perform optimally and when you have overreached those boundaries. Taking gasping, shallow breaths through your mouth triggers an emergency response in your body to produce adrenaline to save you from a potentially life-threatening situation. This is a wonderful coping mechanism that our bodies developed back in the caveman days to save our lives as we were running away from the saber-toothed tigers, but we are not meant to live every day as if we are in an emergency that results in gasping for air through our mouths. This adrenaline response depletes our systems and leaves our body thinking we are fighting off an emergency every day of our lives. Our body in turn creates stress-fighting hormones called free radicals, which are acidic and cancer causing, to mitigate against this stressful lifestyle created by breathing improperly. Breathing through one's nose is the first step in learning to exercise effortlessly. When we learn to breath into the calming receptors in the lower lobes of our lungs, we can learn to exercise and compete from the "eye of the hurricane," also known as the "runner's high." This is a place of meditative calm where exercise becomes effortless and you perform at your personal best (174).

So, the final takeaway? Dedicate one hour a day to play! This goes hand in hand with and is JUST as important as eating the right food for optimal physical health. The good food is the yin energy (what you take in); the sleep and exercise is the yang energy (what you put out). Now you have the foundation for physical health, for your earth element. Now, let's go to the next chapter and dive into all the other wonderful parts of you—your water, your fire, and your air!

Chapter 6

Classical Elements
of Holistic Health

Classical Elements of Holistic Health

"Everything passes. Both soaring joys and crushing sorrows fade away like a dream. However, the knowledge of having lived one's life to the fullest never disappears."

~Daisaku Ikeda

Okay, my friend, so hopefully this has been an informative journey for you on how to actively take responsibility for your personal best physical health—by eating the best healing foods for your body, eating mindfully, eating at the proper time of day and with the seasons, by looking at food as the first and primary source of healing rather than medicine. Also, I have suggested to you that food and eating are only half the equation. Food is the intake; exercise is the outtake. You cannot do one without the other if you desire your best physical health. This is the basis, the foundation, of Whole Earth Diet—a whole-foods, plant-based diet and a fitness program that incorporates exercising all four of our elements—earth, wind, fire, and air. But wait, we are not done. We do not stop with the body, as most diets do. Whole Earth Diet has taught you to rethink your nutrition by transitioning to a plant-based diet and to remake your lifestyle with self-care and exercise, and now we want to give you the tools to create a healthy life.

In this chapter, we are going to begin to explore how the health of the mind, the health of the heart, and the health of the soul are intimately connected with the body's physical health. If any one of these parts of the whole is out of alignment, is weak and not functioning properly, then all parts suffer, and the self can only be as strong as the weakest link. For example, you can eat the best foods, exercise daily, have a good family life, and go to church every week, but if your mind is unhappy, if you have a job or a career that you hate and that doesn't serve your higher purpose, then your health will fail. If you cannot function emotionally because you cannot love yourself, then your health will suffer as you binge eat and self-sabotage yourself every step of the way. If you have everything going for you, but you have no spiritual connection to God and you are in that state of spiritual vacuum, then all of this is for nothing as you will live in fear and emptiness. BUT when all of this is working together, when the health of one aspect of self feeds into and fosters the health of the next and the other, until the entire self is working together toward better health, the result is a happy life.

So how do we find true health and happiness? By actively working on all parts of our self simultaneously. The growth must be balanced and equal to avoid imbalances in the psyche and the self. I have dedicated several chapters to finding perfect physical health for your physical body, your earth element. There should be, and will be, separate books in the Whole Earth Wellness Series that will be dedicated exclusively to mental, emotional, and spiritual health, but here I just want to give you an idea of where we should head with mental, emotional, and spiritual wellness, all necessary elements of a happy life.

Recreate Your Life Purpose ~ Flow Into Your Dharma

"Don't get set into one form, adapt it and build your own, and let it grow, be like water. Empty your mind, be formless, shapeless — like water. If you put water in a cup it becomes the cup, if you put into a bottle it becomes the bottle. You put water into a teapot it becomes the teapot. Now, water can flow or it can crash. Be water, my friend." ~ Bruce Lee

As your physical body is represented by the earth element, as the basis and foundation for your body's health, your mind is represented by water—ideally fluid, energized, and adaptable, yet strong, calm, and quiet. We have already talked a bit about water as a nutrient, water as a form of fitness through yoga, and now water as it represents your mind. So how should you seek to grow the health of your mind? Just as the health of your body is determined primarily (or at the foundation) through a combination of food and fitness, so the health of your mind is determined by a combination of education/lifelong learning and career. Your current career and education are intricately connected. As a child you probably began your educational process in primary school, continued through high school, perhaps college, perhaps even graduate school, and today you probably have a job or a career that is intimately connected to your education.

But like a river winding its way through a valley—at times a rushing river, at times a still lake, at times a lazy, winding stream—your career and your education may, will, and should change as you move through life's cycles and changes. People are living much longer and retiring much later than they ever have (if they retire at all), so the idea or notion that you must choose your life work at age eighteen as soon as you're out of high school is ludicrous. You may want to shift your thinking now. Perhaps begin to think of your life's purpose not as a single career, but as a series of careers, perhaps related, perhaps not, but all driven by one motivation—your passions and commitments.

Education and Lifelong Learning

Just as the health of the body starts with the food that you eat, the health of the mind starts with the information you feed it! When we speak of education, we are not speaking of education in terms of what you learned in school as a child or young adult. Education is never ending, a lifelong process, where every day you learn new things—not just ONE new thing, but lots of new things. Particularly in this day and age, with many of us on the Internet for most of our day, we have information at our fingertips 24/7 in ways that no one in the past has ever had. We are living in a time of an educational overload explosion! And so it is critical that what we feed our mind is healthy and not diseased, biased, or tainted. We choose every day what to read, watch, and listen to. Be sure that it passes the Whole Earth Wellness checklist. Be sure that it:

1) Is information based on facts, science, and unbiased research, rather than opinions;

2) Is something that helps you to grow physically, mentally, emotionally, spiritually;

3) Is something that promotes love and not hate, unity not division;

4) Teaches you something that you care passionately about.

Research during the 1990s, a decade of pioneering brain research, proved that a stimulated mind promotes a healthy brain. These studies were conducted at many research facilities including Harvard, Duke, and Johns Hopkins Universities. They showed that keeping older brains stimulated helps retain mental alertness as people age. The brain's physical anatomy actually responds to enriching mental activities. Scientists have discovered that the brain, even an aging brain, can grow new connections and pathways when challenged and stimulated.

In the words of Dr. Paul Nussbaum, director of the Aging Research and Education Center in Pittsburgh, Pennsylvania, "Every time your heart beats, 25 percent of that blood goes right to the brain. But while exercise is critical, it may be education that is more important. In the twenty-first century, education and information may become for the brain what exercise is for the heart." Just like the human heart, our brains need to be nurtured. So lifelong learning can be considered a health club for our minds. (175)

Making lifelong learning part of your life also fosters a sense of personal empowerment and increased self-esteem. It ensures continued growth and intellectual stimulation, leading to a more fulfilling, enjoyable, and enriched lifestyle. It helps develop natural abilities, immerse people in the wonders of life, stimulate natural curiosity about the world, increase wisdom, enable people to use their experience to make the world a better place, and help older adults face the inevitable changes of society.

Let's return our thoughts to the last chapter where we discussed the relationship between the body and the mind that is fostered by the practice of yoga, and how that corresponds to the water element of physical fitness. Yoga keeps the fluids moving in the body, and lifelong learning keeps the fluids moving in the brain. Yoga and lifelong learning are truly the anecdotes to the stiffness and rigidity that can come with old age; as the body locks up and becomes inflexible, so too does the mind.

Your Career Path and Finding Your Dharma

So now you are at least thinking about some ways to keep your mind healthy. Keep learning. Keep flexible. And so wherever you are on life's journey, maybe you are still a young person with a multitude of options ahead of you, maybe you are an older person with a more limited range in some respects, but you have the wisdom now to truly know yourself, which in fact is a huge advantage. Wherever you are, continue to feed your mind with enriching information and with healthy food that stimulates your mind in a positive way.

It just may be that you find yourself now, as an adult, pulled toward learning something completely new and different from what you have been educated to do, completely out of alignment with your current career. Maybe the universe has given you a good thumping and you are without a job or a career at the moment, so you find yourself at crossroads. This, my friend, is the universe not just whispering to you but shouting at you to take the road less traveled. To follow with your mind where your heart is leading. We talk a lot about the mind/body connection. Equally important is the mind/heart connection. You must love what you do. You must be so excited to get up every morning and go to work that you can't stand the weekends. In fact, you find yourself working on weekends happily. If this is you, then you are following your dharma.

What is your purpose here? What is your dharma? "Dharma" is a Sanskrit word that means "that which upholds, supports, or maintains the regulatory order of the universe" (176). It is both abstract and concrete and refers to ideas such as duty, vocation, religion, and everything that is considered correct, proper, or decent behavior. Bringing the idea of dharma into supporting our whole health, you must learn to discern what the universe wants you to do. The universe is calling you to a higher purpose, to bring your own very unique and individual gifts and talents and knowledge to the world. You must discern exactly what that calling is. If you remain trapped in a job that you hate, doing something that is not contributing to the higher good, you will never be happy, and your mind will never be healthy. Seek your purpose. We all have one; we were all born for a distinct and unique reason. There is no other you.

Start with educating yourself toward what it is that you love, then start on the path to your purpose. Not sure what your higher passion is? Then spend time with yourself and explore what drives and motivates you. Keep the money aside for a few days and ask yourself, if you didn't have to worry about earning, what would you ideally be? When we follow our passion and excel at it, money also flows in that direction. Initially, we must have the courage to follow our heart's passion. It all begins with the first step—being clear about what you truly are passionate about and committed to at each stage of your life.

I hear some of you thinking, *"Yeah, right, well, I need to earn a living. I can't just up and walk away from a paycheck, even if I hate the work."* I get it. You have a couple options. Start to train yourself for a different career through your education, start to quietly lay it out after-hours so that you can start to build your own business in your spare time, and gradually transition into turning your dharma first into a part-time job, then finally into a full-time job. The other option might be that your dharma lies in volunteering for a non-profit organization on weekends or after-hours, allowing you to keep your safe, full-time job, but pursuing your dharma on weekends. Maybe your dharma lies at home, in neither a career or with a charity. Maybe your dharma is to stay at home and care for children or aging parents or handicapped siblings. All work is honorable and good, even if you feel that you did not select your dharma; sometimes the universe hands you your dharma. But recognize that no matter what, you should embrace all work, whether chosen or not, with love. I just found this quote from Kahlil Gibran on the Internet this morning, so I will close with this:

"Work is love made visible. And if you cannot work with love but only with distaste, it is better that you should leave your work and sit at the gate of the temple and take alms of those who work with joy. For if you bake bread with indifference, you bake a bitter bread that feeds but half man's hunger. And if you grudge the crushing of the grapes, your grudge distills a poison in the wine. And if you sing though as angels, and love not the singing, you muffle man's ears to the voices of the day and the voices of the night." – Kahlil Gibran

Revive Your Passion ~ Ignite Your Heart

"To love oneself is the beginning of a lifelong romance."
~ Oscar Wilde

One of the key ingredients to having a healthy and happy life is in the area of relationships—with yourself, your loved ones, your fellow man, your fellow earthlings, and with your planet. When one does not have healthy and fulfilling relationships, it is nearly impossible to be a truly healthy person. One of the most common reasons for poor health is emotional distress caused by negative relationships with yourself and/or with others, which leads to emotional overeating, under-eating or binge eating, and other self-destructive behaviors, such as smoking, drinking, taking drugs, or mindfully sabotaging your diet or workout routine. No matter how dedicated your mind may be to eat good food and work out daily, if your heart is not in it, if you are not happy in your emotional life—your fire aspect of self—you will never get to the level of health and happiness you deserve.

Love Yourself

It is human nature for us to be attracted to members of our species who exude confidence. An air of confidence can overcome any kind of physical deficiency. We are not talking about arrogance or overconfidence, which manifests in an overbearing manner and superior attitude and makes others around them feel inferior or unimportant. We are talking about the confidence that comes from one's own internal happiness and balance, and in fact these people often seek to make others around them feel important as well. Actually this is also true in the animal kingdom; it is always the proud, confident animals that attract members of the opposite sex. So, in order to have a healthy heart, in order to have healthy emotional relationships, you need to begin by "falling in love" with yourself! You may be thinking, "What? Fall in love with myself? But I am so undesirable ... no one wants me!" Talk about an internal dialogue that creates a vicious cycle. Of course no one else would love you because you don't love yourself first. You must take responsibility for your own emotional well-being by falling in love with that incredible person that is uniquely you.

Once you start down this road of holistic health, it is the opposite of a vicious negative cycle; it becomes a rolling snowball of happiness, growing bigger and bigger with every turn. As you begin to work on your foundation, your earth, by eating good food and exercising daily, your physical body will start to change into something stronger, healthier, and happier—in effect, more lovable! You will find yourself checking out your new, thinner shape; your newly defined muscles that are starting to show on your arms and legs; your healthier and glowing skin, hair, and nails; and you'll think, "Man, I love the person I am becoming." As you work on your spirit, your soul, and your relationship with God/Universe through daily meditation, you will find yourself more at peace and with a growing creativity in your soul and a growing feeling of love for others—for everyone and everything—that you may not have ever experienced before. As you grow your mind through a change in career to something that is more fitting for your life's calling and through a continual pursuit of knowledge, and as your yoga brings your mind and body into harmony more and more every day, you just may find yourself falling in love—with yourself!

To celebrate this new, wonderful relationship with self, you must learn to pamper yourself and treat yourself as if you were the most perfect mother in the universe taking care of her only, precious child; you are that mother, and you are that same mother's child. You must recognize how precious you are, that your life is a gift and your body a temple to the love/God/universe/life force that lives inside you.

No matter how busy you are, you must take the time to do those things that make you feel loved. The good news is that self-love maps back to some of the important aspects we discussed in our chapter on self-care. Take warm, relaxing baths once a week, treat yourself to a nice massage and a day at the spa once a month and a manicure and pedicure once a month, and give yourself a vacation from work at least once a year. (Even if you cannot afford to go anywhere, treat yourself to a vacation at home with nothing to do and no place to go except wherever you decide that day.) These are the things that rejuvenate the heart and turn up the internal flame of the heart fire. Unless your heart fire is burning with love for self, you will never be able to share love with others in a healthy way. Finally, realize that it is not even you, really, who is loving yourself; it is the God, the spirit, the energy source—whatever you call it—that lives within you that is loving you.

Once you have created this incredible love affair with self, you will find incredible things happening. As the sun gives life and love to the Earth without expecting anything in return, so you too will be like the sun, giving love to everyone you know, to everyone you meet, to all of Earth's creatures great and small, to the Earth's natural beauty, without expecting anything in return. Don't be surprised if this new increase in love manifests itself as a completely new life direction for you—perhaps a change in career or a change in an existing relationship. Perhaps you will notice that you no longer rely on someone else to make you feel loved and special. And when you've got that all figured out, just like the mother who adopts a child only to find out she's pregnant, you just "may" meet the love of your life, your soul mate, just as you've gotten yourself to the point where it no longer matters. What has happened is that you have made yourself so full of self-love and self-confidence—giving and beautiful—that people will stand in line for a chance at the opportunity to spend the rest of their lives beside you.

Love for Strangers = Agape = Compassion for All

Other amazing things will start to happen as your heart heals and fills with love for yourself and for your loved ones around you. Much of this flows also from the karma you are receiving from living a purely cruelty-free life, an authentic life of pure love, not causing harm to anyone or anything. You will notice also your love for people that you have never met, for people that are very different from you, from different cultures and backgrounds. Every bit you do to raise your own consciousness contributes to the level of global consciousness.

You will start to understand the meaning of the word "agape." Agape is a Greek word that means love, but more specifically love for mankind. Once one is on the path to complete holistic health—eating right, exercising, and living a purposeful life—once one has fostered self-love and love for one's friends and family, one cannot help but flow into the next step of a healthy heart, which is the peace that comes from agape, from a growing surge of brotherly love. Sometimes this love for mankind will result in a peaceful feeling, but oftentimes it does not. When one begins to love everyone, one cannot help but be awakened to compassion, which can actually be a painful experience.

Now, you may have always been a good person before. You may have been empathetic toward others less fortunate than you. But there is a big difference between empathy and compassion. Empathy is merely "the capacity to recognize feelings that are being experienced by another sentient being." It is an understanding based and seated purely in the mind. "Compassion" means "to suffer together." It is a deeper understanding and feeling for the suffering of others, an understanding no longer in the mind but felt in the heart. So here we have been growing in love for ourselves, and for those close to us, but now this healthy heart has taken a strange turn for the worse. All of a sudden, we are filled with pain and anguish for the suffering of others. Compassion gives rise to an active desire to alleviate another's suffering; we can no longer sit idly by and ignore it. Once we understand that, as blessed as we are, as long as there are others who are suffering, we can never truly be happy because we sincerely know and feel their pain.

This is what drives us to do great things, impossible things. Compassion in every major religious tradition is called the greatest of virtues because it is loving outside your own self and following through and acting on that love.

Love for All Beings

We are not talking about love only for fellow human beings, but love for all fellow earthlings. Once you have switched over to a plant-based diet, you will also notice the depth of your compassion extending not just to fellow human beings, but also to other sentient beings, particularly animals. Most of us have or have had cats and dogs, birds and fish, hamsters and rabbits. We are all capable of loving these animals, and in return feeling the love they give back to us. We know in our hearts that, though they are not human, they are fully capable of feeling love, fear, happiness, loneliness, or abandonment. There is no difference between a pig and a dog, between a cow and a cat. When you stop eating animals, and as you grow in love, it will soon become impossible to ever consider going back to eating meat or dairy again.

Renew Your Spirit ~ Discover Your Source

"I love all religions but I am in love with my own religion."
~ Mother Teresa

The Whole Earth Wellness philosophy is very deeply rooted in religion and spirituality, but it is purely nondenominational, 100 percent interfaith, and NOT a cult! I am a Catholic, and though I am in love with my religion, I truly love all the others as well. I also do not find my religion infallible or perfect, nor do I see the others that way. You can still love imperfection and still believe in change and transformation. We have so much to learn from each other. My intent is not to convert anyone to any religion, but to ask people to look inside themselves for all the answers and to express those truths outwardly through their own traditional religions. Trying to convert someone else to your religion, regardless of what many religions tell you to do (including my own), seems to me the ultimate negative expression of ego. So I just don't do it even though it's what I have been told to do. As you already know by now, I do tend to think for myself and sometimes balk at the strict confines of my traditional faith. I not only think outside the box, I sometimes blow up the box completely, but at least I am not afraid to say so. I hope that if enough of us speak up and push for change and reform within, then change will come. I love traditional religions, though I think all of them need to take a big step forward, change with the times, and embrace a more progressive philosophy on all things. God may not ever change, but the earthbound, man-made traditions must.

Anyways, we have talked about a healthy body, and a healthy mind, and a healthy heart, and it is possible to have all of these "three aspects of self" healthy and functioning at their optimal levels, but yet still not feel 100 percent happy, not quite complete. We have heard it said that everyone has a God-shaped hole in their heart, and that we are never quite complete until that hole is filled with God, or Yahweh, or Krishna, or the Universe, whatever you want to call it. We will never be complete until we fill that hole, and it is true. I know so many lovely vegan atheists who are wonderful people, but they have an anger and a dislike for other people and for the world that is so entirely unhealthy, and mostly, so sad. It seems that they are just very unhappy people at their core. And here is where the true secret to happiness comes— with a real, true relationship with God.

So let's talk about religion and spirituality.

First of all, let's come right out and say that religion has gotten a pretty bad rap lately. It seems that so many of world's problems in the twenty-first century are being caused by wars, created by traditional religions gone extreme, and getting mixed up with aggressive unhealthy politics. Religious extremism was the root cause of September 11 and all the wars that followed. Terrorism is on the rise under the guise of being Islamic, but the truth is it is a completely warped and evil version of Islam that is not pure, accurate, or true. For this and many other reasons, people who have been brought up in a certain faith have rejected the religion of their childhood because of the abhorrent, hypocritical, and sometimes downright evil behavior of people who claim to be religious yet lack any true morality or spirituality. In this new age, many younger people who feel that pull toward the unknown and the sacred are looking toward more new-age spirituality than toward the religion of their youth, their family, or their ancestors.

The Whole Earth Wellness philosophy is that religion (masculine) and spirituality (feminine) are the yin and the yang of our deepest need to understand the unknowable, to find meaning in our lives. One without the other is incomplete and unbalanced. Religion is the outward expression of a culture to try to find the meaning of life, to make sense of the sacred by giving it a human story and wrapping it in outward manifestations of things that we otherwise could not see; spirituality is the inner expression of an individual to try to find the meaning of life, to make sense of the sacred by turning inward with reflection and meditation.

Religions are not bad. Religions are beautiful even if imperfect. It's religion without its feminine side of inner spirituality that can make it empty, hollow, devoid of true meaning, and at times even dangerous.

To have a fulfilled soul in this life, we need to pursue both paths simultaneously as one feeds from and sustains the other. Belonging to a traditional religion is like being a part of a larger family, and we can all benefit from being part of something larger than ourselves. It allows for the expression of wonderful traditions and celebrations, and life would just be so empty without religious holidays and festivities. All religions that advocate for brotherly love are contributing to the greater good. No one should ever try to convert or condemn another because they have a different religious background. I believe that interfaith understanding, respect, and love, will lead the world to peace. If you pursue an individual spiritual path without the boundaries of a religious faith tradition, without the support and camaraderie of others all working together for the common good, without having others around to keep you in check to make sure you don't cause more harm than good, then you can easily go down a path that leads nowhere or worse, into a real cult or some other strange situation.

The traditional religions of the world need those of us who are growing in our inner spirituality and enlightenment to bring this new hope and energy to our dusty old religions and make them new again. Let's not turn our backs on the past; let's bring the past forward with us into the future. I would encourage all of you to return to the religion of your youth, of your ancestors, or maybe even to explore something new that you've always wanted to learn more about. You may want to join an interfaith organization so that we can all learn to not only understand and tolerate one another, but respect and love one another. I love this quote from Gandhi when, late in his life, he was asked whether he was a Hindu, he replied, "Yes I am. I am also a Christian, a Muslim, a Buddhist and a Jew."

Developing Inner Spirituality

So now maybe we return to religion. Maybe we start going through the motions of being a religious person. Maybe we are never missing any masses or services, but until we deepen our inner spirituality, we are like a hollow icing without the cake. In fact, we should bake our cake (which is our spirituality) before we even think about going back to church (the icing on the cake).

What is spirituality? Spirituality exists wherever we struggle with the issues of how our lives fit into the greater scheme of things. This is true when our questions never give way to specific answers or give rise to specific practices such as prayer or meditation. We encounter spiritual issues every time we wonder where the universe comes from, why we are here, or what happens when we die. We also become spiritual when we become moved by values such as beauty, love, or creativity that seem to reveal a meaning or power beyond our visible world. An idea or practice is "spiritual" when it reveals our personal desire to establish a felt-relationship with the deepest meanings or powers governing life.

How does one deepen their inner spirituality? Whatever you believe in, whether it is God, the Universe, Buddha, or just an un-nameable life force, spirituality is that inner path toward connecting with that divinity and discovering the deeper meaning in life. While religion always implies a particular faith tradition and therefore divides us into different camps, spirituality (the underlying meaning) is not bound to any particular faith, is universal across religions, and therefore so important not only for individuals but also for societies and the world as a whole. It is an imperative for us to be healthy individuals, and in an even broader and perhaps more important sense, it is imperative for us to be spiritual in order for us to have a healthy, peaceful Earth.

What are some ways we can develop our inner spirituality?

Meditation: I encourage you to meditate daily, even if it is for only five minutes a day. Meditation teaches you how to quiet your mind so that you can listen to messages from God/Universe.

Prayer: While meditation is listening to God, prayer is actively talking to God. This is an equally important side of the equation. Prayer helps you to activate a real, powerful relationship with God. It can be formal or spontaneous. Focus more on prayers of gratitude and praise instead of petitions and asking for things.

Silence: We are bombarded daily with sounds and voices. You need to look for opportunities for silence, such as walking alone early in the morning; sitting in a tub in the evening without any noise or distraction, only candlelight; going for a silent retreat. From Mother Teresa: "In the silence of the heart God speaks. If you face God in prayer and silence, God will speak to you. Then you will know that you are nothing. It is only when you realize your nothingness, your emptiness, that God can fill you with Himself. Souls of prayer are souls of great silence."

Fasting: "Fasting will bring spiritual rebirth to those of you who cleanse and purify your bodies. The light of the world will illuminate within you when you fast and purify yourself. What the eyes are for the outer world, fasts are for the inner." – Mahatma Gandhi.

Breathing: "Pranayama" is Sanskrit meaning "extension of prana (life force) or breath." "Prana" is the breath (the life force, vital energy, or soul); "ayama" means to extend or draw out. On a physical level, it is the extension of the breath; on a deeper level, it is the extension of life. When one thinks about the breath as being the life force, the Universe, or God, one has a much deeper appreciation of the value of breathing (177).

Plant-based diet: There is a definite correlation between your food choices and violence in the world. When you eat meat, you are eating fear, anger, anxiety, violence, and death. It is no accident that all the world's greatest spiritual leaders have been vegetarians (Buddha, Gandhi, Krishna, Mother Theresa), or at very least pescetarians (Jesus). When you eat peace, you become peaceful and more spiritual. It is the law of karma.

Yoga: Yoga was actually developed 5,000 years ago in India as a way for the practitioner to achieve spiritual enlightenment. Yoga is not just a series of poses; it is a way of learning to control and silence the chatter of the mind and allow for deeper spirituality.

Reading: Reading spiritual writings and holy books, reading what others have written who perhaps devoted their entire lives to deepening their inner spirituality, is a great way to deepen spirituality. One of my current projects is to read all the sacred texts of the world's great religions—the Bible, Bhagavad Gita of Hinduism, the Qur'an of Islam, the Tao Te Ching of Taoism, the Dhammapada of Buddhism, and the writings of Christian mystic saints. Education and knowledge at the level of the mind leads to deepening of the soul.

Living a purposeful life/volunteer: Spend time either with a career serving others or helping to change the world, or volunteering to serve others or help to change the world. Living a purposeful life is key to living a spiritual life. Actively engaging in charity and doing for others with no expectation is one of the most profound ways to lead a spiritual life.

Love: Self-love, leading to loving others, leading to agape, is almost synonymous with spirituality. The only difference is that love without spirituality, as wonderful as it is, can be hollow unless you realize that the source of your ability to give and receive love is not your own self, but of the God/Life Force/Universe that lives inside you.

This brings us to the close of the topics that round out the Whole Earth Diet, which is not truly a diet at all but a lifestyle aimed at healing body, mind, heart, and soul, and not just healing them, but fostering and growing health and wellness in all four parts of self, to be the very best that you can be in this lifetime. Why? What is the point of all this? True happiness and bliss in this lifetime. So our next chapter takes this down to ten practical, simple steps that you can take to create an abundance of happiness in your life.

Chapter 7

10 Simple Steps to Happy Life

10 Simple Steps to Happy Life

"Each morning when I open my eyes I say to myself: I, not events, have the power to make me happy or unhappy today. I can choose which it shall be. Yesterday is dead, tomorrow hasn't arrived yet. I have just one day, today, and I'm going to be happy in it."

~Groucho Marx

Okay, we have covered a lot of ground here so far. In the first part of this book, we focused on the Whole Earth Diet—why it makes the most sense for your health, for the animals, and for the planet. We talked nutrition and gave you some pretty detailed, practical instructions on how to make the Whole Earth Diet happen for you, a step-by-step guide to rethinking your diet and nutrition to create your most perfect physical health. In this second part of the book, we've been talking holistic wellness because the key word that is missing from any other diet book is HAPPINESS. Unless we are happy, we cannot and will not stick to any diet or exercise program.

The Whole Earth Diet will lead you to physical health, but if we want this health to be sustainable, we need to bring the whole self along for the ride. And the formula is simple: a healthy, powerful body from food and fitness leads to a passionate heart from loving yourself and loving others, which leads to a constantly learning and expanding mind that turns new knowledge into purpose, which leads to a soul that grows in both inner spirit and outer faith and comes into communion with God. All of this together is what leads ultimately to a joyful life. To real happiness.

It really is a simple, step-by-step process. You can have a life of pure joy, no matter what your current life circumstances are today, by following these ten steps. But what is most important is that you give this a chance to work. You must be patient. These steps are simple, BUT they must be maintained for at least six months to start to really see and feel the results. Those six months won't be perfect. I'm not saying you won't fail from time to time, but everytime you fall off that horse, you need to climb right back on without judgement or self-criticism. Give yourself a hug and climb right back on.

Six months sounds like a long time, but it takes six months to ingrain any new diet and/or lifestyle pattern into your brain. Once it is done though, you are good to go for the next 100 years!

Let's start!

Step #1: Eat Healthy Food

The obvious first step: Eat real, plant-based foods. Once you really get into this new way of eating, you are going to notice a different relationship with food that will consistently bring you joy and happiness instead of guilt and anguish. Now that you know the secret to eating real, plant-based foods—foods you can go ahead and eat like crazy without gaining weight or feeling guilty—you can lose the negative relationship you had with food, and just start EATING! And the beautiful thing is, you are about to discover a whole new world of food – new tastes and textures, all good, no guilt on any level. Never worry about food ever again, as long as you just remember these simple Food Rules:

- Don't eat anything that had a face.

- Don't eat anything that came OUT of anything that had a face.

- Don't eat anything from a box with ingredients containing unpronounceable words.

- Don't eat anything with high fructose corn syrup or hydrogenated vegetable oils.

- Don't drink anything with artificial sweeteners, artificial colors or artificial flavors.

- Don't eat fried foods and don't cook with oils.

- Don't eat anything made with white flour or white sugar.

- Do eat all the colorful fresh fruit you want.

- Do eat all the colorful veggies you want—cooked or raw, fresh or frozen.

- Do eat all the beans you want. From bulk or from cans, just eat 'em.

- Do eat all the healthy whole grains you want: quinoa, oats, brown, black and wild rice.

- Do drink all the herbal teas you want.

- Drink tons of water always.

- Enjoy in moderation whole grain breads and pastas; grain-based "meats" and "cheeses", tofu, and tempeh;

organic black coffee, matcha green tea, red wine, organic beer, dark chocolate.

- 90/10 Rule: Eat right 90 percent of the time; 10 percent of the time you can cheat with the occasional vegan red-velvet cupcake or sweet potato fries (except on rules #1 and #2—no meat or dairy ever— no cheats allowed there!). If you are going to "cheat," do so mindfully, publicly, and without guilt, sitting at the table, eating slowly. It is okay as long as it is done only once in a while and in the full light of day, mindfully.

- Take your B12 and omega-3 oil supplement daily.

- Get at least 1 tablespoon of green protein powder daily.

- If you're over fifty, take D2/calcium/magnesium/zinc daily.

- Don't smoke or do drugs.

- Always eat mindfully, slowly, and with gratitude.

Step #2: Exercise Your Four Elements

Exercise is key to physical wellness, but also mental, emotional, and spiritual wellness. Power and strength training specifically for physical health, yoga for mental and spiritual health, dance or martial arts or rock climbing or whatever thrills you for emotional health, cardiovascular and breathing for mental and spiritual health—all forms of fitness nourish all parts of self in some way or other.

So this is Rule #2 for happiness:

Each and every morning for the rest of your life, do one of these and mix it up across the week:

- EARTH: Strength training; weight lifting at gym; power lifting or power yoga classes; boot-camp classes; interval training (increases physical strength and power)

- WATER: Yoga—personal practice at home or classes at the studio—preferably yin, restorative, or calming/slow stretching classes; (increases mental and physical flexibility, fluidity and purpose)

- FIRE: Dance classes, martial arts, zumba classes, going out dancing, anything that makes you excited and laugh-out-loud happy; (increases feel-good hormones, self-esteem, happiness and passion)

- AIR: Walking, running, hiking, rowing, bike riding, treadmills or other cardio machines at gym, breathing exercises, meditation; (increases connection with breath, spirit, God, prayer)

If you are one of those folks who LOVES exercise, great. The only thing you need to do is add in some variety. If you are one of those folks who HATES exercise, you need to just rethink what you call it. Instead of calling it "exercise", call it "play." Studies show that physical activity stimulates various brain chemicals that leave you feeling happier and more relaxed. You will also feel better about your appearance every day, which will boost confidence and self-esteem. Exercise increases happiness. If you don't know where to begin, the one element that increases happiness immediately is your Fire element. Sign up for some dance classes, or zumba, or go out line dancing, or belly dancing, or just anything that just makes you laugh-out-loud happy even at the thought. Simple. But whether you drag yourself out there or trot happily out there every morning, it doesn't matter. Just do it. You may not be happy when the alarm goes off, you may even curse me on that dark, cold early morning drive to the gym! BUT I promise you will always be happy on the drive home, basking in your warm, happy sweat. You'll start every day being happy that your exercise is DONE, and you'll end every day happy that you are feeling so good about the new body, the new energy, and the new happiness that have come into your life. Then … you will thank me.

Step #3: Create Routines

Now I know at first glance this doesn't sound like fun, but studies actually show that folks that follow a regular routine live longer, healthier, happier lives. When you don't have a routine, the chances that you will not eat correctly, that you will forget to find time to exercise, not get enough sleep, not find time to meditate, forget to take your daily supplements, will add up. Also, having a regular routine helps to alleviate a lot of stress. When you know what is coming next, you can be prepared and relaxed, but if every day and every hour brings unexpected events, our bodies will stay in a stressful mode. It's better to have our days fairly well planned, but to also find that comfortable balance between living an overly scheduled life and allowing for a little bit of spontaneity and surprise. Allow for flexibility when the mood strikes, or if something unexpected and wonderful comes up. It is okay to stray. Again, pull out the old 90/10 rule here too when it comes to lifestyle. Adhere to your routine 90 percent of the time, but allow for spontaneity and flexibility 10 percent of the time, and you should be golden.

Here is an example of a routine:

DAILY:

Morning:

4:30: Drink full glass of water, then meditate

5:00: Hot coffee ritual; feed birds

5:30: Ready for gym

6:00: Exercise: M/W/F: Cardio/Strength; T/Th: Yoga

7:15: Chop fresh fruits

7:30: Read paper & enjoy breakfast smoothie (with supplements)

8:00: Clean up kitchen, dishes, laundry, trash

8:30: Shower and get ready for day

9:00–1:00: Work (drink liter of water)

Lunchtime:

1:00–1:30: Eat lunch outside in sun; soak up vit D; mini-meditation

1:30–5:30: Work (drink liter of water)

Evening:

5:30: Chop fresh veggies; prepare dinner

6:00–6:30: Eat dinner mindfully

6:30: Clean up kitchen, dishes, laundry, trash

7:00: Watch TV & relax

8:00: Upstairs, into PJs and into bed, read, write in gratitude journal

8:30: Lights out

WEEKEND:

Friday Night: Date night or movie night

Saturday Morning: Farmers' market; shopping for the week; fill up car/car wash

Saturday Afternoon: Fitness ~ outdoor activity, dance class, housecleaning

Saturday Night: Out with friends

Sunday Morning: Church

Sunday Afternoon: Self-care ~ hair, nails, massage, beach, or _____

Sunday Night: Family or friends over for dinner

ONCE/MONTH:

Massage

Facial

Manicure/pedicure

Deep housecleaning

Car wash

<u>ONCE/SEASON:</u>

Clothes shopping

Hair appointment

Cleanse/detox

Weekend escape

ONCE/YEAR:

Jan: Prepare taxes

Feb: Doctor appts

May: Graduations

Summer: Family vacation

Oct: Anniversary vacation

Dec: Strategic planning for next year

This is an example, but please create your own. Put these things into your smart phone calendar, hang daily to-do lists on your refrigerator, set reminder beepers and whistles and tweets—do whatever you need to do to make sure you actually do these things cosistently. Create them all as appointments with yourself, and treat them as if they are every bit as important as a meeting with your boss or client. They are not to be moved, changed, or cancelled (unless of course something REALLY fun and unexpected comes your way!).

Having a routine will also help you get into good financial shape too, since you can figure a dollar amount for all of these activities, which will help you create a budget for yourself. Creating and sticking to a budget are also great stress relievers tied directly to having a routine. A routine will help your financial wellness, which in turn will also increase your happiness. There is no happiness like the feeling of being debt free and living eithin your means financially, with even some money left to go into savings! All of this stems from routine.

A routine will increase your happiness because it is only after months of consistent action that you will start to see positive results in any area of your life, and it is only by having a routine that you will get the consistency you need to effect those results. I know this may not appeal to some of you, my spontaneous butterfly types, having to live by any strict routine, but the sooner you can get into this groove, the faster you will start to see results with your physical, mental, emotional, and spiritual well-being. I am not making this stuff up. The rishis in India made this stuff up 5,000 years ago, and modern studies are proving they were right. So stop questioning, and just do it. It will make you so much happier.

Step #4: Laughter and Sleep

There is an old Irish Proverb that says, "A good laugh and a long sleep are the two best cures for everything." And the more studies that are done on the health benefits of both laughter and a good sleep, the more we are starting to prove the wisdom in this old proverb.

Try to find a reason to laugh every single day. The things that make one person angry would make another person laugh. Be that person who sees the levity in every situation, who can laugh at yourself and laugh equally with (not at!) others. People who take everything very seriously are putting too much stress into their lives. Laughter is key to enjoying and living a long life. Laughing lowers blood pressure; reduces stress hormone levels; improves your cardiac health; boosts your immune system; triggers the release of those happy, feel-good hormones called endorphins, which help ease chronic pain; and it also gives your abdominal muscles a workout! But perhaps most importantly, daily laughter increases your overall sense of well-being and your happiness. Find a reason to laugh every day, and you will increase your happiness quotient tenfold and improve the overall quality of your life (178).

Just as important as daily laughter is nightly sleep. The latest studies on sleep show that both quantity and quality of sleep are important. You need 7-9 hours of uninterrupted sleep to be fully rejuvenated because our bodies go through cycles while they sleep, rather like a washing machine. If you stop it halfway through, your clothes are not going to be rinsed clean! When we sleep, we go first into Stage 1 NREM (non-rapid eye movement) sleep, which is about the first six hours. You begin with a light sleep, then a deep sleep, finally the deepest sleep yet, where your blood pressure drops, your heart rate slows, your muscles are totally relaxed, and hormones are released. It is during this deep sleep phase that your body is hard at work repairing tissues and fighting off inflammation. In the last two hours of the night, as sunrise approaches, you enter into REM (rapid eye movement) sleep, where your brain is fairly active and dreaming, and your eyes dart back and forth under your eyelids. It is during REM sleep that your body is releasing healthy hormones to support growth, development, immune system functioning, as well as appetite control. REM sleep helps consolidate memory and emotion, as blood flow rises sharply in several brain areas linked to processing memories and emotional experiences(179).

What can we do to ensure a good full night's sleep? Get to bed early, and if you are having trouble sleeping, try these things:

- No caffeine after noon
- No eating food after 6:30 p.m.
- No more than one glass of red wine with dinner, if that, weekends only
- No more than one glass of water after dinner, if that, as needed only
- Have a glass of water by your bed at night and sip it as needed
- Drink a full glass of water as soon as you wake up.
- Drink two to three liters of water all day

We spend one-third of our lives sleeping but it is not a wasted time. Sleep contributes directly to how full, energetic, and successful the other sixteen hours of the day can be, and how happy overall our lives can be!

Step #5: Pamper Yourself Weekly

This is the big one. I see so many people who are unhappy and do not feel worthy of love because they do not love themselves. The very first step to emotional wellness, crucial to happiness, is to learn to love yourself. None of this will do any good if you don't love yourself, if you feel you don't deserve to live a healthy, happy life. You know the right foods to eat, but you will sabotage yourself, eating what you know isn't good. You know you should get out of bed and exercise, but you don't do it because you don't really deserve to be fit and toned. You know you need more sleep, but you don't deserve it; you need to work harder. You're lonely without a partner, and you think you don't deserve love anyways, so you overeat the wrong foods. Or you drink too much alcohol. Or you binge on sugar or fast food, trying to heal your heart with food. There is a direct connection between emotional wellness and physical wellness, between the heart and the body. If your heart is empty, you will make poor choices for your physical health. You must learn to love yourself as if you were your own perfect parent. And the great thing is, this goes beyond just eating right and exercising! We are talking here about spoiling yourself rotten because that's just how precious you are. Even if you don't feel it or you don't believe, you need to start living as if you truly loved yourself silly. Just start acting this way,you're your heart and your brain will follow. You need to plug into your calendar a couple hours each week for self-care. Pick whatever day of the week and however much time you need, as long as it is not any less than one hour per week. During that time, find ways to pamper yourself, and it doesn't have to be expensive either.

Here are some ideas of how to pamper yourself weekly:

- Spend an hour out in nature or in the library, whatever you prefer.
- Go for a slow walk or lie on a park bench reading a good book.
- Go visit a farm sanctuary and play with the animals.
- Go for a massage (and you should get a massage for your health at least once each month).

- Go get a manicure/pedicure, and ask for extra massage time on those hard-working hands and feet.
- Go shopping and buy yourself a small treat, whatever makes you happy and is in your budget!
- Give yourself a total makeover with a new hairstyle and makeup.
- Cook yourself a romantic candlelit gourmet meal.
- Pick up a new hobby, or return to an old one that you once loved.
- Take a long, luxurious bath soaking in lavendar oils and minerals.
- Have a movie night at home with popcorn and fuzzy slippers.

You need to treat yourself to whatever makes you happy and makes you feel spoiled, at least once a week. So stop what you are doing now, put down this book, and make an appointment for next Friday morning or Sunday afternoon in your calendar. Where are you going to go? What are you going to do? Whatever it is, show yourself some love.

Step #6: Love Your Family

Once you have mastered self-love, then you will be capable of loving others. You cannot give love away to someone else before you fill yourself up, so focus first on pampering and loving yourself, then you can choose who you want to give your love to. You can create your family and never have to be alone. People are naturally social, and to be happy you need to have close relationships with others. You need to create and love your family. We tend to think about others as simply "family" or "friends". However, I would like to blur our black-and-white thinking here and toss out the old definitions. It's possible that friends can become family;

it's even possible that our animals can become family! Family is not only about sharing DNA anymore!

First, there is the family you were born into, your original family—your mom and dad and possibly siblings. You should love and honor those family bonds with all your heart and soul, no matter what you receive, or don't receive, in return. Being close to the family you were given, being close and connected to your roots, will create happiness.

And then there is the family you create— your significant other and possibly children (hairy or hairless!). We cannot expect everyone to get married and have lots of babies anymore. I once had a very traditional view of family, but I evolved right outside that box! My new definition of family is at least two beating hearts that love each other and are living under one roof. A single man and his dog = a family, a family that is just as valid and can be just as rewarding as a traditional family with a man, a woman, and two children. Living with an animal in your home has proven health benefits, like lowering your blood pressure and increasing your lifespan (178). There is nothing that creates as much happiness as an animal that you have rescued and whose life you have saved; they seem to know it and will love you more than life for the rest of their life. And that is an abundant source of happiness.

The bottom line: don't live alone and feel lonely. Create your family, however you want to define it on your own terms, and fill your house with love and happiness. Have love surrounding you under your roof, in your home, no matter what your circumstance. There is no excuse not to. This may be the single biggest thing you can do to create your happy life.

Step #7: Develop Mental Fitness

We now have stepped through the process for a healthy body and a healthy heart, but to be able to stick with this program long-term, to make it sustainable and truly create the happy life we deserve, we must look at building mental fitness—a mind that can easily alternate between laser focus one minute and soft quietness the next. How does one develop mental fitness, and how will it make life happier?

Mental fitness is developed by a combination of learning (enhancing) and meditation (relaxing). Just as the ideal way to exercise is with interval training the body—alternating between hard exercise and rest—to develop mental fitness you need to "interval train the brain"! Especially as we grow older, it's important to keep our mind alert, fresh, and strong, exercising the mind just like we exercise the body. Studies show that in older people their mental functioning remains high and alert, and they can avoid Alzheimer's and senility if they keep exercising their minds (180).

Techniques for enhancing your brain power, keeping in mind that the brain is a muscle that need to be worked:

- Start to read and study things that interest you.
- Work daily crossword puzzles.
- Play virtual chess online.
- Do the Sudoku puzzles in your newspaper.
- Learn to play a musical instrument.
- Take a class at your local community college.
- Learn a new language.
- Learn something new everyday on Wikipedia:Random.
- Write with a pen and paper instead of always on a keyboard.

- Download the Luminosity app for special brain-training activities.

Remember, if you don't use it, you will lose it, whether we're talking about muscles, or the brain.

Mental wellness is more than just exercising your brain. You also need to find time to relax your mind, cut out the chatter and chaos.

Here are some ideas for how to relax your brain:

- Daily meditation, ideally 20-30 mins/day
- Take a tech break daily, leave your cell phone behind and go for a walk alone, even if just for five minutes.
- Take a daily afternoon nap, eyes closed, legs elevated, no technology nearby, even if just for five minutes.
- Listen to calming music while stretching
- Do progressive deep relaxation exercises, relaxing each muscle group, while deep breathing with eyes closed

When you realize that your body, your mind, and your emotions are all interconnected, and when you are growing your mind into a more powerful tool through alternating exercise and relaxation, you will notice more mental strength overall—and this is critical for happiness. Mental strength, willpower—call it what you will. When you develop a more heightened mental strength, you will be better able to just say "no" to the temptations that brought you down before. Instead of eating that sweet, sugary snack on a whim, you can think about what you are doing and just say "no." Instead of buying that cute little thing online or in the store, you can just say "no" and save your bank account from being drained or your credit card bill from keep getting larger and larger. It is something called "delayed gratification", and something our society seems to have lost touch with altogether. The source of many of our problems in life are the day-to-day little temptations we cave into every single day that seem so small, but always add up to something big: the little nibble here, the little spending there ... and before we know it, our weight has gone way up, and our bank account has gone way down! All because we didn't have the mental strength to stop ourselves. So get rid of that debt, get rid of that extra weight, have a strong and healthy mind, watch your weight go down and your bank account go up, and find true joy!

Step #8: Find Your Purpose

You are the author of your own life. No one else is writing this novel but you. Sure, there are plot twists and turns that are not of your creation that are thrown at you, and everything that happens to you—the good, the bad, and the ugly—happens for a reason. But ultimately YOU are the creator of your life story. And life goes very quickly. We are here only for a short while, so you really need to pay attention to what I am about to say. You are here for a reason. At birth you were given a secret special assignment, and the meaning of life is to discover what that assignment is, and act on it. In Hinduism they call this your "dharma," your life work. It is the reason you are here.

As long as you live without discovering and fulfilling your purpose, the more unhealthy and unhappy you will be. You must discover your dharma. How? Keep asking. Every time you meditate, you need to ask yourself these questions:

- "Why am I here?" Listen quietly to receive the message. Often God does not speak in words but in pictures or in emotions. Often He will show you your purpose by showing you your pain.
- Where is your wound? What causes you the most grief? How can you help yourself heal from this? How can you help others heal? You are the salve, the ointment, the medicine that is needed for this ill. It may be a wound that is personal; a societal ill; the pain of certain animals, children, or women; or people suffering from a certain illness—physical, mental, emotional, or spiritual.
- What is the source of your deepest pain? Therein lies the answer to your purpose.

The key is to develop a fierce and fearless creativity to your life. You are here for a reason, you have a precious gift to share, and you MUST allow this spirit to flow through you. Discover what your creative gift is, whether it is writing, art, dance, cooking, or whatever it is. No matter what your new path, it will involve a certain amount of creativity, even if it is writing computer programs or creating a non-profit to solve a need. Maybe you will need to get creative in how to survive on less money or how to re-prioritize your life, but whatever you do, never give up. If you are in alignment with your purpose, God and the Universe will conspire to make it happen for you, always. Fully, finally, live the reason you were born.

Happiness will flow, guaranteed.

Step #9: Meditation and Prayer

Daily meditation is the other half of creating mental wellness, but it is just as important for spiritual wellness as well. Meditation allows the mind to relax, so that you can get your mind out of the way and allow for a deeper communication with God. For thousands of years, people have used meditation to move beyond the mind's stress-inducing thoughts and emotional upsets into the peace and clarity of present-moment awareness. The variety of meditation techniques, traditions, and technologies is nearly infinite, but the essence of meditation is singular: the cultivation of mindful awareness and expanded consciousness.

These are the ultimate gifts of meditation, yet people are initially drawn to meditation for many different reasons. Some begin meditating because of a doctor's recommendation, seeking the health benefits of lowered blood pressure, stress reduction, and restful sleep. Others come to meditation seeking relief from the fearful, angry, or painful thoughts that constantly flood their minds. Still others come to meditation to find greater self-understanding, to increase their intuitive powers, or to improve their ability to concentrate.

It is accurate to say that the purpose of meditation depends on the meditator, but it is also true that anyone who meditates regularly receives profound benefits on all of levels—physical, mental, emotional, and spiritual.

Here are just a few of the proven benefits (181):

- Relief from stress and anxiety (meditation mitigates

the effects of the "fight-or-flight" response, decreasing the production of stress hormones such as cortisol and adrenaline)

- Decreased blood pressure and hypertension
- Lower cholesterol levels
- More efficient oxygen use by the body
- Increased production of the antiaging hormone DHEA
- Restful sleep
- Restores brain growth in the areas of memory, empathy, sense of self and stress regulation,
- Reduces depression, anger, and anxiety
- Promotes happiness

When you begin to meditate, you first learn to focus your mind on the present moment. There are many ways to do this, but the important thing is that you stop your thoughts from wandering and begin to relax your body and observe your breath. Try and push all thoughts away. When you do this, you automatically lose sight of the things that are making you upset, and you experience the simple joy of being alive. The more you experience the present moment, the happier you become. According to Lao Tzu, "If you are depressed you are living in the past. If you are anxious you are living in the future. If you are at peace you are living in the present." Start meditating and get in touch with your present moments of happiness, one moment at a time.

While meditation will help you to find inner peace and grow your own personal inner spirituality, it is not all you need to do to have a healthy soul. You also need daily prayer. Where meditation is quietly listening for God, prayer is actively speaking with Him. And just as His voice may not come to you in words but as pictures or feelings, so too your prayer to Him doesn't need to be in the form of spoken words.

In fact, He will listen better if you use the language of your heart, which is the language of feelings, or the language of your actions since you are God on Earth. Prayer can be as simple as feeling grateful every day, maybe even keeping a gratitude journal. It can simply be that feeling of awe that you get when you see a beautiful sunset. Prayer is the goose bumps you get when you hear about something amazing. Prayer can be expressed through music or art or writing. Prayer can be spoken out loud in a group or whispered quietly inside the mind. Prayer for you might be volunteering at a soup kitchen or going overseas and volunteering to help people devastated by a natural disaster.

Prayer is simply the knowledge that God is real and that your life purpose is to serve Him by serving others, through your vocation, through your creativity, through your talent, through your charity, through your compassion, through your life. There is a great prayer by St. Francis that says: "Preach the gospel at all times. When necessary use words." Our lives are meant to be lived as if every action was a prayer. When you get this, really get this, you will know the last and ultimate stage of real happiness, which is the deepest peace and unending joy that comes only with living a life where every moment is a prayer, and God is a very real presence in your life.

Step #10: Engaged in Community

All of this is well and good for developing happiness inside ourselves; for nourishing our four elements of earth, water, fire, and air; and for nurturing our physical, mental, emotional, and spiritual wellness; but we still haven't talked about perhaps the most important piece for happiness—nourishing our fifth element. No man is an island, and as we recall from studying the blue zones of the world where the most centenarians are found, one thing they all had in common was high levels of social engagement in their communities.

In the next section we will talk about a peaceful world that really is all about YOUR engagement with the world—how you relate to and engage with your local community and your global community. We will give you ten ways to create a peaceful world, all of which revolve around social engagement because without social engagement, you cannot be happy, and without social engagement we will never have world peace, so read on. The next section may perhaps be the most important section yet.

PART THREE:

PEACEFUL WORLD ~ THE WHOLE EARTH VISION

"As long as there are slaughterhouses there will always be battlefields."

~ Leo Tolstoy, Russian novelist (1828–1910)

Chapter 8

Christianity & the Plant-Based Diet

Christianity & the Plant-Based Diet

---•●•---

"Do you not know that your body is a temple of the Holy Spirit, who is in you, whom you have received from God? You are not your own; you were bought at a price. Therefore honor God with your body."

~1 Corinthians 6:19-20

Here in part three of this book, I will attempt to make the case for this much bigger vision. That crazy idea that world peace begins on your plate! This notion may sound like a real stretch to you now, but I hope that after a couple chapters I will have you with me on this. Part three is really about understanding that religion and spirituality are not only a cause but an effect of eating a cruelty-free diet, and that it is our only hope for a peaceful world.

Part three will address my two tribes separately. First, the more intimate subgroup, my own fellow Catholic Warriors for Peace. Then, the larger interfaith coalition of Rainbow Warriors for Peace.

Starting with the folks who are nearest and dearest to my heart, my larger family: my fellow Catholics, and all Christians really. For those of you readers who are not Catholic or Christian, feel free to skip this chapter or read it as you wish. But I would feel like a huge piece of this book was missing if I did not include this message to Christians—the reason that I will never give up this diet, or decide to follow some other type of "healthy eating" plan. For me, it really all comes down to this.

Becoming the Lamb of God

"Behold what you are, become what you receive."

~ St Augustine.

I looked this quote up after mass one Sunday when we sang this beautiful tune, *"Amen, el cuerpo de Cristo, amen, el sangre del Senor."* It means, "This is my body, this is my blood, you become what you receive, amen." I was particularly moved by the line, "We become what we receive," as we were going up to Communion, and I actually fought back tears in church. The weight and meaning of those words really hit me, being a health coach who daily preaches, "You are what you eat." I looked up the origin of the lyrics to the song and to that line in particular. I found it credited to St. Augustine, a first-century Christian theologian who was very influential in the development of early Christianity and who wrote frequently on the Sacrament of the Eucharist. He was reminding us that we are eating the body and blood of Christ, and that when we eat this, we will actually become one with Christ. We are what we eat.

As a practicing Catholic, I guess you could say that the only flesh and blood I eat is during the Eucharist, and I don't take eating flesh lightly! Just the thought of eating any flesh creates a huge psychic ripple through my soul. It has a tremendous impact on me, much more so than folks who eat flesh regularly and don't give it a second thought. Just as I now physically feel the pain of the millions of animals suffering every minute of every day to become our food, when I take Communion, I also am now more physically aware of the pain that Christ endured when he died. If we are what we eat, then I am now composed of lots and lots of fruits, veggies, beans, and legumes (okay, and a glass of red wine and a vegan dark chocolate cupcake or two) ... and then also the flesh and blood of Christ. There must be some pretty amazing alchemy happening in my body these days!

But then I also thought, sadly, that no wonder there are so few Catholics who are 100 percent plant-based. Every Sunday we kneel before a crucifix, a reminder of the final agony of Jesus' life. If Christ died and we eat HIM every Sunday, then why should we ever feel the slightest twinge of sympathy or mercy for farm animals who die for us? Besides, weren't animals put here for us to eat? Shouldn't we just be NUMB when it comes to the suffering of animals since there is just so much suffering in the world? Well, I beg to differ—vehemently and loudly. Jesus said repeatedly that He was the last sacrifice, that He was the last Lamb of God, and yet somehow Christians seem to be deaf to this final, most important message that He left with us at His Last Supper. Throughout the mass, we call repeatedly to the Lamb of God to have mercy on us, but yet we can find no mercy in our hearts for the baby lambs that we kill without mercy or compassion for our meals. After praying to the Lamb, we often go home after mass to a supper with lamb on the table.

Sometimes I feel a little bit like John the Baptist, like the crazy, lonely voice of one calling in the wilderness. I have many Catholic, Christian, and religious friends—very good people whom I love dearly and I know have a profound love for and faith in God—but most of them eat meat and animal products, maybe because they are blessed with loving, traditional families who have grown up eating meat at every holiday, and they feel it is God's will for us to eat the animals. It's always been this way, and anyways, the Bible tells us it's okay! To stop eating meat and dairy would be a huge upset to the family dynamic, to family tradition, and it does not make any sense to them; they see no reason to stop. The "compassion light bulb" just hasn't gone off for them yet. I have lost Christian friends over my crazy, extremist views on food.

So I turn toward my many plant-based group of friends—very good people whom I love dearly and I know have a deep love and compassion in their hearts for all living creatures, even the smallest of birds and tiniest of baby bees and spiders—but most of them don't recognize that the profound love, compassion, and empathy they feel toward the animals is actually the true and living proof of God working in and through them. They call themselves atheists, agnostics, or humanists, but they are often filled with more of the true Spirit of God than many of my "religious" friends. They are just people that, like the apostle Thomas after the resurrection, until they see it with their own eyes, they just don't believe it, and so they call God by another name—"Love" or "Compassion." They are good people, but the "spiritual light bulb" hasn't gone off for them. I have also lost lots of these friends too, when they catch wind that I am one of those religious nutcases (and I may lose a couple more after they read this chapter!).

So I pivot to the very small group of friends (I can count them on one hand) that have made the connection between Christianity and a plant-based diet. I am not sure which comes first, the spiritual chicken or the vegan egg, but I do know that throughout history, the most spiritual people, the ones most completely devoted to God, did not eat animal products. I'm not sure if their spirituality led to their diet, or the diet to their spirituality.

Maybe it works both ways, though for me, my healthy and compassionate diet led to mental health and happiness through my career change, which led to emotional health and happiness, which then led to the fanning of the inner flame of spirituality. So if any of you are struggling with your faith or your spirituality, if you are having doubts about the existence of God, if you are feeling stuck on your spiritual path, one of the little-known but perhaps most precious gifts that comes from giving up meat and dairy is the overwhelming knowledge that there is a God,that the world is in the process of a tremendous spiritual evolution, and that the sooner we all stop eating meat, the sooner the world will change for the better.

I am not one of those who believes that we are in the end times, or that the world is about to end, as some Christians maintain. Rather, I do believe that the world as we know it is about to end for sure, but that it is going to be a beautiful thing. I see a future world that has the best of everything—a newfound worldwide peace and profound spirituality, stemming from a global cruelty-free diet and intercultural friendships linked via technology. A world where we maintain all the diverse, lovely, and ancient religions, traditions, and faiths, but evolved beyond all that causes pain, violence, discrimination, torture, and war still done today in the name of religion. I see a return to the simplicity and peace of the Garden of Eden, but with really cool technology tying us all together across the world as one family. Crazy? Maybe. Naïve? Probably. But it's my dream and

I'm sticking to it, and I will actively push to see it become a reality for as long as I live.

Changing the Way We Think

The end of the world as we know it. *Change.* I know this word scares a lot of people. But change is a necessary part of human life on this planet. Change is not only inevitable, it's also a good thing. But this doesn't mean that everything needs to change. We can keep the good stuff and just get rid of that which no longer makes sense. It no longer makes sense to eat meat and dairy. We are not living in the frozen Ice Age tundra anymore. Eating a meat- and dairy-free diet is better for your health, better for the environment, and well, certainly better for the 3,000 animals that die EVERY SECOND for a flavor that we favor. There are so many delicious meat and dairy substitutes now that this old paradigm needs to change. That being said, we can still have our big family holidays and our cultural and religious festivities; we need only to make some very simple substitutions to the old family recipes. THAT'S IT. So simple.

Why do it at all? you ask. Because I promise you when you give up the meat and dairy, not only are you going to experience the anticipated benefits to your physical health, to the physical environment of our planet, and to the physical well-being of animals everywhere, you are going to witness some amazing, perhaps unexpected, not-so-easily-measured changes in yourself, and then in those around you, and I am convinced that when the ripple effect spreads far enough and wide enough, that we together will change the world. How do I know this? Because it happened to me, and I am actively supporting and seeing this change in so many of my clients right now. One person at a time, we are all becoming the change we wish to see in the world.

How does eating plants make you more peaceful? There is an ancient science that describes the energetics of food (182), that all food contains energy and provides you with energy when you eat. Root vegetables provide a grounding quality for when you feel scattered. Springtime sprouts and baby veggies provide youthful, light energy. Meat provides a negative, violent, dark energy. Once you stop eating the brutal death and violence and blood of animals, you feel more at peace, more relaxed, happier, less anxious. In my experience, once I stopped eating meat and dairy, I noticed more love in my heart for others—for myself, for my family and friends, for strangers, and for animals at whom I could now look with a completely clear conscience, knowing I was no longer personally responsible for any of their brethren's deaths.

My new calm and deepening spirituality that stemmed from my diet led to my return to Catholic church, the religion of my youth. I had drifted away from my church because of what I perceived around me - the bad behaviors of Catholics and Christians in general, living hypocritical lives devoid of true spirituality or compassion, too concerned with power and politics instead of the true teachings of Jesus. I returned to church nonetheless, wanting to be a part of a larger faith-based family again. I had experienced for the first time what it meant to be completely filled with the Holy Spirit, with sudden and unimaginable blasts of pure bliss that come from out of nowhere, and it was and is unlike anything I could imagine. I felt compelled to bring back this newfound inner spirituality, the Holy Spirit, to the dusty old religion of my youth, not to go away from it and wish for a religion-free world with some sort of a global, new-age, generic, white-washed spirituality where we all look alike and act alike. I wanted to go back and reinvigorate the deeper sights, sounds, colors, smells, tastes, and textures of my ancient faith as best I could.

Just as I don't want to give up my Scottish great-grandma's shepherd's pie recipe if all I have to do is make a couple minor tweaks to the recipe to swap out the meat (and it is still just as delicious), so too I don't want to see my Catholic faith disappear into the dustbin of history. I am much too fond of my history, my ancestors, my culture, my family traditions and recipes, to give it all up because there is an element that spoils. I believe that we need to surgically change our past traditions with a scalpel, not with a machete. I know my Catholic faith is not perfect, and I know I am not a perfect Catholic either. I do insist on thinking for myself and thinking outside the box, as we all should. No one should be a mindless sheep. I have views that run counter to what the church teaches, but that is okay because the church, every church, every faith, does needs to change with the times. God may be perfect and eternal, but man-made faith traditions are neither, and need to gently and gradually change with the times. And I hope we can all be a part of that change.

Was Jesus a vegetarian?

So maybe you are still thinking, "Well, the Bible tells me it is okay to eat meat, and it's the way it has always been done. There are contradictory studies on both sides to support or deny health benefits of a plant-based diet, so I still see no reason to change anything based on Laura Robinson Oatman's subjective and anecdotal experience promising me some sort of a new spiritual high! I mean really ...."

Okay, okay, then I guess I have to pull out the big guns. Maybe this will sway you: There is much controversy today about whether or not Jesus was actually a vegetarian himself. Across the globe, there is a small handful of vegetarian Christians who assert that He was, in fact, a vegetarian. The Bible and other sources seem to possibly support this belief. I am not 100 percent convinced either way, but let me tell you what I've learned that just may point to a plant-based Jesus.

1. Many believe that vegetarianism is not without precedent in the Christian faith. Many early church fathers were vegetarian, including St. Basil, St. John Chrysostom, and St. Francis of Assisi, and these beliefs may have been passed down from Jesus Christ Himself (183).

2. There are multiple references in the Bible that Jesus was from Nazareth. Many biblical scholars believe Jesus was a member of the Nazarene Essenes, a Jewish religious sect that typically followed a vegetarian diet and rejected animal sacrifices. Jesus was loved by some, hated by others, and accused of blasphemy by the priests of His time because He claimed to be the Jewish Messiah, the "Nazarene," that was prophesized about in the Old Testament (184).

3. The Old Testament prophesized a vegetarian Messiah. Isaiah 7:14-15: "Therefore the Lord himself shall give you a sign; Behold, a virgin shall conceive, and bear a son, and shall call His name Immanuel. Butter and honey shall He eat, so that He may know to refuse the evil, and choose the good." What does eating butter and honey have to do with knowing how to choose between good and evil? Well, throughout history there have been many vegetarian Jews. Even today,

only India has more faith-based vegetarians than Israel. These vegetarian Jews believed meat corrupted your soul. In fact, just like alcohol, the Bible teaches that meat makes you "stumble" and corrupts your heart. That is why the anticipated Messiah would be seen as eating butter and honey, instead of meat, so that His heart would not be corrupted. If Jesus ate meat, then He would not have fit the Messianic prophesy of the Jews (185).

4. Nowhere in the Bible does it ever mention Jesus eating meat, only bread and wine. We see Him passing out fish to the multitudes to eat, but never does it mention that He Himself was partaking. And when it comes to red meat, there is only reference to Jesus becoming very angry in the temple when He sees that they are selling goats and lambs for sacrifice/eating.

5. He was adamantly against animal sacrifice. He quoted Hosea 6:6, saying, "For I desire mercy, not sacrifice, and acknowledgment of God rather than burnt offerings" (186).

6. And then finally we have the story of the Last Supper where there is no mention of lamb or meat as would have been common for most traditional Jewish Passover meals (and still is); there was only bread and wine and some kind of dip (perhaps a nice chickpea hummus or olive tapenade??). This was a very typical supper for the early Jewish vegetarians at that time. Jesus also refers to Himself as the Paschal Lamb, as the last and ultimate sacrifice. He distinctly asks that people eat bread and drink wine in His memory, not slaughter and eat lamb in His memory (187). All of this points to a vegetarian Jesus.

Now, knowing that the Bible never mentions Him eating meat and that He was a Nazarene Essene, considering the obvious omission of lamb on the table during His last Passover meal, and taking into account that He taught nothing but pure love and kindness, how hard is it to assume He just might have been a vegetarian? There is no way we will ever know for certain now, but it is some "food for thought."

Early Vegetarian Monks

Next, we have a long list of some pretty amazing early Christian monks and saints, all followers of Jesus, who lived a vegetarian life. There are really too many to mention here (and most likely the basis of another book I need to start soon!), but let me just mention a couple of notable early Christian ascetics:

- Origen (185–254, Alexandria), the "man of steel" who developed the *lectio divina* (188). and who studied Plato and Socrates (both vegetarian Greek philosophers). His message in two words was, "Be transformed!" He was a hard ascetic who ate nothing but bread and water, who believed in total denial of physical comforts to allow a body to be transformed and ready for the resurrection. The goal was to live a passionless existence to overcome the limitations of the body (189).
- Anthony of the Desert, (251–356, Egypt), a wealthy young man who gave it all away and became the first desert monk to go into the wilderness for his entire life, the father of all monks who came afterwards. The desert became for him a place of healing, not only for him but also for all who came to visit him. It was said

that even in his very last year (and he would have been 105 years old), he came to radiate such magnetic charm and openness to all that any stranger who came upon him, surrounded by crowds of disciples, would know him at once. Anthony was the one whose heart had achieved total transparency to others (190).

- Evagrius (345–399) took the insights and philosophy of Origen and the example of desert asceticism from Anthony of the Desert and developed from them a theory of monastic life that would be passed down through the ages until today. In his book *The Practice*, he explains that we must eliminate evil thoughts (later known as the seven deadly sins—gluttony, lust, covetousness, anger, sloth, envy, and pride). Gluttony would always lead the list; it was his belief that food fuels the passions of the body, so the only remedy to overcome the evil of gluttony was fasting and a simple vegetarian diet (191).

All of these early Christian monks provide insights for us today to understand the true meaning of food, that it should be used to fuel the body, not as an obsession or desire. When mindful vegetarian eating is focused on the soul and its transformation, the body naturally, physically follows. The insight they gave us was the body can be seen as the "text" of the soul, the medium for reading the inner workings of the human person. Your body is the outward manifestation of your inner spirituality, so what is it that you are broadcasting to the world about your inner life? The early desert monks taught us that faith must ALWAYS come down to the body level, if it is real, that it is only through fasting that one can achieve a deep connection to God. Fasting and a simple vegetarian diet deepens faith.

St. Augustine spent much of his life studying his "disordered desires" for things he shouldn't have. He found his heart perpetually unstable, always tumbling off balance toward what it wanted, in a state of being out of control (sound familiar?). The cure for this comes ONLY by God's grace, when we are able to love God above all and to love God in others. The body can be seen as either a temple or a tomb—a temple for worship and glory to God or a tomb ... and of course I cannot help but think in terms of nutrition here as well.

If you had a temple, you would fill it with sweet flowers, fruits, and incense. If you had a tomb, it would be filled with dead bodies. When you eat meat, you are eating death and violence. Your body becomes a tomb. When you eat living foods, your body becomes a temple.

I know I have probably not convinced all of you. Some of you may still believe that eating animals is part of God's plan because that's the way it was done in biblical times, and that's the way it has always been done since. Well, there are also plenty of references to slavery and stoning in the Bible as well, and thankfully we as a nation, as human beings, decided to pray to God for the right thing to do instead of picking and choosing quotes from the Bible that condone actions no longer valid in today's world. Humanity has evolved, and continues to evolve, spiritually. It is my most fervent wish that the same thing will happen for the animals, that we will stop looking at eating animals as something that is condoned by God because meat and animal sacrifice is included in Bible stories from ancient times. I don't think that God intended to freeze history right then and there because He sent His son to the world in a certain time in history. I don't think that God intended that we should not evolve as human beings further or that because the Bible was written 2,000 years ago that we should forever remain locked into lifestyle of that age forever. We have happily let go of slavery, of stoning, of animal sacrifice. It is not time to let go of eating animals now as well. It is time to pray to God again to ask what is the right thing to do.

Meat as Gluttony

There are many things that were done in biblical times that no longer apply to today's world. Today we know we don't need animals to survive; in fact, we thrive on a plant-based diet from a health perspective. All Christians should look inside their hearts and answer these questions: Would God really want any animals in His kingdom to suffer and die needlessly as they are today? Does the eating of animals today fall under the vice of gluttony as defined by Evagrius – the overindulgence of food to the point of extravagance or waste? It seems to me that continuing to eat meat and dairy when it is completely unnecessary just because we like the taste, when it is unhealthy, and when it is cruel is the ultimate vice of gluttony.

It's time to do two things, if you dare. First, go online and watch a slaughterhouse video, any slaughterhouse video. Better yet, watch "Earthlings" online, if you dare. Then look at yourself in the mirror, in the eyes, and ask yourself, ask God who lives inside of you, what He would have you do.

I think you would hear the words that Jesus spoke, the final and only commandment that really counts, "Love one another. As I have loved you, so you must love one another." How hard is it to imagine that the Lamb of God was also speaking of the lambs themselves? True spirituality, inner peace, and world peace can come only when you give up eating violence and death. Let's all stop the talk about an apocalypse coming with the rebuilding of the temple and bringing back animal sacrifice again, seriously. Let's stop the drumbeat about the end of the world being at hand. Let's stop the drumbeat of going to war against the "bad guys" (other religions, other cultures, other political groups) fueled by our flesh-eating violent energy;. Let's extract ourselves from politics and divisive social issues fueled by self-righteousness and misunderstanding. These ideas are not moving our world in the direction it needs to go! Let the Body of Christ be the only flesh you eat, let the rest be plants, and reach out in peace to try to understand and respect those you might disagree with. Let's take responsibility for making this Earth and all who live here the peaceful Garden of Eden it was meant to be.

I'll close this chapter with the words of Jesus in the Sermon on the Mount from the gospel of Matthew. Please read it, and while you do, picture the animals—the sheep, the pigs, the cows, the goats, the chickens—who are pleading for our mercy:

> *"Blessed are the poor in spirit,*
> *for theirs is the kingdom of heaven.*
> *Blessed are those who mourn,*
> *for they will be comforted.*
> *Blessed are the meek,*
> *for they will inherit the earth.*
> *Blessed are those who hunger and thirst for righteousness,*
> *for they will be filled.*
> *Blessed are the merciful,*
> *for they will be shown mercy.*

Blessed are the pure in heart,
for they will see God.
Blessed are the peacemakers,
for they will be called children of God.
Blessed are those who are persecuted because of righteousness,
for theirs is the kingdom of heaven.
Blessed are you when people insult you, persecute you and
falsely say all kinds of evil against you because of me.
Rejoice and be glad, because great is your reward in heaven,
for in the same way they persecuted the prophets who were
before you."

~ Matthew 5:3-12

Chapter 9

The Fifth Element – What Connects Us

The Fifth Element – What Connects Us

"At times I feel as if I am spread out over the landscape and inside of things, and am myself living in every tree, in the splashing of waves, in the clouds and the animals that come and go, in the procession of the seasons."

~ Carl Jung

In the last chapter I spoke from my heart to my Catholic and Christian community. In this chapter I want to speak from my heart to literally everyone. To the Whole Earth. In this final third section of the book, we are talking about a peaceful planet, and so we must shft our focus upwards, to a higher level—to God, religion, and spirituality—because without God, there can never be peace. I know there are many atheists who will disagree with that statement, feeling as they do (and understandably so) that all our current global violence stems from religion. But God is love and God is peace, and what is passing for "religion" often has nothing to do with God or religion for that matter. And I have plenty of anecdotes about atheists doing horrible things too, which there is really no need to go into. Evil is not being caused by religion but it certainly loves to masquerade as such, being as evil as evil is! So even if you are an atheist, please stay with me until the end. Hopefully I can at least open your mind to the idea that perhaps there is a universal force for good, call it whatever you want —God/ Universe/ Creator/ Beloved/

Love/ Goodness/ the "Fifth Element"—that it is in all of us regardless of our faith or lack thereof, and that without this universal force for good, there can be no peace on Earth. Don't confuse religion with God—and I'm talking now to both atheists who hate religion and so don't believe in God, and religious folks who think God is found only with their faith. Don't confuse religion with God.

The last chapter was devoted exclusively to Catholicism and Christianity because as a Catholic I feel compelled to send a targeted message to this very beloved part of our Rainbow Warrior tribe. However, our Rainbow Tribe includes everyone—atheists, Christians, Muslims, Jews, Buddhists, Hindu. All faiths are true and all are equally beloved by God. Even those people who don't believe in God are equally loved by God. This may go against what the traditionalists of my faith believe, but it is what I believe. Whenever I explain how I can believe this, I love to recount the story of the blind men and the elephant, originally from India. (I actually heard this story for the first time in my Catholic high school, in my favorite religion class that was taught there on comparative religions.) The parable implies that one's experience can be true, and it can be completely different from someone else's experience that is different but also equally true. For me, the parable is the best explanation of the unknowable nature of God, and that all religion is just our own incomplete version of the whole Truth based on where we were born and where we stand. If anyone claims to have all the answers, then they are not telling the truth. No one can have all the answers to that which is unknowable.

The Parable of the Blind Men and the Elephant

A number of blind men came upon an elephant. Somebody told them that it was an elephant. The blind men asked, "What is the elephant like?" and they began to touch its body to see what they could discover. One of them touched its leg and said, "It is like a pillar." Another man touched its ear and said, "The elephant is like a basket." Similarly, the one who touched its trunk thought it was like a hose, the one who touched its tusk thought it was like a pipe, and the one who touched its belly thought it was like a wall. In the same way, he who has seen the Lord in a particular way from a particular life experience limits the Lord to that alone, and thinks that He is nothing else (192), and that everyone else is wrong.

Anyone who claims to know the "only truth" suffers from the same blindness as these men. I cannot have a conversation with someone who claims to be so religious that they completely know and understand that which is unknowable. I know this goes contrary to what many Christians and some other faiths teach, but as a Catholic, I learned to be a bit more ecumenical and openminded. We were always taught that there are many more mysteries than answers, and as I said in the beginning, I refuse to fit into a box I am not comfortable with. I will not blindly mimic dogma that doesn't make sense, doesn't promote love, or that goes against science. If more people of faith would do the same, if more people of faith would not be afraid to step outside their boxes, perhaps the atheists would stop laughing at us.

So in this chapter, I expand out to the broadest definition of religion and spirituality to encompass everyone, the fifth element, that spark of divine that exists inside all of us regardless of faith or no faith, whether you like it or not!

Our Biggest Challenge Lies Just Ahead

So this is the problem: Our world is suffering from disease, poverty, and war. At the time of this writing, the news is inundated with fear. Fear over the latest health epidemic, be it measles or Ebola. Fear stemming from fighting, hatred, and division within families, within societies, and across the world. Fear of an enormous existential threat in the form of religious extremism as terrorism, beheading innocent people, raping young women, and burning people alive in cages. There is something horribly wrong with our world. But if we feel that torture of humans is awful, but pigs and chickens being thrown into vats of scalding water in a slaughterhouse while still conscious is not, or if we sit at our family dinner table or in a restaurant, laughing, talking, and celebrating our lives' milestones while eating the tortured remains of animals is okay, then it's time for a check-in with the truth—and with our souls—to be sure they're still attached to us. Because the question is not: Do animals have souls? The question is: When will humans regain theirs? It all starts when we wake up and really see our food for what it is. When we are able to turn a blind eye to the torture of animals for food, how much easier to turn a blind eye to the suffering of humans? When humans become so numb to compassion that they can slit an animal's throat without any emotion, how much easier to learn how to slit a human's throat without any emotion as well? Killing animals for food is how we all learn to turn off our natural, God-given compassion and empathy, whether we are doing the klling ourselves, or payig someone else to do it for us. If we could not look an animal in the eyes and kill the animal with our bare hands, how dare we pay someone else to do our dirty work?

What Do We Do?

So the reality is, how do we fight the evil that seems to be growing on this Earth if we hope to achieve world peace? Here I am writing this Pollyanna book that implies that all of this can be changed if everyone were to read this book, to stop eating meat and dairy and junk, and to start living a holistically healthy life. World peace begins with a plant-based diet. Does this all sound a bit naïve to you? I don't blame you if you think so, but let me at least lay out my case for why the Whole Earth Diet is going to save the world.

1. We are eating death and violence. Food is our most intense connection both with the living natural order of our environment, and with our culture and society. By eating the plants and animals of our surroundings, we literally incorporate them into our bodies and make our very cells from them. It is also through this act of eating that we partake of our culture's values and paradigms at the most primal levels. It is becoming increasingly obvious, however, that the choices we make about our food are leading to environmental degradation, enormous human health problems, and unimaginable cruelty toward our fellow creatures. When we eat meat and dairy, we are eating death and violence and rape, and it is becoming who we are. When we eat violence, we become violent. It is no surprise that the human beheadings that seem to come so easily to Daesh have been practiced hundreds of times killing their own animals for food, publicly letting the blood run in the streets. When we

allow life to be taken away without mercy or compassion from a four-legged animal, it is good practice for taking away life from a two-legged animal. When we eat the pure, peaceful energy of plants, we will become purer and more peaceful.

2. We are eating unconsciously, brainwashed into willing complacency and blindness. By reducing vast expanses of our precious forests and prairies to toxic monocultures, where only one species is allowed to grow in order to feed the mistreated animals whose flesh and secretions we are all pressured into eating, we create the ongoing conditions of psychological, ethical, ecological, cultural, and spiritual disconnectedness. These prevent us, as a society, from understanding the roots of our unyielding dilemmas. It is way beyond time for all of us in our culture to look behind the curtain of institutional denial and bring the light of compassion and awareness to our meals and what our meals require. When we take off the blinders and look at what our food choices are causing—the devastation of the Earth, the suffering of the animals—we will grow in compassion and start to feel compassion and concern for the whole world - all people, and all animals, and all of nature.

3. A lot of the ills of society are interconnected with poor food choices, and once we start to eat with integrity and authenticity, a lot of these problems will go away. When we buy the cheaper food that comes from Monsanto, we are helping to put small farmers around the world out of business. When we buy meat, we are contributing to the destruction of the rainforest. When the world eats crap, there is a global health crisis that fuels a diseased psyche for the planet. The

grain that we feed to our factory-farmed animals for meat could feed the starving children around the world ten times over. As long as the world is suffering, this toxicity leaks into the world's psyche, and there is unrest, unhappiness, and terrorism.

4. Whole Earth Diet is more than just a diet. It is a lifestyle that suggests that we as a species must take steps toward a more conscious enlightenment. By shedding some of the toxic divisions that come from black-and-white thinking, we can all become freer to evolve our thinking outside the old boxes we have been locked into, and become more intelligent, more loving, and happier. Divisions, whether they are political or religious, come from black-and-white thinking inside the box. We encourage nuanced thought and shades of grey outside the box. We look always for what unites us, not what divides us, because what unites us—our love for our family, our friends, and our country; our desire for a long, healthy life for ourselves and our loved ones; the desire for world peace and an end to war; a desire to spend less money on sickness and more money on fun; freedom to live our lives as we please—is so much more meaningful than the petty politics. We are all one, no matter what they tell you!

We are all one. That is what the fifth element is.

I know there are many of you who know me as an architect and perhaps are wondering what in the heck I could possibly know about any of this. I don't blame you for your doubts. But those of you who know me also know that I have an unquenchable thirst for knowledge and that I am constantly learning and educating myself about things that are important. When the economy crashed and I found myself wondering what to do with my life, my first concern was getting my health back, and in doing so I needed to educate myself about health and nutrition and the definite link between what you eat and the state of your health, which I guess should be obvious but so many people are oblivious. It is a group delusion almost, so that it becomes not so obvious at all. I was as blind as anyone else. I started off on this journey just wanting to lose some weight, and I ended up here, wanting to save the world, because the trail that I followed just kept leading me around one mind-blowing corner to the next to the next. And so I am now forming my tribe of Warriors for peace, and trust me—I am not alone here. This tribe started to form WAY before I woke up, in fact, WAY before I was born. This tribe was born within our common fifth element that we all share, which has finally ripened as the time has come. Want to know who else is in our rainbow Warrior tribe?

Meet Our Tribe

Here are some quotes from just a few heroes of our tribe:

"For as long as men massacre animals, they will kill each other. Indeed, he who sows the seed of murder and pain cannot reap joy and love." ~ Pythagoras

"But for the sake of some little mouthful of flesh we deprive a soul of the sun and light, and of that proportion of life and time it had been born into the world to enjoy." ~ Plutarch

"It is more important to prevent animal suffering, rather than sit to contemplate the evils of the universe praying in the company of priests." ~ Buddha

"The time will come when men such as I will look upon the murder of animals as they now look upon the murder of men." ~ Leonardo Da Vinci

"Non-violence leads to the highest ethics, which is the goal of all evolution. Until we stop harming all other living beings, we are still savages." ~ Thomas Edison

"I hold that the more helpless a creature, the more entitled it is to protection by man from the cruelty of man." ~ Mohandas Gandhi

"I will not kill or hurt any living creature needlessly, nor destroy any beautiful thing, but will strive to save and comfort all gentle life, and guard and perfect all natural beauty upon the earth." ~ John Ruskin

"Not to hurt our humble brethren (the animals) is our first duty to them, but to stop there is not enough. We have a higher mission—to be of service to them whenever they require it. ... If you have men who will exclude any of God's creatures from the shelter of compassion and pity, you will have men who will deal likewise with their fellow men." ~ St Francis of Assisi

"Ethics, too, are nothing but reverence for life. That is what gives me the fundamental principle of morality, namely, that good consists in maintaining, promoting, and enhancing life, and that destroying, injuring, and limiting life are evil." ~ Albert Schweitzer

"The worst sin toward our fellow creatures is not to hate them, but to be indifferent to them: that's the essence of inhumanity." ~ George Bernard Shaw

"As long as people will shed the blood of innocent creatures there can be no peace, no liberty, no harmony between people. Slaughter and justice cannot dwell together." ~ Isaac Bashevis Singer, writer and Nobel laureate

"A man can live and be healthy without killing animals for food; therefore, if he eats meat, he participates in taking animal life merely for the sake of his appetite. And to act so is immoral." ~ Leo Tolstoy

"People often say that humans have always eaten animals, as if this is a justification for continuing to the practice. According to this logic, we should not try to prevent people from murdering other people, since this has also been done since the earliest of times." ~ Isaac Bashevis Singer

Most of these people of course have passed, but even today there are mighty Warriors for peace that are aligning on the right side of history.

"There is no way to overstate the magnitude of the collective spiritual transformation that will occur when we shift from food of violent oppression to food of gentleness and compassion." ~ Will Tuttle, World Peace Diet

"I became a vegetarian after realizing that animals feel afraid, cold, hungry and unhappy like we do. I feel very deeply about vegetarianism and the animal kingdom. It was my dog Boycott who led me to question the right of humans to eat other sentient beings." ~ Cesar Chavez

"We do not need to eat animals, wear animals, or use animals for entertainment purposes, and our only defense of these uses is our pleasure, amusement, and convenience." ~ Gary L. Francione

"Every time we make a dining choice, we make a choice between compassion and cruelty, a choice between the law of the jungle and the law of higher moral consciousness." ~ Kathy Freston

"I refuse to believe that no one cares. Because the problem is you've been programmed not to care. Brainwashed to be a good little consumer of animal body parts. ... It can't be that difficult to understand that each animal values his or her life as much as you value yours. You might not care about cows and pigs and chickens and fish, but when your thoughts are prejudicial, who the hell cares what you think?" ~ Gary Yourofsky

"If slaughterhouses had glass walls, the whole world would be vegetarian." ~ Paul McCartney

"Perhaps in the back of our minds we already understand, without all the science I've discussed, that something terribly wrong is happening. Our sustenance now comes from misery. We know that if someone offers to show us a film on how our meat is produced, it will be a horror film. We perhaps know more than we care to admit, keeping it down in the dark places of our memory—disavowed. When we eat factory-farmed meat we live, literally, on tortured flesh. Increasingly, that tortured flesh is becoming our own." ~ Jonathan Safran Foer, Eating Animals

"It was all so very businesslike that one watched it fascinated. It was pork-making by machinery, pork-making by applied mathematics. And yet somehow the most matter-of-fact person could not help thinking of the hogs; they were so innocent, they came so very trustingly; and they were so very human in their protests—and so perfectly within their rights! They had done nothing to deserve it; and it was adding insult to injury, as the thing was done here, swinging them up in this cold-blooded, impersonal way, without pretence at apology, without the homage of a tear." ~ Upton Sinclair

"The path of the norm is the path of least resistance; it is the route we take when we're on auto-pilot and don't even realize we're following a course of action that we haven't consciously chosen. Most people who eat meat have no idea that they're behaving in accordance with the tenets of a system that has defined many of their values, preferences, and behaviors. What they call 'free choice' is, in fact, the result of a narrowly obstructed set of options that have been chosen for them. They don't realize, for instance, that they have been taught to value human life so far above certain forms of nonhuman life that it seems appropriate for their taste preferences to supersede other species' preference for survival." ~Melanie Joy, *Why We Love Dogs, Eat Pigs, and Wear Cows: An Introduction to Carnism: The Belief System That Enables Us to Eat Some Animals and Not Others*

"Being vegetarian here also means that we do not consume dairy and egg products, because they are products of the meat industry. If we stop consuming, they will stop producing. Only collective awakening can create enough determination for action." ~ Thích Nhất Hạnh, *The Fruitful Darkness: A Journey Through Buddhist Practice and Tribal Wisdom*

"Nobody can possibly be so hungry that they need to take a life in order to feel satisfied—they don't after all, take a human life, so why take the life of an animal? Both are conscious beings with the same determination to survive. It is habit, and laziness and nothing else." ~ Morrissey, *Autobiography*

"If your meals consistently revolve around corpse multiple times daily, you might become one sooner than you planned." ~ *Kris Carr, Crazy Sexy Diet: Eat Your Veggies, Ignite Your Spark, and Live Like You Mean It!*

"Cruelty to animals is an enormous injustice; so is expecting those on the lowest rung of the economic ladder to do the dangerous, soul-numbing work of slaughtering sentient beings on our behalf." ~ Victoria Moran, *Main Street Vegan: Everything You Need to Know to Eat Healthfully and Live Compassionately in the Real World*

"The vegan lifestyle is a compassionate way to live that supports life, supports fairness and equality, and promotes freedom." ~ Robert Cheeke, *Vegan Bodybuilding & Fitness: The Complete Guide to Building Your Body on a Plant-Based Diet*

"Without pushing an agenda (okay, maybe I've pushed a bit), I've spread a little veganism wherever I've gone. I've become friends with chefs at the meatiest restaurants you can imagine, and shown them a few things that opened their minds (and their menus) to vegan options. It's easy to be convincing when the food is delicious. It doesn't feel like a sacrifice—it feels like a step up." ~ Tal Ronnen, *The Conscious Cook: Delicious Meatless Recipes That Will Change the Way You Eat*

"Never forget there is no such things as 'humane slaughter.' I never saw an animal clicking its heels going to the slaughterhouse, saying 'Yippee, skippy, I'm going to be a McDonald's Burger tomorrow!' There is always fear in their eyes. They know exactly what is going to happen. So for anyone to claim there is such a thing as 'humane slaughter,' well, that's the greatest oxymoron in the world." ~ Howard Lyman, former fourth-generation cattle rancher turned vegan and activist

"I've had an epiphany recently. ... I want to challenge all of you as people of deep conscience, people who are environment stewards of the earth and oceans. ... By changing what you eat, you will change the entire contract between the human species and the natural world." ~ James Cameron, Director

"You know the world has gone mad when those who have enlightened, compassionate views and future visions, are accused of borderline insanity, ridiculed and criticised for thinking positively." ~ Mango Wodzak, Destination Eden

"Don't wait for a better world. Start now to create a world of harmony and peace. It is up to you, and it always has been. You may even find the solution at the end of your fork." ~ Sharon Gannon, Yoga and Vegetarianism: The Path to Greater Health and Happiness

So I guess all of this was my way of showing you that I am not a lone, crazy voice crying out in the wilderness, though at times I certainly feel like I am. The WE that I refer to is the communal soul I feel from my brothers and sisters who have already seen the light, who have awakened, either coming at it from a health perspective or a spiritual perspective. It is really impossible to keep the two separate for long, to not let one evolve into the other. Once you make the connection, it becomes so much more than one individual's physical, mental, emotional, or spiritual health; it becomes about the health of the communal soul, the WE. The ether. The fifth element. The ripple effect as one individual influences another individual who influences another individual, and one by one, one at a time, we will change the world.

There is just no other greater cause in our lifetimes than this one. This is why we were born today—now, today—not last century, not next century. It is an amazing time to be alive as one tide washes out and a new one washes in—a bit turbulent, not always smooth, but at the end we will have our Garden of Eden back again. This is all our assignments—to put an end to this madness that is destroying our health, destroying our planet, and destroying our communal soul. Join the tribe, and let's do this together.

Chapter 10

10 Simple Steps to Save the World

10 Simple Steps to Save the World

"The love of awakened motherhood is a love and compassion felt not only towards one's own children, but towards all people, animals and plants, rocks and rivers—a love extended to all of nature, to all beings. Indeed, to a woman in whom the state of true motherhood has awakened, all creatures are her children."

~ Amma (Mata Amritanandamayi)

So let's do this. This is really what it's all about. For any diet to work, it must really be a lifestyle change, and for any lifestyle change to work, it must be about something bigger than yourself. This is not just about you anymore. It is about the animals. It is about the future of our planet. It is about all the rest of us. It is about being part of a tribe of Warriors, Warriors of light out to change the world for the better for their children and their children's children, Warriors really out to save the world, without exaggeration. I think we all know that if we don't swing this ship hard around, it is going to go over the falls. This is not about one or two of us going off the cliff anymore. It is about the salvation of humankind.

So what simple, practical steps can we take to save the world? How does one join the tribe of wellness Warriors for peace? It's easy. Huge change can come when a small group of people feel passionately about something, and I can tell you for certain that once you start to follow the Whole Earth Diet, you too will become a passionate Warrior for Peace.

Step #1: Promote Whole Earth Diet.

Tell everyone that you are "on the Whole Earth Diet." Spread the word about eating real, whole, plant-based foods. Nothing processed. No meat and dairy. Gift everyone you know a copy of this book! The more people that start eating food that creates health, the more we will see a reduction in number of killer diseases (obesity, cancer, heart disease, diabetes) until they are eliminated completely. There will be cleaner air and water, oceans filled again with fish and marine life, forests teeming with wildlife. And the net result of all of this—the reduction of violence thru a peace-based, cruelty-free, compassionate diet—is global hunger, malnutrition, and war shall cease.

World peace begins on your plate, and will become a reality when you consistently eat peace instead of violence, and become the role model for others to do the same.

Step #2: Create a Play Group!

Get outside and play with others. Join or create an outdoor club around your favorite recreational activity. Daily exercise releases endorphins, releases tensions and negativity, and creates better physical health and less disease, which leads to a world full of healthier people with better mental health, and who are less of a burden on the health care system. Reconnect with nature, soak up some sunshine, maybe go barefoot in the sand or the grass. Join a sports team, a football club, a rock-climbing group, a hiking group, whatever. Just get outside and have fun with others. When you join a group based on a common outdoor interest, often you'll find yourself with a new group of friends of various ethnicities, political beliefs, religious backgrounds, from different cultures. When you have diverse friendships, then you're more likely to begin respecting all cultures, all races, all religions. We're only afraid of what is unfamiliar. So go find a playgroup to join or create your own if you don't find what you are looking for! And this is key: do not take yourselves too seriously! Have FUN! Don't get all competitive. Just have fun and laugh a lot. Laugh especially at yourself.

World peace will become a reality when you go out, play, laugh, have fun, maybe even have a beer with people that come from diverse backgrounds and different cultures that live in your local community.

Step #3: Go on Adventures.

You need to travel outside your little corner of the world. This may sound very elitist, but it's not. There are lots of ways to travel, no matter your economic means. You can go on an adventure travel outing to another state or another country where you might sleep in tents under the stars and cook your meals over a fire. There are many organizations that offer volunteering opportunities where you will volunteer your time and expertise in a specific location and they will pay for your lodging and food, sometimes even your flights to get there. There are now ways to save money when traveling with a house swap or by couch surfing. You can sublet an apartment for a week or two in another city somewhere and save lots of money. Travel is not just for the well-heeled, and it is probably the best education there is when it comes to learning about and understanding different cultures, people, and places. Travel will also increase your happiness, which is always a good thing.

World peace will become a reality when you travel to other lands and develop an understanding, respect, and love for other cultures that comes only from seeing and experiencing with your own eyes.

Step #4: Donate to Nondenominational Charities.

Donate your time and your money to charities and non-profits OUTSIDE your own faith. I see well-meaning people everywhere donating all their time and money to their own particular faith-based organizations. Of course, it is your right to do with your time and money as you please, BUT if we are trying to create world peace, we have to do more than this. If all that we do is donate to our own church, we are further reinforcing the idea of separate tribes. We love our tribes, but we need to love and support other tribes as well! We want to bust down the boxes we create when we donate only to our own church, synagogue, temple, or mosque. Donate your time and money to your own faith, sure, but also make sure you have enough to give to interfaith or non–faith-based organizations.

World peace will become a reality when you reach out beyond your own "tribe" to give to others outside your tribe, without any motive other than unconditional love and compassion.

Step #5: Stay Current AND Positive; Avoid Labels.

In this new Internet age, we have at our fingertips access to more information than we have ever had in the past, and it can be overwhelming. You can find scientific studies, polls, research, to prove "without a doubt" two completely contradictory conclusions with regard to the same question. Then you turn on the TV to get caught up on the current-event news of the day, and you get completely different spins on those stories depending on what news channel you watch. People are becoming so polarized based on which news channel they watch and what their tribe is telling them is happening. It doesn't matter which side of the aisle you are on or what country you live in; no one is safe from this current trend of fear and divisiveness. So what should we do?

- TV: Watch a different news channel each day. Try CNN, MSNBC, Fox News. Watch some international news: BBC, Al Jazeera, NHK Japan. Watch Comedy Central, and the Mormon Newsroom. Watch your local news too. We need to keep an open mind to all sides of every story always, whether national or international news.

- Newspaper: Support your local newspaper and have it delivered to your home. There is nothing like having a cup of coffee in the morning and reading a good old-fashioned newspaper. This is one old tradition I hope I never have to learn to live without. If your local area is divided politically, be sure to have both papers delivered.

- Internet: Surf the web every day. It is an amazing tool. The Internet can be entertaining, but if something really sparks your interest, fact-check it. Snopes.com is a great place to start. But here's a rule of thumb: search reliable sources for your facts, such as prominent medical institutions, universities, and non-profit groups. Don't look at everything you see or read on the internet as fact.

- Primary sources: If a politician has just given a speech, listen to the speech; don't listen to someone else's interpretation of the speech. Always go to the primary source to learn, and create your own opinion before someone tells you what your opinion should be. Focus on the positive, do your homework, and fact-check.

The bottom line: let's all stop the "us vs. them" thinking. Don't label people and place them in a box based on their politics, profession, body type, handicap, race, culture, or religion. Be outside the box yourself, and assume others have stepped outside the box as well. The more people that think for themselves, the sooner we will be out of this chaos caused by Paleolithic tribalism (probably fueled by the currently popular Palo diet!).

World peace will become a reality when we stop labeling others, step outside our boxes, and develop an open mind and a positive attitude.

Step #6: Use Internet for Good.

This is the first century where geography no longer contains us. We are not limited to social interaction with just those folks in our community. Now, no matter where we are in the world, we have the ability to reach out to everyone in the world, or at least to those people that have Internet access or are on social media. There are about 7 billion people in the world, and according to a recent study, 42 percent have access to the Internet. It is simply amazing that with technology today, we can send a communication out over the Internet to someone on the other side of the world in an instant. It is truly the physical manifestation of the fifth element that unites all of us, and it is a thing of amazing beauty when used properly and to promote goodness, peace, and goodwill.

We can use the Internet as a tool for our conscious evolution, and a pretty efficient tool at that. Use this tool for its highest purpose! When you have friends on the Internet from every walk of life, of all political persuasions and religious beliefs, from all over the world, you can learn from them. Let's make the internet a place where goodness can spread and know no bounds. Reach out to friends and strangers online and around the world with random words of kindness and senseless acts of beauty.

World peace will begin when you start to fully utilize the collective consciousness of the web as a force for collective evolution, for peace, for conversation, for getting to know those that are different from you ... And it all starts with you, today. What energy will you send out into the world today?

Step #7: Create Plant-Based Faith Group.

Just as your personal journey toward health and happiness started with a plant-based diet, so the first step in the journey of evolution for traditional faiths must start with embracing a plant-based diet as well. This is not going to be easy. But I think if there are enough of us pushing from within, from wherever we are located in our corner of the world, in whatever faith, change will come. I outlined the reasons why Catholics or Christians should consider giving up meat and dairy. There are equally compelling reasons why Jews, Muslims, Hindu, and Buddhists should also stop eating meat. When you stop eating meat and you start eating a purely plant-based diet, your energy shifts from violence to peace and your relationship to God is deepened. Any serious faith group must believe that God would prefer for us to eat peace rather than violence and death. People of goodwill everywhere should be repulsed by the idea of eating meat and dairy, if they would really look at the facts behind those industries.

Create a plant-based faith group within your congregation, whatever your faith. Help to spread the information you have read in this book, perhaps by forming a study group or a book club. Start with this book, then read some of the other recommended reading in Appendix C. Get together once a month at someone's home for a plant-based potluck, movie night, or book club discussion. Spread the message, and support one another.

World peace will begin when people of faith and goodwill everywhere across the world start to espouse a plant-based diet for moral, ethical, and spiritual reasons. It will start with you, forming an education and support group around plant-based eating in your local congregation, and starting to spread the word.

Step #8: Create Interfaith Prayer Group.

Think globally and act locally, right? That's what they always say. There may not be something like this in your area, but if not, create an interfaith prayer group. Reach out to the leader of a different faith in your community and get together to chat about interfaith relations. Figure out ways that you can sit in on one another's religious services. Put together a live network of friends from different faith groups, and create a prayer and study group. You can take turns presenting scripture or readings from the other holy book and have a group discussion. Focus on world peace. Imagine if these interfaith prayer groups and subsequent friendships sprang up in all corners of the Earth. World peace would become a reality, not just a fantasy. And if you happen to live in a small town somewhere without a lot of interfaith opportunities, you can also do the same thing via technology, meeting via Skype or other virtual meeting spaces.

World peace begins when people of other faiths and cultures become true friends. It will start with you, joining or forming an interfaith prayer group in your local area, or online, today.

Step #9: Visualize World Peace.

Have you seen those bumper stickers that say "Visualize World Peace"? What exactly does this mean? Well, if we "see" peace in the world, peace will be reflected back to us. Our inner thoughts and perceptions are reflected back to us. If we "see" peace, if we envision peace, we create peace. All the war that we are currently experiencing is a manifestation of our collective unhealthy psyche. We are seeing the world filled with evil, and so the evil is coming to life.

It reminds me of this great story I heard about a hall of mirrors. There was this hall covered with mirrors. Mirrors on all the walls, on the ceiling, and on the floor. One day a dog entered the hall of mirrors and immediately became defensive and angry when he saw himself surrounded by all these other dogs. The dog started to growl and bark. As he barked and snarled, all the other dogs barked and snarled back. The dog barked louder and louder and became more vicious. The other dogs became just as vicious. The dog eventually died of exhaustion trying to fend off the other dogs. Then a monk entered the hall. He noticed all the other peaceful-looking monks around him. He smiled, and all the other monks smiled back at him. He was so ecstatic to see himself surrounded by all these wonderful beings that he at that point in time reached enlightenment.

Situations such as war, violence, hatred, and illness are human manifestations. They are situations that occur in this human form. But they are not who we are. We change our experience by bringing our attention back to our true essence, by remembering who we are. Einstein said, "You can't solve a problem from the same level of thinking that created the problem." War and violence are problems that arise at the basest, lowest level of the human consciousness. Meeting them at the same level will not solve the problem; only a shift and an elevation in consciousness will transform the situation.

You need to believe in world peace, and it will happen. Instead of fighting a situation or trying to make something happen, just manifest it happening, and so it will be. You need to simply be the change you wish to see in the world.

Step #10: Become a Warrior for Peace.

Well, I warned you this was no ordinary diet book, didn't I? It's the most holistic diet program ever, nurturing you not only physically, but mentally, emotionally, and spiritually as well; not only making you healthy, but making you happy too—and not only you, but the whole Earth. So this is where it gets tricky. Even though we know we are spiritual beings having a human experience, we still have this very human side. We will never be perfect as long as we're still human, so we will always have challenges and setbacks. There will be times when we feel weak, want to give up, feel like the task is impossible. This is again where the fifth element steps in. We are a community.

I know that at a very base level, somehow we need to feel grounded within a tribe. We want to cling to our warrior stories and tribal affiliations. There is glory in war, and bravery, and deep beauty in defending those you love with your very life. I know the warrior heart beats within all of us, wanting to define the good guys vs. the bad guys, wanting to defend our loved ones, wanting to defend our tribe. We need evil to know good. We need bad guys. We want to fight. It's strange, but it is a part of who we are. The dark side. The part of ourselves that still carries the memory of war, of heroic and epic battle. This is why we create these artificial divides between our various tribes, why we bond with those that are like us and make enemies (or at least strangers) of those from different tribes, different skin colors, different cultures, different religions, different politics. Up until now, they have been the "bad guys."

But I would ask you to consider elevating your thinking to a whole new breathtaking level. We can still be Warriors, grounded within our tribe, but our definition of tribe has changed. We are not separated by things like race, religion, and politics. We are Warriors from many tribes, all faiths, all cultures, all races, all religions, from all around the world. It is a coalition of good, enlightened spirits in earthly bodies that have stopped viewing people through a human lens and have started to view them through God's lens. And please, don't think for a minute this is a cult or a religion. It is something that cannot so easily be defined.

Whole Earth Wellness is creating a tribe of Warriors for the truth, for the light, for the good side, for the common spirit of God that lives inside all of us. And just because we are good does not mean we are weak. We are fiercely committed to good. Together we are on the hero's journey.

And to fight for good against evil, we must take on a Warrior spirit. We are soldiers of the light. We need to rise to the same level of intensity and passion as those who are manifesting darkness through bloodshed and violence. The difference is our weapons are not swords; they are words and deeds, but we wield them with the exact same precision and intensity. There is no question there are bad things happening in this world today, but we must and we will shift the energy to peace. We just need to be strong, firm, and never back down from what we know to be the truth. Peace begins on your plate, and every individual has the power and the responsibility to change the world.

Join our Whole Earth Wellness Warrior Tribe. This is not just a book you have read. This is a real world tribe you have joined. You are not alone. There are online virtual and live group programs you can attend, and there are international live retreats you can attend. I will come and do speaking engagements for you anywhere in the world, attend peace conferences, help you save a baby goat—you name it. It is all equally important. There is a growing online presence that is Whole Earth Wellness that is working for truth, justice, and peace, starting with what we put onto our plates. You can reach out to me personally at any time. I am here to help support you on your journey. We have the power to change the world. Starting now.

Conclusion:

Be the Change You Wish to See in the World

---

*"Never doubt that a small group of thoughtful, committed
citizens can change the world;
indeed, it's the only thing that ever has."*

~ Margaret Mead

I warned you this was much more than just another a diet book! And I have a confession to make that actually might help you. The goal with a diet, any diet, is not to get skinny, but to get healthy. As you start to put this all to practical use, as you start eating a plant-based diet, lose the need to count calories or worry about nutrients, though that was a big part of what we talked about at first. Just concentrate on eating three beautiful meals a day and making them the best meals that you can because you are the alchemist creating your body every time you eat. The goal is not to get into skinny jeans. The goal is to lose our antagonistic and troubled relationship with food, and our antagonistic and troubled body image. If we never get back into those skinny jeans, really, at the end of the day, does it matter? As long as you feel good, strong, and are healthy, little love handles can be just adorable, so learn to love yourself always, no matter what. Focus on one day at a time, making every day your very best day, putting in good food, putting out good energy. Being strong and healthy is not a destination, it is a daily journey.

What started with a diet ends with an inspired action to change the world. We started with your health, took you through your whole self to a more holistic vision for personal wellness, then took to see how your personal choices can impact the world. The idea that some lives matter less is the root of all the evil in the world. The inability to feel compassion is the source of all our pain. Once we realize this, the shift is easy, and it's imperative.

In our current world, as people's health, finances, careers, and spirituality are all going through major upheavals, it can be difficult to have hope, look toward the future, or feel that one person can make a difference. But the future is made up of a series of moments—one after another—and each moment is a decision, an opportunity, a potential for joy and change. And if each of us begins to recognize the power of each individual at each single moment, we can start to see how all of us together can bring about the change we wish to see in the world, by BEING as we wish others would be—starting with being our best possible self at this moment.

We started this book by challenging you to completely rethink nutrition, to understand that food and fitness are the foundation to transforming and living one's life to its highest potential. This is the starting point. Following the food and nutrition principles outlined in this book, excess weight will begin to go, but you will also begin to feel healthy, energetic, and capable of living the life you always dreamed of. And it starts with your food. Give up the processed fake foods. Give up the tainted meat and dairy.

The biggest leap of faith we are asking you to make, of course, is the meat and dairy. Health is becoming big business now. Health coaches everywhere in the workplace advocate a "lean protein" diet of fish and chicken, and of course the fruits and veggies. Some are even brave enough to suggest their clients give up the red meat. Give up the processed foods, yes—on this subject almost every diet agrees. This is more socially acceptable to the mainstream. This is what "sells." But almost everyone is afraid to advocate giving up meat and dairy altogether.

So why listen to me and other health professionals that are telling you to give up your meat and dairy when it is the last thing you want to do, not the easiest thing to do, and certainly not what the loudest "noise" is telling you to do? Just like with any good mystery, you have to look for motive. I am not saying there is ANYTHING wrong with making money or making a profit. There are many admirable, ethical companies making huge profits, and trust me, I don't see any problem with making a buck myself. I am not a crazy liberal. I do believe that capitalism at its best works, and works very well. That being said, just because it is profitable doesn't make it automatically admirable or virtuous. If the profit comes at the expense of others' health, happiness, or even their life, it is obviously wrong. And all lives matter.

So you hear A LOT of noise from the one side saying you need A LITTLE meat and dairy to be healthy, all to the tune of a BIG profit. And people gladly listen to this message, not only because of the amplitude, but because people love being told that their favorite bad habits are okay and they can continue eating what they enjoy. And so many health coaches and professionals continue to say that you can eat "just a little" meat and dairy. But wait ... meat and dairy are so bad for you that you must trim it back to "just a little." Why not omit it altogether? Obviously the profit inherent in a message that has been watered down enough to allow just a bit of the bad stuff.

So what drives those of us on the other side, the thin sliver of folks screaming and yelling at you to back away from your meat and dairy? Well, it is certainly not profit. It is not fame and glory. It is not because our voices are being sponsored by any of the big industries in this country. It is not because the medical studies on our side are paid for by big meat, big dairy, or big food lobbyists. It is not because we don't love our country. In fact, quite the opposite. We have seeing what is happening to our country. What drives us? PASSION and COMPASSION. Money? Profit? Power? Furthest things from our minds. If we were worried about this, we would go silent.

We do it because we are PASSIONATE about the rights of life, liberty and the pursuit of happiness for each and every individual on planet Earth regardless of their color, creed, nationality, or species—not for profit, not for attention. And we are driven to this passion because we have developed a particularly painful and very real form of COMPASSION. We quite literally feel another's pain. Com Passion. With Pain. If we see a young person suffering from diabetes or heart failure, we can feel exactly what pain that person is in. If we see an animal waiting its turn in line to be executed, we literally feel the staggering, nauseous fear of impending doom that the poor animal is experiencing. And we know that all of this pain is completely unnecessary. We have seen the light and we want to shout it to the mountaintops because it is the solution to all the world's problems, and that is no exaggeration. These are our motives. You know, if I never make a dime on this book or my business, I don't care. For me, success means watching one person at a time wake up, and stop suffering, and stop causing suffering, and discover health and happiness. Watching one farm animal at a time be rescued and set free into a green field. Watching the world change right before my eyes as premature death rates from cancer, heart disease, and diabetes start to drop; as world hunger and child starvation become things of the past; as peace begins to settle over the Earth. These are my motives, the same as many others like me.

Which motive will you listen to? Whose motive will you believe? Profit, or passion?

You cannot call yourself a health advocate and continue to eat cruelty, saturated fat, and cholesterol. You are only doing so because you are either still brainwashed, asleep, or lying to yourself. Everyone can succeed at this by tweaking their plant-based diet to what works for them.

You cannot call yourself an animal lover, treating your dogs and cats with as much love as your own children, while turning a blind eye to the brutal lives and torturous deaths of millions of cows, pigs, goats, sheep, and chickens.

You cannot call yourself an environmentalist who cares about the planet while you continue to choose to eat that which causes land and water pollution, contributes to global warming, and uses far more energy and water than any plant-based foods.

You cannot claim to love humankind if you continue to take the grains away from the mouth of a hungry child so that you can feed it to the cattle for your burger.

You can't call yourself a spiritual leader and turn a blind eye to suffering of any kind—and not just turning a blind eye, but being the cause of suffering. No God would condone this kind of evil being inflicted on animals, on His precious creation, when it is no longer necessary for human health or life.

If everyone on Earth were to adopt a cruelty-free diet, if everyone on Earth started down this same path together toward being not only physically well, but mentally, emotionally, and spiritually healthy and happy, if everyone on Earth knocked down the superficial barriers and partitions that divide us into competing groups and saw at the end that we are all truly one, if everyone took a personal vow to do no harm to man nor beast, then the world would make a dramatic and enormous shift into the new enlightened age. A healthier, happier, peaceful world awaits us. We are all already on this journey; some of you just don't know it. Some are farther along the path, some are farther behind, but we are all on the path nonetheless. It is our mission to help ourselves first, then look back and lend a guiding light and a gentle helping hand to those who follow, so that together we can all lift each other up and help each other toward our ultimate goal—a peaceable kingdom here in Earth. We do believe this is possible. We do believe this is coming. And we don't plan to stop striving for this with every fiber of our being until it comes to pass, and it will, within my lifetime. I'm not going anywhere until it does.

And so it will be.

Are you ready to become a Warrior for Peace?

Are you in?

Let's ride.

Xoxox

Laura

Appendix A – 21-Day Jump-Start & Recipes

21-Day Jumpstart Sample Menu

Day 1: Sunday:

Brunch: Swiss Chard Frittata & Fruit Salad

Dinner: Lemon Orzo Primavera & Salad

Day 2: Monday:

Breakfast: Superfood Green Smoothie

Lunch: Big Salad, or Subway Vegan Sandwich

Dinner: Mega-Veggie Burritos & Salad

Day 3: Tuesday:

Breakfast: Oatman's Oatmeal

Lunch: Leftovers, Big Salad, or Native Foods Bowl, Salad, or Wrap

Dinner: Thai Coconut Milk Soup & Salad

Day 4: Wednesday:

Breakfast: Forever A Kid Cereal

Lunch: Leftovers, Big Salad, or Chipotle Sofritas Bowl, Salad, or Burrito

Dinner: Rainbow Greek Salad

Day 5: Thursday:

Breakfast: Amazing Fruit Salad

Lunch: Leftovers, Big Salad, or Veggie Grill Bowl, Salad, or Wrap

Dinner: Simple Spaghetti Squash & Salad

Day 6: Friday:

Breakfast: Breakfast Toastie

Lunch: Out with Friends (www.happycow.net)

Dinner: Out with Friends (www.happycow.net)

Day 7: Saturday:

Brunch: Blueberry Flax Pancakes & Leftover Fruits Smoothie

Dinner: Out with Friends (www.happycow.net)

Day 8: Sunday:

Brunch: Potato Kale Squares & Fruit Salad

Dinner: Moroccan Lentil Stew & Salad

Day 9: Monday:

Breakfast: Superfood Green Smoothie

Lunch: Big Salad, or Quiznos Vegan Sandwich

Dinner: Tuscan Pasta & Salad

Day 10: Tuesday:

Breakfast: Oatman's Oatmeal

Lunch: Leftovers, Big Salad, or Native Foods Bowl, Salad, or Wrap

Dinner: Papaya Avocado Salad

Day 11: Wednesday:

Breakfast: Forever A Kid Cereal

Lunch: Leftovers, Big Salad, or Panera Vegan Soup & ½ Bagel

Dinner: Tex-Mex Chili

Day 12: Thursday:

Breakfast: Amazing Fruit Salad

Lunch: Leftovers, Big Salad, or Veggie Grill Bowl, Salad, or Wrap

Dinner: Lazy California Bowl & Salad

Day 13: Friday:

Breakfast: Breakfast Toastie

Lunch: Out with Friends (www.happycow.net)

Dinner: Out with Friends (www.happycow.net)

Day 14: Saturday:

Brunch: Lavender Blueberry Scones & Leftover Fruits Smoothie

Dinner: Out with Friends (www.happycow.net)

Day 15: Sunday:

Brunch: Southwest Tofu Scramble & Fruit Salad

Dinner: Irish Stew & Salad

Day 16: Monday:

Breakfast: Superfood Green Smoothie

Lunch: Leftovers, Big Salad, or Subway Vegan Sandwich

Dinner: Rainbow Stir-Fry & Salad

Day 17: Tuesday:

Breakfast: Oatman's Oatmeal

Lunch: Leftovers, Big Salad, or Native Foods Bowl, Salad, or Wrap

Dinner: Mexicali Chopped Salad

Day 18: Wednesday:

Breakfast: Forever A Kid Cereal

Lunch: Leftovers, Big Salad, or Z Pizza Berkeley Pizza (gluten-free)

Dinner: Indian Kicharee & Salad

Day 19: Thursday:

Breakfast: Amazing Fruit Salad

Lunch: Leftovers, Big Salad, or Veggie Grill Bowl, Salad, or Wrap

Dinner: Sweet Potato Black Bean Salad

Day 20: Friday:

Breakfast: Breakfast Toastie

Lunch: Out with Friends (www.happycow.net)

Dinner: Out with Friends (www.happycow.net)

Day 21: Saturday:

Brunch: Lemon Poppy-Seed Muffins & Leftover Fruits Smoothie

Dinner: Out with Friends (www.happycow.net)

BREAKFAST RECIPES:

SWISS CHARD FRITTATA
Prep Time: 20 mins
Cook Time: 20 mins
Serves 4

INGREDIENTS
1/8 cup low-sodium veggie broth
6 garlic cloves, thinly sliced
1 bunch red Swiss chard, stems removed, chopped (about 4 cups)
2 tsp dried oregano
1 pound extra-firm tofu
1 Tbsp nama shoyu or tamari
1 tsp Dijon mustard
1/4 tsp dry turmeric
Fresh black pepper
1/8 cup nutritional yeast
Celtic sea salt, to taste
Coconut oil (for greasing the pan!)

DIRECTIONS
Preheat oven to 400 degrees. Preheat a large pan over medium-low heat. Add the broth and garlic and cook for about 3 minutes, or until garlic turns a light amber color. Add the chard and oregano and turn up to medium-high heat. Sauté for about 5 minutes until chard is wilted.

While chard is cooking, prepare the frittata base. Give the tofu a squeeze over sink to remove some water. Use your hands to crumble into a bowl and squeeze until it has the consistency of ricotta. Add the nama shoyu or tamari, mustard, turmeric, black pepper, and yeast to the tofu and mix well.

When chard is ready, incorporate into the tofu (and be sure to get all the garlic but none of the extra water). Taste for salt, pepper.

Lightly grease an 8-inch pie plate with coconut oil, and firmly press the frittata mixture into it. Bake for 20 minutes until the frittata is firm and lightly browned on top. Let cool for about 3 minutes, then invert onto a plate and serve.

***

SUPERFOOD GREEN SMOOTHIE
Prep Time: 10 mins
Cook Time: 0 mins
Serves 2

INGREDIENTS
8 oz. young coconut water
8 oz. pure water
4 oz. fresh organic blueberries
1 apple
1 banana
1 tropical or citrus fruit of choice
1/2 avocado
1 inch ginger root

½ inch turmeric root (use 1 tsp powdered if root not available)
Juice from ½ lime or lemon
2 cups chopped/shredded dark leafy greens of choice (kale, spinach, collards)
2 Tbsp all-green protein powder
1-2 Tbsp raw cacao powder - optional
1-2 tsp maca powder - optional
1-2 tsp hemp seeds, flax seeds, or chia seeds - optional
1-2 tsp raw cacao nibs - optional
Natural sweetener to taste (agave or maple syrup, xylitol, stevia)

DIRECTIONS
Blend together all fruits, roots, greens, and liquids first, until smooth.

Then add the superfood powders and seeds and blend again.

Add extra water to desired smoothie consistency.

Add sweetener a little at a time until the taste is just right.

***

OATMAN'S OATMEAL
Prep Time: 3 mins
Cook Time: 5-30 mins (depending if quick-cooking oats)
Serves 2

INGREDIENTS
1 cup steel-cut oats
3 cups water
1 tsp organic vanilla extract
1 tsp cinnamon
1 tsp nutmeg
1 tsp shaved raw ginger root
1 tsp shaved raw turmeric root

Optional raw organic nuts: crumbled walnuts, chopped almonds or pecans
Optional raw organic seeds: 1 tsp hemp seeds, chia seeds, or ground flaxseeds
Optional fruits: raisins, cranberries, finely chopped apples or pears
Other options: coconut shreds, cacao nibs, goji berries, plant-based milk, 1 Tbsp green protein powder
Natural sweetener to taste (agave or maple syrup, xylitol, stevia)
Pinch of Celtic sea salt
Drizzle of DHA/EPA omega-3 oil

DIRECTIONS
Bring water to a boil, and stir in oats. Reduce heat and cook for 5-7 minutes, stirring occasionally. Add vanilla, cinnamon, and nutmeg in last minute of cooking. Remove from heat and scoop into a bowl. (Mix in green protein powder now if you have just worked out and like green oatmeal!) Sprinkle lightly with more cinnamon and nutmeg. Shave raw ginger root and turmeric root on top. Add nuts or seeds of choice. Add dried or fresh fruit of choice. Add other options of choice. Lightly salt, drizzle oil, and enjoy.

NOTE: Eat 2 servings of raw fruit this morning in addition to your oatmeal, separately, to make sure you are getting your daily fruit.

***

FOREVER A KID CEREAL
Prep Time: 5 mins
Cook Time: 0 mins
Serves 1

INGREDIENTS
2 cups organic cereal like granola or muesli, gluten-free as needed

1/2 banana, sliced
1/4 cup mixed fresh berries (strawberries, blueberries, raspberries)
1 tsp shaved raw ginger
Dash of cinnamon, nutmeg, and/or allspice
Drizzle of agave syrup
½ cup plant-based milk or yoghurt

DIRECTIONS
Throw in a bowl and enjoy!

***

AMAZING FRUIT SALAD
Prep Time: 10 mins
Cook Time: 0 mins
Serves 2

INGREDIENTS
1 banana, sliced
1 cup mixed fresh berries (strawberries, blueberries, raspberries)
1 apple, chopped
½ tropical fruit of choice (papaya, pineapple, mango, or kiwi)
½ avocado
handful of walnuts
1 Tbsp of hemp seeds
1 Tbsp shaved raw ginger
1 Tbsp shaved raw turmeric
Dash of cinnamon, nutmeg, and/or allspice
Drizzle of agave syrup
Juice from ½ lime
1 Tbsp fresh chopped mint or cilantro, optional

DIRECTIONS
Chop it all up and enjoy!

***

BREAKFAST TOASTIES
Prep Time: 5 mins
Cook Time: 0 mins
Serves 1

INGREDIENTS
2 slices of whole grain sprouted wheat OR gluten-free bread, toasted

Options:
PB&J: 1 Tbsp peanut butter, 1 Tbsp no-sugar-added fruit jam
AB&F: 1 Tbsp almond butter, thinly sliced fresh fruit (apple, pear, or banana), cinnamon
Blueberry Toastie: 1 Tbsp peanut/almond butter, cover butter with blueberries
Surfer Toastie: 1 Tbsp peanut/almond butter, banana slices, drizzle agave syrup
California Toastie: ½ avocado sliced thin, sunflower seeds, paprika, sea salt, black pepper
Hippie Toastie: ½ avocado, hemp seeds, mushrooms, thinly sliced tomato, sea salt, black pepper
Warrior Toastie: vegan sausage or bacon, raw spinach, thinly sliced tomato, sea salt, black pepper
Foodie Toastie: ½ avocado, rosemary marcona almonds, chopped cilantro, sea salt, black pepper

DIRECTIONS
Toast 2 pieces of bread. After toasted, spread your nut butter or avo on one piece, stack the other things on top, sprinkle your seasonings, and top with second piece of toast. Enjoy!

***

BLUEBERRY FLAX PANCAKES
Prep Time: 10 mins
Cook Time: 10 mins
Serves 8

INGREDIENTS
1 ½ cups all-purpose gluten-free flour
2 tsp aluminum-free baking powder
½ tsp Celtic sea salt
1 tsp ground cinnamon (optional)
½ cup flax seed meal
2 Tbsp canola oil
1/3 cup water
1 to 1 ¼ cups plain rice or almond milk
2 Tbsp pure maple syrup
1 tsp pure vanilla extract
1 cup fresh or thawed blueberries

DIRECTIONS
Set a cast-iron or stainless-steel skillet over medium heat.

In a medium bowl, stir together the flour, baking soda, salt, cinnamon, and flax seed meal. Make a well in the center and pour in the oil, water, milk, maple syrup, and vanilla. Stir just until moistened.

Spray the pan with a light coat of cooking spray or light coat of coconut oil. Spoon 1/4 cupfuls of batter onto the hot skillet. Sprinkle with as many blueberries as desired. Cook until bubbles appear on the surface, then flip and cook until browned on the other side. Serve and enjoy!

***

POTATO & KALE SQUARES
Prep Time: 15 mins
Cook Time: 30 mins
Makes 16 squares

INGREDIENTS
3 pounds potatoes, cut into ½-inch chunks
1/4 cup nutritional yeast
1/4 cup olive oil

1 bunch black kale, stems removed, leaves chopped into bits
2 Tbsp chopped fresh oregano
1 Tbsp chopped fresh dill
2 Tbsp fresh lemon juice
Lemon zest from 1 lemon
1 1/2 tsp Celtic sea salt
Black pepper to taste
1 1/4 cups gluten-free breadcrumbs
Paprika
Fresh oregano for garnish (optional)

DIRECTIONS

In a large cast-iron pot, cover potatoes with water and bring to a boil. Lower heat to simmer for 20 minutes. Drain and place potatoes in large mixing bowl. Preheat oven to 400 degrees F.

Use a potato masher and mash the potatoes. Add nutritional yeast and oil and mash until creamy. Combine kale with potatoes. Add oregano, dill, lemon juice, zest, and several dashes of pepper to taste. Mix in 1 cup of breadcrumbs. Taste and adjust salt, pepper to taste.

Lightly grease a 9x13 baking pan with coconut oil. Spread potatoes in evenly and cover with ¼ cup breadcrumbs and a few dashes of paprika. Lightly drizzle breadcrumbs with olive oil to barely moisten. Bake for 30 minutes, and let cool for at least 10 minutes before cutting into squares. Let cool completely before serving, and sprinkle with fresh oregano as garnish. Serve with fresh tomatillo salsa on the side for a spicy kick.

***

LAVENDER BLUEBERRY SCONES
Prep Time: 10 mins
Cook Time: 20 mins
Makes 12 scones

INGREDIENTS
1 ¼ cups almond milk, unsweetened
2 tsp apple-cider vinegar
3 cups gluten-free coconut flour
2 Tbsp aluminum-free baking powder
½ tsp Celtic sea salt
½ cup raw organic sugar, plus extra for sprinkling
¼ cup finely chopped fresh culinary lavender
½ cup nonhydrogenated vegetable shortening
2 cups blueberries
2 Tbsp canola oil
1 tsp pure vanilla extract

DIRECTIONS
Preheat oven to 375 degrees F. Lightly grease a baking sheet with coconut oil or line with parchment paper. Measure out the milk in a measuring cup and add the vinegar to it. Set aside to curdle.

Combine the flour, baking powder, salt, sugar, and lavender in a large mixing bowl. Add the shortening in small spoonfuls, then use your (clean!) fingers to knead the shortening into the flour until the dough has a pebble-like consistency. Add the milk mixture, oil, and vanilla. Mix with a wooden spoon until all ingredients are just moistened, taking care not to over-mix (a couple dry spots here and there are fine). Fold in the blueberries. Spray a small measuring cup with cooking spray and use the cup to scoop scones onto baking sheet.

Dust the tops of scones with sugar and bake for 18-22 mins, or until tops are lightly browned. Cool on a cooling rack, but try to eat at least one still warm from the oven with a cup of tea!

***

SOUTHWESTERN TOFU SCRAMBLE
Prep Time: 20 mins

Cook Time: 15 mins
Serves: 6

INGREDIENTS
1/8 cup low-sodium veggie broth
1 medium red bell pepper, diced (about 1 cup)
1 small carrot, diced (about ½ cup)
4 green onions, chopped (about ½ cup)
1 clove garlic, minced (about 1 tsp)
½ tsp ground cumin
¼ tsp ground turmeric
1 14-oz. pkg. medium tofu, drained and crumbled
½ tsp hot sauce
2 Tbsp chopped cilantro
salsa, for garnish

DIRECTIONS
Heat 1/8 cup broth in large cast-iron skillet over medium heat. Add bell pepper and carrot, and cook 7 minutes, or until just tender. Stir in green onions, garlic, cumin, and turmeric, and cook 1 minute more. Add tofu and hot sauce, and cook 5 minutes, or until heated through and all liquid has cooked off. Stir in cilantro, and serve with salsa.

***

LEMON POPPY-SEED MUFFINS
Prep Time: 10 mins
Cook Time: 25 mins
Makes 12 muffins

INGREDIENTS
2 cups coconut flour
2/3 cup raw sugar
1 Tbsp aluminum-free baking powder
5 tsp poppy seeds
½ tsp Celtic sea salt
1 cup almond milk

¼ cup fresh lemon juice
1/2 cup canola oil
2 Tbsp lemon zest
2 tsp pure vanilla extract

DIRECTIONS
Preheat oven to 375 degrees F. Lightly grease a muffin tin with coconut oil.

In a large mixing bowl, blend the flour, sugar, baking powder, poppy seeds, and salt. Add the milk, lemon juice, canola oil, zest, and vanilla and stir.

Scoop batter into muffin tins, almost filling each cup. Bake for 23-27 minutes, or until a toothpick inserted into center comes out clean. Let cool on rack and enjoy.

***

DINNER RECIPES:

LEMON ORZO PRIMAVERA
Prep Time: 15 mins
Cook Time: 15 mins
Serves 4

INGREDIENTS
1/8 cup low-sodium veggie broth
1 cup uncooked orzo pasta
1 clove garlic, crushed
1 medium zucchini, shredded
1 medium carrot, shredded
14 oz. low-sodium veggie broth
1 lemon, zested
1 Tbsp chopped fresh thyme + sprigs for garnish
1/8 cup nutritional yeast

DIRECTIONS

Heat 1/8 cup broth in a pot over medium heat. Stir in orzo, and cook 2 minutes, until golden. Stir in garlic, zucchini, and carrot, and cook 2 minutes. Pour in the rest of the broth and mix in lemon zest. Bring to a boil. Reduce heat to low and simmer 10 minutes, or until liquid has been absorbed and orzo is tender. Season with thyme and top with nutritional yeast and a sprig of thyme to serve.

***

MEGA VEGGIE BURRITOS
Prep Time: 90 mins
Cook Time: 10 mins
Serves 4

INGREDIENTS
1/8 cup low-sodium veggie broth
8 oz. organic baked savory tofu, thinly sliced
1/2 cup organic corn kernels, rinsed and drained
1/2 cup organic black beans, rinsed and drained
1/2 cup diced brown mushrooms
1 large green bell pepper, seeded and diced
4 tomatillos, diced
1 cup organic salsa
1 tsp ground cumin
Sea salt and freshly ground black pepper
1/2 cup + 4 Tbsp chopped fresh cilantro, divided
2 cups shredded vegan cheddar cheese, optional
1 jalapeño chili, minced, optional
4 10-inch, round flour tortillas (gluten-free as needed)
1 avocado, peeled and diced
2 limes

DIRECTIONS
Preheat broiler. Heat large skillet over medium heat, and add veggie broth. When hot, place tofu slices in broth, and sauté 2 to 3 minutes. Add corn, beans, mushrooms, green pepper, tomatillos, salsa, cumin, salt and pepper. Reduce heat to

medium-low, and cook 10 minutes, stirring occasionally. Stir in 1/2 cup cilantro, and remove from heat.

Meanwhile, sprinkle 1/2 cup cheese and one-quarter amount of jalapeño, if using, on tortilla, and broil until cheese melts and bubbles. Remove from broiler, spoon on tempeh mixture, sprinkle with one-quarter avocado, 1 Tbsp chopped fresh cilantro, squeeze of fresh lime, and wrap. Repeat with remaining ingredients until used up. Serve while hot.

***

THAI COCONUT MILK SOUP
Prep Time: 15 mins
Cook Time: 20 mins
Serves 4

INGREDIENTS
1/8 cup low-sodium veggie broth
1/2 onion, sliced
2 carrots, peeled and cut into matchsticks
1 cup shiitake mushrooms, sliced
3 cloves garlic, chopped
1–2 red Thai (or jalapeño) peppers, seeded and finely chopped
1 1/2 cups low-sodium veggie broth
1 12-oz. can coconut milk
1 Tbsp grated ginger
1 4-inch piece of lemon grass, cut into very thin (1/16 inch) slices on the diagonal
1 tsp grated lime zest
Juice of 1 lime
1 16-oz. pkg. extra-firm tofu, raw, fried, or baked, and diced
Sea Salt (optional) and black pepper to taste
2 Tbsp chopped cilantro
Lime wedges

DIRECTIONS

In a medium saucepan, bring 1/8 cup veggie broth to medium heat. Add the onion, carrots, and shiitake mushrooms and sauté for 3 minutes. Add the garlic and peppers and sauté for another minute.

Pour in 1 ½ cups veggie broth and coconut milk. Stir in the ginger, lemon grass, lime zest, lime juice, and tofu, then bring to a simmer. Reduce the heat to low and cook for 15 minutes.

Remove from the heat and season with salt, if desired. Add the cilantro, then serve with a lime wedge.

***

GREEK SALAD
Prep Time: 15 mins
Cook Time: 0 mins
Serves: 4

INGREDIENTS
1 garlic clove, chopped
¼ small cucumber, peeled, quartered
Celtic or Himalayan sea salt
½ container coconut-milk yogurt
Fresh squeezed lemon or lime juice (3 wedges)
1 Tbsp chopped fresh dill, mint, or Italian parsley (or a mix of the 3)
Fresh ground black pepper
3 oz. organic baked savory tofu, diced
1/2 tsp dried oregano
1/2 tsp dried rosemary
1/2 Tbsp olive oil
1 Tbsp red-wine vinegar
½ medium-sized head romaine lettuce, finely chopped (about 3 cups)
1 celery stalk, finely chopped
1 medium heirloom tomato, finely chopped
1/4 cup purple onions, finely chopped
1/2 red bell pepper, finely chopped

1/2 orange bell pepper, finely chopped
1/8 cup Kalamata olives

DIRECTIONS
In a food processor or high-speed blender, combine the garlic, cucumber and ¼ tsp salt. Process to a paste. Add the yogurt, 1 wedge lemon juice, dill, salt and pepper to taste. Process until well blended.

In a bowl, combine the tofu, oregano, rosemary, juice from 2 lemon wedges, oil and vinegar, tossing to coat.

Put lettuce into large serving bowl. Add the tofu mixture, onion, celery, tomato, onions, bell peppers, and olives. Drizzle on the yogurt dressing, toss and enjoy!

***

SIMPLE SPAGHETTI SQUASH
Prep Time: 10 mins
Cook Time: 40 mins
Serves 2

INGREDIENTS
1 medium spaghetti squash
Coconut oil
Sea salt and black pepper
Italian herbs mix
1 jar organic marinara sauce
1 vegan Italian sausage, chopped (optional)
Fresh basil leaves
Nutritional yeast
Fresh lime

DIRECTIONS
Preheat oven to 400 degrees. Microwave spaghetti squash for one minute to make it easier to cut in half. Chop spaghetti squash in half and scrape out seeds. Season with coconut oil, salt, pepper, and Italian herbs. Place flesh side down on a foil-

lined baking tray and roast for 30-40 minutes until fully cooked. Remove from oven and let rest until cool enough to handle.

Meanwhile, heat organic marinara sauce of choice in a sauté pan. When squash is cool enough to handle, use a large kitchen fork or spoon to scrape the strands of squash from inside the skin into a large pot on low heat. Pour in MOST of the marinara sauce (reserve some on side), throw in some fresh basil leaves, salt and pepper to taste, and toss all together. Serve garnished with extra sauce, some fresh basil leaves, a sprinkle of nutritional yeast (for a parmesan cheese–like flavor), and a squeeze of fresh lemon or lime. Enjoy!

***

MOROCCAN LENTIL STEW w/RAISINS
Prep Time: 10 mins
Cook Time: 30 mins
Serves 4

INGREDIENTS
1/8 cup low-sodium veggie broth
1/2 cup chopped onion
2 cloves garlic, minced
1 14-oz. can crushed tomatoes
1 18.2-oz. carton prepared lentil soup, such as Dr. McDougall's or Trader Joe's
1/2 15-oz. can chickpeas, rinsed and drained
1/4 cup raisins or dried currants
1 tsp ground cinnamon, or more to taste
1 tsp ground cumin
1/4 tsp red pepper flakes, or to taste
3 Tbsp plain nonfat coconut or soy yogurt, optional
1 Tbsp chopped cilantro, optional

DIRECTIONS
Heat 1/8 cup broth in medium saucepan over medium heat. Add onion, and sauté 3 minutes, or until softened and translucent. Add garlic, and cook 1 minute, or until garlic is softened, but not browned, stirring constantly.

Stir in tomatoes, soup, chickpeas, raisins, cinnamon, cumin, and red pepper flakes. Season with salt and pepper, if desired. Bring stew to a simmer over medium-high heat, stirring occasionally.

Reduce heat to medium-low, and simmer, uncovered, 20 minutes, or until mixture is reduced and sauce has thickened, stirring often from bottom to prevent sticking. Garnish each serving with 1 Tbsp yogurt and cilantro, if using.

***

TUSCAN PASTA
Prep Time: 15 mins
Cook Time: 15 mins
Serves 4

INGREDIENTS
1 bottle Chianti red wine
Coarse Celtic sea salt
1 pound gluten-free spaghetti
3 Tbsp coconut oil
¼ pound vegan "bacon"
3 Portobello mushroom caps, thinly sliced
2-3 sprigs fresh rosemary, chopped leaves
4 garlic cloves, chopped
2 pinches red pepper flakes
4-5 cups chopped dark greens (choice of chard, escarole, spinach, or kale)
Black pepper, to taste
1/4 tsp freshly grated nutmeg (dried spice ok, but fresh is better!)

Nutritional yeast

<u>DIRECTIONS</u>
Pour the entire bottle of wine into a large pot. Add water and fill the pot up as you would to cook pasta. Bring the wine and water to a boil over high heat. When the liquids boil, add salt and the pasta and cook to al dente per package directions.

While pasta is cooking, heat a large cast-iron skillet over medium heat. Add 2 tablespoons coconut oil, then chop and add the "bacon." Brown the pieces slightly (about 3 mins) then transfer them to a paper-towel-lined plate. Add the mushrooms to the oil in the same skillet, season with the chopped rosemary, and cook until deeply golden, 6-8 mins. Push mushrooms to sides of pan, then add 1 more tablespoon coconut oil to the center. Add the garlic and red pepper flakes and cook for a minute or so, then toss the mushrooms together with the garlic. Add the greens to the pan and season them with salt, pepper, and the nutmeg. When the greens have wilted down (after just a couple minutes or so), add a couple ladles of the pasta cooking liquid to the pan and cook for a minute to reduce.

By this time the pasta should be done. Drain the pasta well and add it to the skillet. Add the bacon. Toss the pasta for a minute or so to allow it to absorb the remaining liquid. Adjust the seasonings and serve with nutritional yeast on side to add a parmesan-like flavor!

***

PAPAYA AVOCADO SALAD
Prep Time: 10 mins
Cook Time: 0 mins
Serves 2

<u>INGREDIENTS</u>
1 Tbsp red onion, chopped
1 Tbsp lime juice

1 medium Hass avocados, diced
1 papaya, diced
1 Tbsp chopped cilantro
Sea salt and pepper to taste

DIRECTIONS
In a small bowl combine onion, lime juice, and salt.

In a medium bowl, combine avocados, papaya, and cilantro. Toss with lime juice and onions and serve immediately.

***

TEX-MEX CHILI
Prep Time: 15 mins
Cook Time: 60 mins
Serves 4

INGREDIENTS
1/8 cup low-sodium veggie broth
1 medium onion, peeled and finely chopped
3 garlic cloves, peeled and finely chopped
1/2 large green pepper, seeds removed and finely chopped
1/4–1 jalapeno pepper, finely chopped
1 chipotle chili, finely chopped
1 1/2 tsp ground cumin seeds
2 tsp paprika
1/2 tsp dried thyme
1/2 tsp dried crumbled sage
1 tsp dried oregano
1/4 tsp cayenne
1 cup lentils, picked over and washed
1 cup cooked drained red kidney beans
2–3 canned plum tomatoes, drained and finely chopped
5 Tbsp chopped fresh cilantro leaves (divided)
Celtic sea salt to taste
1 Tbsp yellow non-GMO cornmeal
Garnishes: fresh cilantro, chopped avocado, squeeze of lime

DIRECTIONS
Put the broth in a large cast-iron pot and set over medium-high heat. When hot, put in the onion, garlic, green pepper, jalapeno, and chipotle. Stir and fry for about 3 minutes, or until the seasonings just start to brown. Turn the heat to medium-low and continue to sauté for another 3 minutes. Now put in the cumin, paprika, thyme, sage, oregano, and cayenne. Stir briskly once or twice and put in the lentils, 4 1/2 cups of water, the red kidney beans, plum tomatoes, 3 Tbsp cilantro leaves, and salt. Bring to a boil. Cover, turn the heat down to low, and cook gently for 50 minutes.

Mix the cornmeal with 3 tablespoons water and then pour the mixture into the chili pot. Stir to mix and bring to a simmer. Cover and simmer gently for 10 minutes, stirring now and then. Serve with chopped fresh cilantro, chopped avocado, and a squeeze of fresh lime.

***

LAZY CALIFORNIA BOWL
Prep Time: 10 mins
Cook Time: 30 mins
Serves 4

INGREDIENTS
1 cup uncooked red quinoa, rinsed and drained
1 15.5-oz. can organic black beans, rinsed and drained 1 garlic clove, minced
1/4 medium yellow onion, chopped
1 cup broccoli, chopped
1 cup carrots, peeled and chopped
1 cup shitake or cremini mushrooms, sliced
1/2 cup chopped cilantro

DIRECTIONS

Place 1 1/2 cups water in a saucepan, add 1/2 tsp salt, and bring to a boil. Add the quinoa, return to a boil, then reduce the heat to a simmer. Cover and cook until the quinoa is tender and the water absorbed, about 15 minutes. Remove from heat and set aside.

In a medium saucepan, sauté the garlic and onion in 1/2 cup water for 5 minutes. Add the carrots and broccoli and simmer 10 minutes over medium heat. Add the mushrooms and cook for 5 minutes more. Pour off any water, then add black beans to pan, heating only until warm. Add salt and pepper to taste.

Put 3/4 cup cooked quinoa into each of 4 bowls, add the beans and veggies mixture, and sprinkle with chopped cilantro.

***

IRISH LAGER STEW

Prep Time: 30 mins
Cook Time: 60 mins
Serves 8

INGREDIENTS

1/8 cup + 1 ½ cups low-sodium veggie broth
8 oz. button or shiitake mushrooms, halved
2 cloves garlic, minced (2 tsp)
1 medium leek, white part only, diced (1 cup)
3 small red potatoes, cut into 1-inch cubes (1 ½ cups)
2 medium carrots, peeled and sliced (2 cups)
2 small parsnips, peeled and sliced (1 ½ cups)
1 ½ tsp tomato paste
1 15-oz. can crushed tomatoes
2 sprigs fresh thyme, tied in bundle, plus 1 tsp chopped fresh thyme, divided
½ cup lager beer
1 ½ Tbsp quick-cooking tapioca

1 cup shredded cabbage
1 Tbsp white miso
2 Tbsp chopped parsley

DIRECTIONS

Heat 1/8 cup veggie broth in large pot over medium heat. Add mushrooms and garlic; sauté 8 minutes, or until mushrooms are browned. Remove from pan. Add remaining 1/2 Tbsp oil to pot. Add leek, and cook 5 minutes. Add potatoes, carrots, parsnips, and tomato paste. Cook 2 minutes. Add tomatoes, broth, and thyme sprigs; bring to a boil. Reduce heat to medium-low, cover, and simmer 40 minutes, stirring occasionally.

Add lager, tapioca, and mushrooms. Simmer 10 to 15 minutes, or until thickened, stirring often. Remove thyme sprigs, stir in cabbage and miso, and simmer 4 to 5 minutes, or until cabbage softens. Stir in chopped thyme and parsley, and season with salt and pepper, if desired.

***

RAINBOW STIR-FRY

Prep Time: 15 mins
Cook Time: 15 mins
Serves 4

INGREDIENTS

3 Tbsp frozen orange juice concentrate
2 Tbsp hoisin sauce
1 Tbsp nama shoyu
1/2 tsp chili-garlic sauce
2 tsp toasted sesame oil
1/2 lb. green beans, halved crosswise
1 cup thinly sliced purple cabbage
1 15-oz. can baby corn, rinsed and drained
1 small red bell pepper, sliced (1 cup)
1 cup frozen, shelled edamame

1 8-oz. can sliced water chestnuts, drained
4 green onions, thinly sliced

DIRECTIONS
Whisk together orange juice concentrate, hoisin sauce, nama shoyu, and chili-garlic sauce in small bowl. Heat oil in wok or large skillet over high heat. Add green beans, and stir-fry 3 minutes. Add 3 Tbsp water; stir-fry 3 minutes more. Add cabbage, baby corn, bell pepper, edamame, and water chestnuts; stir-fry 4 minutes. Stir in green onions and orange juice mixture; cook 1 minute more. Serve over brown rice, with raw, dark-green salad on side.

***

MEXICALI CHOPPED SALAD
Prep Time: 30 mins
Cook Time: 15 mins
Serves 8

INGREDIENTS
Tortilla Strips:
1 ½ tsp sunflower oil
3 6-inch corn tortillas
½ tsp chili powder
¼ tsp maple crystals or sugar
⅛ tsp salt
Dressing
½ cup olive oil
2 cloves garlic, minced (2 tsp)
2 tsp ground cumin
2 tsp ground coriander
1 tsp sugar
1 tsp salt
⅓ cup lime juice
¼ cup chopped green onion
¼ cup cilantro leaves

Pinch cayenne pepper

Salad:
1 head romaine lettuce, sliced (8 cups)
2 medium tomatoes, chopped (2 cups)
1 avocado, diced (1 cup)
3 celery stalks, sliced (1 cup)
1 cucumber, seeded and diced (1 cup)
1 cup fresh or frozen, thawed corn kernels
¾ cup cooked pinto beans
½ cup jarred roasted red bell peppers, rinsed, drained, and sliced
⅓ cup finely chopped red onion

DIRECTIONS
To make tortilla strips: Preheat oven to 350°F. Brush oil on tortillas. Cut in half, then cut into 1/8-inch-wide strips. Spread on baking sheet. Combine chili powder, maple crystals, and salt in bowl. Sprinkle chili powder mixture over strips. Bake 15 minutes, or until crisp. Cool.

To make dressing: heat oil, garlic, cumin, coriander, sugar, and salt in saucepan 2 to 3 minutes over low heat, or until garlic begins to sizzle.

Blend remaining dressing ingredients with garlic oil in blender until smooth.

Toss together all salad ingredients with tortilla strips and 1/4 cup dressing.

***

INDIAN KICHAREE
Prep Time: 15 mins
Cook Time: 90 mins
Serves 4

INGREDIENTS
1 1/2 Tbsp coconut oil
1 medium onion, minced
3 cloves garlic, minced
1 tsp turmeric
2 tsp mustard seed
1 ½ tsp coriander powder
1 ½ tsp cumin
Pinch of asafetida
5 cups purified water
1/2 cup pearl barley
1/4 cup green lentils, or mung beans
1/4 cup quinoa
3 slices fresh ginger, ½" thick
1cup shiitake mushrooms
1 parsnip, thinly sliced
¼ cup chopped parsley
2 Tbsp chopped cilantro
1 cup broccoli, chopped
1/2 cup dandelion greens, sliced
Dash of black or white pepper
Dash of cayenne
Sea salt, Bragg's amino acids, or tamari to taste

DIRECTIONS
Rinse the grains thoroughly.

Sauté garlic and onion in coconut oil in a soup pot or stockpot.

Add turmeric, coriander, cumin, asafetida, and mustard seed. Continue to sauté until seeds begin to pop.

Add water, barley, beans, quinoa, and ginger.

Simmer 50 to 60 minutes on low, stirring occasionally.

Add mushrooms, parsnips, and parsley.

Simmer 25 to 30 minutes. Add another cup of water if needed.

Add broccoli, cilantro, dandelion greens, and pepper.

Stir and cover. Simmer 10 to 12 minutes.

For creamier texture, remove 2 cups soup, and puree. Mix blended portion back into kicharee.

Add salt, aminos, or tamari, to taste.

***

SWEET POTATO AND BLACK BEAN SALAD
Prep Time: 15 mins
Cook Time: 30 mins
Serves: 2

INGREDIENTS:
¾ pounds sweet potatoes, peeled and cut into 1-inch dice
1 ½ Tbsp olive oil, plus more for drizzling
sea salt and fresh ground black pepper
¾ cups cooked black beans or ½ (15.5-oz.) can black beans, rinsed and drained
½ cup fresh or thawed frozen peas
¼ cup unsalted roasted cashews or pecan pieces
1/8 cup dried cranberries
1 celery rib, minced
2 scallions, chopped
1/8 cup fresh squeezed orange juice
½ Tbsp fresh squeezed lemon juice
1 tsp agave syrup (optional)
2 cups chopped romaine

DIRECTIONS
Preheat the oven to 425 degrees. Lightly oil a baking sheet and spread the sweet potatoes on the sheet in a single layer. Drizzle with a little olive oil. Season to taste with salt and

pepper. Roast the sweet potatoes until just tender, about 30 minutes, turning once halfway through. Set aside to cool.

In a large bowl, combine the black beans, peas, cashews, cranberries, celery, and scallions.

In a small bowl, combine the orange juice, lemon juice, agave, pinch of black pepper, and salt to taste. Whisk in the 1 ½ Tbsp olive oil to blend.

Add the cooled sweet potatoes to the bowl containing the vegetables. Pour the dressing over the salad and toss gently to combine. Taste and adjust the seasonings if needed.

Arrange the lettuce leaves in a shallow serving bowl, top with the potato-bean mixture, and serve.

Appendix B – Supplemental Info

────────────────●●●────────────────

TABLE 1 – COMPARATIVE ANATOMY

	Carnivore	Herbivore	Omnivore	Human
Mouth Opening vs. Head Size	Large	Small	Large	Small
Teeth (Incisors)	Short and pointed	Broad, flattened and spade shaped	Short and pointed	Broad, flattened and spade shaped
Teeth (Canines)	Long, sharp and curved	Dull and short or long (for defense), or none	Long, sharp and curved	Short and blunted
Saliva	No digestive enzymes	Carbohydrate digesting enzymes	No digestive enzymes	Carbohydrate digesting enzymes
Stomach Type	Simple	Simple or multiple chambers	Simple	Simple
Stomach Acidity	Less than or equal to pH 1 with food in stomach	pH 4 to 5 with food in stomach	Less than or equal to pH 1 with food in stomach	pH 4 to 5 with food in stomach
Stomach Capacity	60% to 70% of total volume of digestive tract	Less than 30% of total volume of digestive tract	60% to 70% of total volume of digestive tract	21% to 27% of total volume of digestive tract
Length of Small Intestine	3 to 6 times body length	10 to more than 12 times body length	4 to 6 times body length	10 to 11 times body length
Colon	Simple, short and smooth	Long, complex; may be sacculated	Simple, short and smooth	Long, complex; may be sacculated
Nails	Sharp claws	Flattened nails or blunt hooves	Sharp claws	Flattened nails

From *"The Comparative Anatomy of Eating,"* by Dr. Milton R. Mills, M.D. bit.ly/1bGBr45

TABLE 2 – MORTALITY FROM HEART DISEASE, WWII

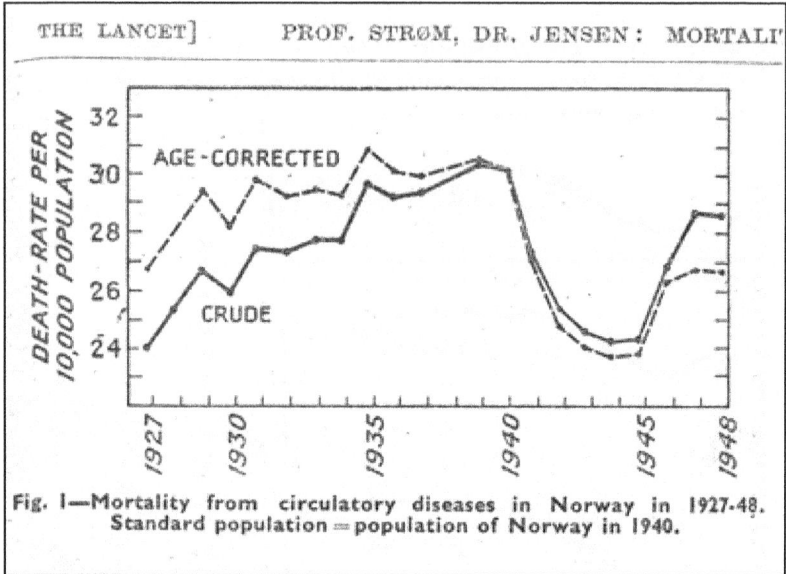

THE LANCET]   PROF. STRØM, DR. JENSEN : MORTALI'

Fig. I—Mortality from circulatory diseases in Norway in 1927-48. Standard population = population of Norway in 1940.

University of Minnesota, Heart Attack Prevention: A History of Cardovascular Epidemiology, Origins: 1900-1940s, *Mortality Statistics* www.epi.umn.edu/cvdepi/history-gallery/mortality-statistics/

TABLE 3 – VITAMINS

Dietary Reference Intakes (DRIs): Recommended Dietary Allowances and Adequate Intakes, Vitamins
Food and Nutrition Board, Institute of Medicine, National Academies

Life-Stage Group	Vitamin A (µg/d)[a]	Vitamin C (mg/d)	Vitamin D (µg/d)[b,c]	Vitamin E (mg/d)[d]	Vitamin K (µg/d)	Thiamin (mg/d)	Riboflavin (mg/d)	Niacin (mg/d)[e]	Vitamin B6 (mg/d)	Folate (µg/d)[f]	Vitamin B12 (µg/d)	Pantothenic Acid (mg/d)	Biotin (µg/d)	Choline (mg/d)[g]
Infants														
0 to 6 mo	400*	40*	10	4*	2.0*	0.2*	0.3*	2*	0.1*	65*	0.4*	1.7*	5*	125*
6 to 12 mo	500*	50*	10	5*	2.5*	0.3*	0.4*	4*	0.3*	80*	0.5*	1.8*	6*	150*
Children														
1–3 y	300	15	15	6	30*	0.5	0.5	6	0.5	150	0.9	2*	8*	200*
4–8 y	400	25	15	7	55*	0.6	0.6	8	0.6	200	1.2	3*	12*	250*
Males														
9–13 y	600	45	15	11	60*	0.9	0.9	12	1.0	300	1.8	4*	20*	375*
14–18 y	900	75	15	15	75*	1.2	1.3	16	1.3	400	2.4	5*	25*	550*
19–30 y	900	90	15	15	120*	1.2	1.3	16	1.3	400	2.4	5*	30*	550*
31–50 y	900	90	15	15	120*	1.2	1.3	16	1.3	400	2.4	5*	30*	550*
51–70 y	900	90	15	15	120*	1.2	1.3	16	1.7	400	2.4[h]	5*	30*	550*
> 70 y	900	90	20	15	120*	1.2	1.3	16	1.7	400	2.4[h]	5*	30*	550*
Females														
9–13 y	600	45	15	11	60*	0.9	0.9	12	1.0	300	1.8	4*	20*	375*
14–18 y	700	65	15	15	75*	1.0	1.0	14	1.2	400[i]	2.4	5*	25*	400*
19–30 y	700	75	15	15	90*	1.1	1.1	14	1.3	400[i]	2.4	5*	30*	425*
31–50 y	700	75	15	15	90*	1.1	1.1	14	1.3	400[i]	2.4	5*	30*	425*
51–70 y	700	75	15	15	90*	1.1	1.1	14	1.5	400	2.4[h]	5*	30*	425*
> 70 y	700	75	20	15	90*	1.1	1.1	14	1.5	400	2.4[h]	5*	30*	425*
Pregnancy														
14–18 y	750	80	15	15	75*	1.4	1.4	18	1.9	600[i]	2.6	6*	30*	450*
19–30 y	770	85	15	15	90*	1.4	1.4	18	1.9	600[i]	2.6	6*	30*	450*
31–50 y	770	85	15	15	90*	1.4	1.4	18	1.9	600[i]	2.6	6*	30*	450*
Lactation														
14–18 y	1,200	115	15	19	75*	1.4	1.6	17	2.0	500	2.8	7*	35*	550*
19–30 y	1,300	120	15	19	90*	1.4	1.6	17	2.0	500	2.8	7*	35*	550*
31–50 y	1,300	120	15	19	90*	1.4	1.6	17	2.0	500	2.8	7*	35*	550*

NOTE: This table (taken from the DRI reports, see www.nap.edu) presents Recommended Dietary Allowances (RDAs) in **bold type** and Adequate Intakes (AIs) in ordinary type followed by an asterisk (*). An RDA is the average daily dietary intake level; sufficient to meet the nutrient requirements of nearly all (97-98 percent) healthy individuals in a group. It is calculated from an Estimated Average Requirement (EAR). If sufficient scientific evidence is not available to establish an EAR, and thus calculate an RDA, an AI is usually developed. For healthy breastfed infants, an AI is the mean intake. The AI for other life stage and gender groups is believed to cover the needs of all healthy individuals in the groups, but lack of data or uncertainty in the data prevent being able to specify with confidence the percentage of individuals covered by this intake.

[a] As retinol activity equivalents (RAEs). 1 RAE = 1 µg retinol, 12 µg β-carotene, 24 µg α-carotene, or 24 µg β-cryptoxanthin. The RAE for dietary provitamin A carotenoids is two-fold greater than retinol equivalents (RE), whereas the RAE for preformed vitamin A is the same as RE.

[b] As cholecalciferol. 1 µg cholecalciferol = 40 IU vitamin D.

[c] Under the assumption of minimal sunlight.

[d] As α-tocopherol. α-Tocopherol includes RRR-α-tocopherol, the only form of α-tocopherol that occurs naturally in foods, and the $2R$-stereoisomeric forms of α-tocopherol (RRR-, RSR-, RRS-, and RSS-α-tocopherol) that occur in fortified foods and supplements. It does not include the $2S$-stereoisomeric forms of α-tocopherol (SRR-, SSR-, SRS-, and SSS-α-tocopherol), also found in fortified foods and supplements.

[e] As niacin equivalents (NE). 1 mg of niacin = 60 mg of tryptophan; 0–6 months = preformed niacin (not NE).

[f] As dietary folate equivalents (DFE). 1 DFE = 1 µg food folate = 0.6 µg of folic acid from fortified food or as a supplement consumed with food = 0.5 µg of a supplement taken on an empty stomach.

[g] Although AIs have been set for choline, there are few data to assess whether a dietary supply of choline is needed at all stages of the life cycle, and it may be that the choline requirement can be met by endogenous synthesis at some of these stages.

[h] Because 10 to 30 percent of older people may malabsorb food-bound B_{12}, it is advisable for those older than 50 years to meet their RDA mainly by consuming foods fortified with B_{12} or a supplement containing B_{12}.

[i] In view of evidence linking folate intake with neural tube defects in the fetus, it is recommended that all women capable of becoming pregnant consume 400 µg from supplements or fortified foods in addition to intake of food folate from a varied diet.

TABLE 4 – MINERALS

Dietary Reference Intakes (DRIs): Recommended Intakes for Individuals, Elements
Food and Nutrition Board, Institute of Medicine, National Academies

Life Stage Group	Calcium (mg/d)	Chromium (µg/d)	Copper (µg/d)	Fluoride (mg/d)	Iodine (µg/d)	Iron (mg/d)	Magnesium (mg/d)	Manganese (mg/d)	Molybdenum (µg/d)	Phosphorus (mg/d)	Selenium (µg/d)	Zinc (mg/d)	Potassium (g/d)	Sodium (g/d)	Chloride (g/d)
Infants															
0–6 mo	210*	0.2*	200*	0.01*	110*	0.27*	30*	0.003*	2*	100*	15*	2*	0.4*	0.12*	0.18*
7–12 mo	270*	5.5*	220*	0.5*	130*	11	75*	0.6*	3*	275*	20*	3	0.7*	0.37*	0.57*
Children															
1–3 y	500*	11*	340	0.7*	90	7	80	1.2*	17	460	20	3	3.0*	1.0*	1.5*
4–8 y	800*	15*	440	1*	90	10	130	1.5*	22	500	30	5	3.8*	1.2*	1.9*
Males															
9–13 y	1,300*	25*	700	2*	120	8	240	1.9*	34	1,250	40	8	4.5*	1.5*	2.3*
14–18 y	1,300*	35*	890	3*	150	11	410	2.2*	43	1,250	55	11	4.7*	1.5*	2.3*
19–30 y	1,000*	35*	900	4*	150	8	400	2.3*	45	700	55	11	4.7*	1.5*	2.3*
31–50 y	1,000*	35*	900	4*	150	8	420	2.3*	45	700	55	11	4.7*	1.5*	2.3*
51–70 y	1,200*	30*	900	4*	150	8	420	2.3*	45	700	55	11	4.7*	1.3*	2.0*
>70 y	1,200*	30*	900	4*	150	8	420	2.3*	45	700	55	11	4.7*	1.2*	1.8*
Females															
9–13 y	1,300*	21*	700	2*	120	8	240	1.6*	34	1,250	40	8	4.5*	1.5*	2.3*
14–18 y	1,300*	24*	890	3*	150	15	360	1.6*	43	1,250	55	9	4.7*	1.5*	2.3*
19–30 y	1,000*	25*	900	3*	150	18	310	1.8*	45	700	55	8	4.7*	1.5*	2.3*
31–50 y	1,000*	25*	900	3*	150	18	320	1.8*	45	700	55	8	4.7*	1.5*	2.3*
51–70 y	1,200*	20*	900	3*	150	8	320	1.8*	45	700	55	8	4.7*	1.3*	2.0*
>70 y	1,200*	20*	900	3*	150	8	320	1.8*	45	700	55	8	4.7*	1.2*	1.8*
Pregnancy															
14–18 y	1,300*	29*	1,000	3*	220	27	400	2.0*	50	1,250	60	12	4.7*	1.5*	2.3*
19–30 y	1,000*	30*	1,000	3*	220	27	350	2.0*	50	700	60	11	4.7*	1.5*	2.3*
31–50 y	1,000*	30*	1,000	3*	220	27	360	2.0*	50	700	60	11	4.7*	1.5*	2.3*
Lactation															
14–18 y	1,300*	44*	1,300	3*	290	10	360	2.6*	50	1,250	70	13	5.1*	1.5*	2.3*
19–30 y	1,000*	45*	1,300	3*	290	9	310	2.6*	50	700	70	12	5.1*	1.5*	2.3*
31–50 y	1,000*	45*	1,300	3*	290	9	320	2.6*	50	700	70	12	5.1*	1.5*	2.3*

NOTE: This table presents Recommended Dietary Allowances (RDAs) in bold type and Adequate Intakes (AIs) in ordinary type followed by an asterisk (*). RDAs and AIs may both be used as goals for individual intake. RDAs are set to meet the needs of almost all (97 to 98 percent) individuals in a group. For healthy breastfed infants, the AI is the mean intake. The AI for other life stage and gender groups is believed to cover needs of all individuals in the group, but lack of data or uncertainty in the data prevent being able to specify with confidence the percentage of individuals covered by this intake.

SOURCES: Dietary Reference Intakes for Calcium, Phosphorus, Magnesium, Vitamin D, and Fluoride (1997); Dietary Reference Intakes for Thiamine, Riboflavin, Niacin, Vitamin B₆, Folate, Vitamin B₁₂, Pantothenic Acid, Biotin, and Choline (1998); Dietary Reference Intakes for Vitamin C, Vitamin E, Selenium, and Carotenoids (2000); Dietary Reference Intakes for Vitamin A, Vitamin K, Arsenic, Boron, Chromium, Copper, Iodine, Iron, Manganese, Molybdenum, Nickel, Silicon, Vanadium, and Zinc (2001); and Dietary Reference Intakes for Water, Potassium, Sodium, Chloride, and Sulfate (2004). These reports may be accessed via http://www.nap.edu.

TABLE 5 – ACID / ALKALINE FOODS

Food & Chemical Effects on Acid / Alkaline Body Chemical Balance™

Most Alkaline	More Alkaline	Low Alkaline	Lowest Alkaline	Food Category	Lowest Acid	Low Acid	More Acid	Most Acid
Baking Soda	Spices/Cinnamon Valerian Licorice •Black Cohash Agave	•Herbs (most) Arnica, Bergamot, Echinacea Chrysanthemum, Ephedra, Feverfew, Goldenseal, Lemongrass Aloe Vera Nettle Angelica	White Willow Bark Slippery Elm Artemesia Annua	Spice/Herb	Curry	Vanilla Stevia	Nutmeg	Pudding/Jam/Jelly
Sea Salt Mineral Water	•Kambucha	•Green or Mu Tea	Sulfite Ginger Tea	Preservative	MSG	Benzoate	Aspartame	Table Salt (NaCL)
				Beverage	Kona Coffee	Alcohol Black Tea	Coffee	Beet, 'Soda', Yeast/Hops/Malt
	Molasses Soy Sauce	Rice Syrup Apple Cider Vinegar	•Sucanat •Umeboshi Vinegar	Sweetner Vinegar	Honey/Maple Syrup Rice Vinegar	Balsamic Vinegar	Saccharin Red Wine Vinegar	Sugar/Cocoa White/Acetic Vinegar
•Umeboshi Plum		•Sake	•Algae, Blue Green	Therapeutic		Antihistamines	Psychotropics	Antibiotics
			•Ghee (Clarified Butter)	Processed Dairy	Cream/Butter	Cow Milk	•Casein, Milk Protein, Cottage Cheese	Processed Cheese
			Human Breast Milk	Cow/Human Soy Goat/Sheep	Yogurt Goat/Sheep Cheese	Aged Cheese Soy Cheese Goat Milk	New Cheese Soy Milk	Ice Cream
		•Quail Egg	•Duck Egg	Egg	Chicken Egg			
				Meat	Gelatin/Organs	Lamb/Mutton	Pork/Veal	Beef
				Game	•Venison	Boar/Elk>Game Meat	Bear	
				Fish/Shell Fish	Fish	Mollusks Shell Fish (Whole)	•Mussels/Squid	Shell Fish (Processed) •Lobster
				Fowl	Wild Duck	Goose/Turkey	Chicken	Pheasant
			Oat 'Grain Coffee' •Quinoa Wild Rice •Amaranth Japonica Rice	Grain Cereal Grass	•Triticale Millet Kasha Brown Rice	Buckwheat Wheat •Spelt/Teff/Kamut Farina/Semolina White Rice	Maize Barley Groat Corn Rye Oat Bran	Barley Processed Flour
Pumpkin Seed	Poppy Seed Cashew Chestnut Pepper	Primrose Oil Sesame Seed Cod Liver Oil Almond •Sprout	Avocado Oil Seeds (most) Coconut Oil Olive/Macadamia Oil Linseed/Flax Oil	Nut Seed/Sprout Oil	Pumpkin Seed Oil Grape Seed Oil Sunflower Oil Pine Nut Canola Oil	Almond Oil Sesame Oil Safflower Oil Tapioca •Seitan or Tofu	Pistachio Seed Chestnut Oil Lard Pecan Palm Kernel Oil	•Cottonseed Oil/Meal Hazelnut Walnut Brazil Nut Fried Food
•Hydrogenated Oil								
Lentil Brocoflower •Seaweed •Nori Kombu Wakame Hijiki Onion/Miso •Daikon/Taro Root •Sea Vegetables (other) Dandelion Greens •Burdock/Lotus Root Sweet Potato/Yam	Kohlrabi Parsnip/Taro Garlic Asparagus Kale/Parsley Endive/Arugula Mustard Greens Jerusalem Artichoke Ginger Root Broccoli	Potato/Bell Pepper Mushroom/Fungi Cauliflower Cabbage Rutabaga •Salsify/Ginseng Eggplant Pumpkin Collard Greens	Brussel Sprout Beet Chive/Cilantro Celery/Scallion Okra/Cucumber Turnip Greens Squash Artichoke Lettuce Jicama	Bean Vegetable Legume Pulse Root	Spinach Fava Bean Kidney Bean Black-eyed Pea String/Wax Bean Zucchini Chutney Rhubarb	Split Pea Pinto Bean White Bean Navy/Red Bean Aduki Bean Lima or Mung Bean Chard	Green Pea Peanut Snow Pea Legumes (other) Carrot ChickPea/Garbanzo	Green Pea Soybean Carob
Lime Nectarine Persimmon Raspberry Watermelon Tangerine Pineapple	Grapefruit Canteloupe Honeydew Citrus Olive •Dewberry Loganberry Mango	Lemon Pear Avocado Apple Blackberry Cherry Peach Papaya	Orange Apricot Banana Blueberry Pineapple Juice Raisin, Currant Grape Strawberry	Citrus Fruit Fruit	Coconut Guava •Pickled Fruit Dry Fruit Fig Persimmon Juice •Cherimoya Date	Plum Prune Tomato	Cranberry Pomegranate	

•Therapeutic, gourmet, or exotic items   Italicized items are NOT recommended

TABLE 6 – PCRM'S POWER PLATE

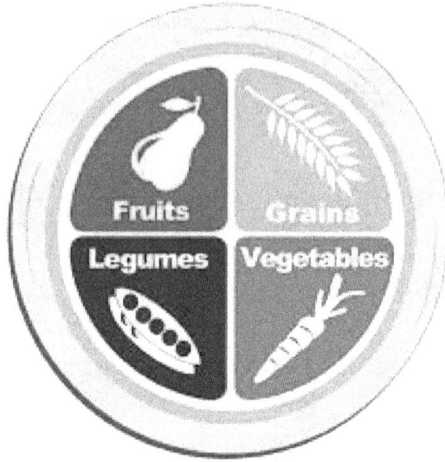

TABLE 7 – COOKING BEANS

Cooking Beans

Beans are a wonderful way to add high-quality, plant-based protein to your diet. They are high in iron, B vitamins and fiber, and are versatile enough that you may never tire of them. Dry beans stay fresh longer when stored in a cool, dark place (rather than on your countertop). Don't use beans that are more than a year old, as their nutrient content and digestibility are much lower. Also, old beans will not soften, even with thorough cooking. One last thing – always keep a variety of canned organic beans in your pantry! If you are running short on time to prepare dinner, there is no shame in opening up a can of canned beans, rinse and drain! Anyways, here are the basic directions for cooking beans from bulk:

1. Check beans for rocks and shriveled or broken pieces, then rinse.
2. Soak for six hours or overnight, with water covering four inches higher than the beans. Small and medium-size beans may require less soaking—about four hours should be enough. Lentils don' require any soaking at all.
   Note: If you've forgotten to presoak the beans, you can bring them to a boil in ample water to cover. Turn off the heat, cover the pot and let stand for one hour.
3. Drain and rinse the beans, discarding the soaking water. Always discard any loose skins before cooking, as this will increase digestibility.
4. Place the beans in a heavy pot and add 3 to 4 cups fresh water.
5. Bring to a full boil and skim off the foam.
6. Add a small piece of kombu (seaweed) and a few bay leaves or garlic cloves for flavor and better digestibility.
7. Cover, lower the temperature and simmer for the suggested time. Check beans 30 minutes before the minimum cooking time. Beans are done when the middle is soft and easy to squeeze.
8. About 10 minutes before the end of cooking time, add 1 teaspoon of unrefined sea salt.
9. Cook until beans are tender.

1 cup dry beans	cooking time
adzuki	45-60 minutes
anasazi	60-90 minutes
black (turtle)	60-90 minutes
black-eyed peas	60 minutes
cannellini	90-120 minutes
chickpeas (garbanzos)	120-180 minutes
cranberry	60-90 minutes
fava	60-90 minutes
great northern	90-120 minutes
kidney	60-90 minutes
lentils*	30-45 minutes
lima beans	60-90 minutes
mung	60 minutes
navy	60-90 minutes
pinto	90 minutes
split peas	45-60 minutes

*do not require soaking

All times are approximate. Cooking lengths depend on how strong the heat is and how hard the water is. A general rule is that small beans cook for approximately 30 minutes, medium beans cook for approximately 60 minutes, and large beans cook for approximately 90 minutes. Be sure to taste the beans to see if they are fully cooked and tender.

TABLE 8 – COOKING GRAINS

Cooking Grains

Whole grains are an excellent source of nutrition, as they contain complex carbohydrates and protein, essential enzymes, iron, dietary fiber, vitamin E and B-complex vitamins. Because the body absorbs grains slowly, they provide sustained and high-quality energy. Remember one cup of dry grain yields enough for 2 to 4 people. You may want to buy bulk canisters for each of these grains and create labels with amount of water and cooking times foe each.

Here are basic directions:

1. Measure the grain and rinse in cold water using a fine mesh strainer.
2. Optional: soak grains for one to eight hours to soften, increase digestibility and eliminate phytic acid. Drain grains and discard the soaking water.
3. Add grains to recommended amount of water and bring to a boil. For variety, try using low sodium veggie broth or coconut water instead of water.
4. A pinch of sea salt may be added to grains to help the cooking process, with the exception of kamut, amaranth and spelt (salt interferes with their cooking time).
5. Reduce heat, cover and simmer for the suggested amount of time, without stirring during the cooking process.
6. After cooking time is complete, uncover, fluff with a fork and eat

1 Cup Grains	Water	Cooking Time	Contains Gluten?
Common Grains:			
Brown rice	2 cups	45-60 minutes	no
Buckwheat (aka kasha)*	2 cups	20-30 minutes	no
Oats (whole groats)	3 cups	75-90 minutes	questionable due to content, contact, or contamination
Oatmeal (rolled oats)	2 cups	20-30 minutes	questionable due to content, contact, or contamination
Alternative Grains:			
Amaranth	3 cups	30 minutes	no
Barley (pearled)	2-3 cups	60 minutes	yes
Barley (hulled)	2-3 cups	90 minutes	yes
Bulgur (cracked wheat)	2 cups	20 minutes	yes
Cornmeal (aka polenta)	3 cups	20 minutes	no
Couscous**	1 cup	5 minutes	yes
Forbidden (black) rice	2 cups	30 minutes	no
Kamut	3 cups	90 minutes	yes
Millet	2 cups	30 minutes	no
Quinoa	2 cups	15-20 minutes	no
Rye berries	3 cups	2 hours	yes
Spelt	3 cups	2 hours	yes
Wheat berries	3 cups	60 minutes	yes
Wild rice	4 cups	60 minutes	no

*The texture of grains can be changed by boiling the water before adding the grains. This will keep the grains separated and prevent a mushy consistency. Do not add kasha to cold water, as it will not cook properly. For a softer, more porridge-like consistency, boil the grain and liquid together.
**Technically not a grain, but a small pasta product made from wheat and does not require soaking.

TABLE 9 – REFRIDGE REMINDER (example)

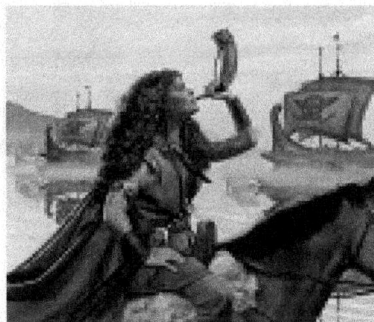

Warriors _ Did you remember to?

- Exercise
- Medidate
- Soak up 15-20 mins
- Dring 2-3 Liter Bottols of Water
- Take Your ~
    - 1 Tbsp DHA/EPA Oil?
    - 500 mcg (Methyl) B12?
    - Super –Greens Power
    - 400IU (Vegan) VIT D3
    - Calcium/ Magnesium / Zinc (2000/1000/50 mg)?
    - Probiotic (Live, Refrigerated)?
    - 1 Tbsp Apple Cider Vinegar?

© 2015 Whole Earth Diet

Appendix C - Resources

Recommended reading:

Becoming Vegan: The Complete Guide to Adopting a Healthy Plant-Based Diet, Brenda Davis and Vesanto Melina ~ As registered dietitians, Davis and Melina are well-qualified to provide the latest information on: how a vegan diet can protect against cancer, heart disease, and other chronic illnesses; getting all the protein you need without meat; meeting your needs for calcium without dairy products; what vegans need to know about B12; why good fats are vital to your health and how to get them; balanced diets for infants, children, and seniors; pregnancy and breast-feeding tips for vegan moms; considerations for those who are overweight, underweight, and who have eating disorders' achieving peak performance as a vegan athlete; and how to deal gracefully with a non-vegan world.

Breaking the Food Seduction: The Hidden Reasons Behind Food Cravings – and 7 Steps to End Them Naturally, Dr. Neal Barnard ~ If sweets and high-fat foods are sabotaging your efforts to lose weight and get healthy, Dr. Neal Barnard has the solution to conquering your food addictions. Backed up by scientific research, *Breaking the Food Seduction* explains that your biochemistry, not your lack of willpower, is the problem. Dr. Barnard reveals the simple dietary and lifestyle changes that can break the stubborn cycle of cravings and make you free to choose healthy and tasty (vegan) foods that can help you lose weight, lower cholesterol, and improve your overall health.

Diet for a Poisoned Planet: How to Choose Safe Foods for You and Your Family, David Steinman ~ *Diet for a Poisoned Planet* took on an entire industry and went on to become a classic work of environmental writing. Now reissued in a new millennium edition, the work's in-depth look at the contaminants in individual food items is updated with the latest Total Diet Study findings. A motivating book, *Diet for a Poisoned Planet* changes people viscerally. Steinman tells his own story of fishing in the Santa Monica Bay as a child and how he went on to testify before Congress as an expert witness on the contamination of his own body by the fish he ate. The book is written by a true expert who has been a member of a National Academy of Sciences committee to advise Congress on seafood safety legislation.

Dominion: The Power of Man, the Suffering of Animals, and the Call to Mercy, Matthew Scully ~ "And God said, Let us make man in our image, after our likeness; and let them have dominion over the fish of the sea, and over the fowl of the air, and over the cattle, and over all the earth, and over every creeping thing that creepeth upon the earth." – Genesis 1:24-26. In this crucial passage from the Old Testament, God grants mankind power over animals. But with this privilege comes the grave responsibility to respect life, to treat animals with simple dignity and compassion. Throughout *Dominion*, Scully counters the hypocritical arguments that attempt to excuse animal abuse: from those who argue that the Bible's message permits mankind to use animals as it pleases, to the hunter's argument that through hunting animal populations are controlled, to the popular and "scientifically proven" notions that animals cannot feel pain, experience no emotions, and are not conscious of their own lives. The result is eye-opening, painful and infuriating, insightful and rewarding.

Eat More, Weigh Less: Dr. Dean Ornish's Life Choice Program for Losing Weight Safely While Eating Abundantly, Dean Ornish, MD ~ You really can eat more and weigh less—if you know what to eat. As this groundbreaking book clearly shows, it's not just how much you eat, it's primarily what you eat. Most diets rely on small portion sizes to reduce calories sufficiently. You feel hungry and deprived. Dr. Ornish's program takes a new approach: abundance rather than deprivation. If you change the type of food, you don't have to be as concerned about the amount of food. You can eat whenever you're hungry, eat more food, and still lose weight and keep it off. In this book, you'll find 250 gourmet recipes from the country's most celebrated chefs. Unlike high-protein diets that may mortgage your well-being, Dr. Ornish's diet and lifestyle program is scientifically proven to help you lose weight and gain health. People not only keep off the weight, they lower their cholesterol and reduce their chances for getting heart disease and such other illnesses as breast, prostate, and colon cancer; diabetes; osteoporosis; and hypertension.

Eat to Live: The Amazing Nutrient-Rich Program for Fast and Sustained Weight Loss, Dr. Joel Fuhrman, MD ~ The *Eat to Live* 2011 revised edition includes updated scientific research supporting Dr. Fuhrman's revolutionary six-week plan and a brand-new chapter highlighting Dr. Fuhrman's discovery of toxic hunger and the role of food addiction in weight issues.

Eating Animals, Jonathan Safran Foer ~ Jonathan

Safran Foer spent much of his teenage and college years oscillating between being an enthusiastic carnivore and an occasional vegetarian. As he became a husband, and then a father, the moral dimensions of eating became increasingly important to him. Faced with the prospect of being unable to explain why we eat some animals and not others, Foer set out to explore the origins of many eating traditions and the fictions involved with creating them. Part memoir and part investigative report, *Eating Animals* is a book that, in the words of the *Los Angeles Times*, places Jonathan Safran Foer "at the table with our greatest philosophers."

Farm Sanctuary: Changing Hearts and Minds About Animals and Food, Gene Baur ~ Leading animal-rights activist Gene Baur examines the real cost of the meat on our plates—for both humans and animals alike—in this provocative and thorough examination of the modern farm industry. In *Farm Sanctuary*, Baur provides a thought-provoking investigation of the ethical questions involved in the production of beef, poultry, pork, milk, and eggs—and what each of us can do to stop the mistreatment of farm animals and promote compassion. He details the triumphs and the disappointments of more than twenty years on the front lines of the animal-protection movement. And he introduces us to some of the special creatures who live at Farm Sanctuary—from Maya the cow to Marmalade the chicken all of whom escaped horrible circumstances to live happier, more peaceful lives.

Fast Food Nation: The Dark Side of the All-American Meal, Eric Schlosser ~ Fast food has hastened the malling of our landscape, widened the chasm between rich and poor, fueled an epidemic of obesity, and propelled American cultural imperialism abroad. That's a lengthy list of charges, but Eric Schlosser makes them stick with an artful mix of first-rate reportage, wry wit, and careful reasoning. Schlosser's myth-shattering survey stretches from California's subdivisions, where the business was born, to the industrial corridor along the New Jersey Turnpike, where many of fast food's flavors are concocted. Along the way, he unearths a trove of fascinating, unsettling truths—from the unholy alliance between fast food and Hollywood to the seismic changes the industry has wrought in food production, popular culture, and even real estate.

Mad Cowboy: Plain Truth from the Cattle Rancher Who Won't Eat Meat, Howard Lyman ~ Told by the man who kicked off the infamous lawsuit between Oprah and the cattlemen, *Mad Cowboy* is an impassioned account of the highly dangerous practices of the cattle and dairy industries. Howard Lyman's testimony on *The Oprah Winfrey Show* revealed the deadly impact of the livestock industry on our well-being. It not only led to Oprah's declaration that she'd never eat a burger again, it sent shock waves through a concerned and vulnerable public. A fourth-generation Montana rancher, Lyman investigated the use of chemicals in agriculture after developing a spinal tumor that nearly paralyzed him. Now a vegetarian, he blasts through the propaganda of beef and dairy interests—and the government agencies that protect them—to expose an animal-based diet as the primary cause of cancer, heart disease, and obesity in this country. He warns that the livestock industry is repeating the mistakes that led to mad cow disease in England while simultaneously causing serious damage to the environment. Persuasive, straightforward, and full of the down-home good humor and optimism of a son of the soil, *Mad Cowboy* is both an inspirational story of personal transformation and a convincing call to action for a plant-based diet—for the good of the planet and the health of us all.

Meat Market: Animals, Ethics & Money, Eric Marcus ~ *Meat Market* elevates the debate over animal agriculture. Erik Marcus exposes and clears away the exaggerated claims and counterclaims put forth by the meat industry and its opponents. In the process, Marcus presents a thorough examination of animal agriculture's cruelties and its far-reaching social costs. Marcus then considers the discouraging progress made by the animal-protection movement. He evaluates where the movement has gone wrong, and how its shortcomings could best be remedied.

Prevent and Reverse Heart Disease: The Revolutionary, Scientifically Proven, Nutrition-Based Cure, Dr. Caldwell Esselstyn ~ Based on the groundbreaking results of a twenty-year nutritional study by Dr. Esselstyn, a preeminent researcher and clinician, this book illustrates that a plant-based, oil-free diet can not only prevent and stop the progression of heart disease but can also reverse its effects.

Skinny Bitch, Rory Freedman and Kim Barnouin ~ Not your typical boring diet book, this is a tart-tongued, no-holds-barred wake-up call to all women who want to be thin. With such blunt advice as, "Soda is liquid Satan" and "You are a total moron if you think the Atkins Diet will make you thin," it's a rallying cry for all savvy women to start eating healthy and looking radiant. Unlike standard diet books, it actually makes the reader laugh out loud with its truthful, smart-mouthed revelations. Behind all the attitude, however, there's solid guidance. *Skinny Bitch* espouses a healthful lifestyle that promotes whole grains, fruits, and vegetables, and encourages women to get excited about feeling "clean and pure and energized." (This was the book that changed my life!)

Slaughterhouse: The Shocking Story of Greed, Neglect, and Inhumane Treatment Inside the US Meat Industry, Gail A. Eisnitz ~ *Slaughterhouse* is the first book of its kind to explore the impact that unprecedented changes in the meatpacking industry over the last twenty-five years— particularly industry consolidation, increased line speeds, and deregulation—have had on workers, animals, and consumers. It is also the first time ever that workers have spoken publicly about what's really taking place behind the closed doors of America's slaughterhouses. In this new paperback edition, author Gail A. Eisnitz brings the story up-to-date since the book's original publication. She describes the ongoing efforts by the Humane Farming Association to improve conditions in the meatpacking industry, media exposés that have prompted reforms resulting in multimillion dollar appropriations by Congress to try to enforce federal inspection laws, and a favorable decision by the Supreme Court to block construction of what was slated to be one of the largest hog factory farms in the country. Nonetheless, Eisnitz makes it clear that abuses continue and much work still needs to be done.

The Beauty Detox Solution: Eat Your Way to Radiant Skin, Renewed Energy and the Body You've Always Wanted, Kimberly Snyder ~ Nutritionist and beauty expert Kimberly Snyder helps dozens of A-list celebrities get red-carpet ready—and now you're getting the star treatment. Kim used to struggle with coarse hair, breakouts, and stubborn belly fat until she traveled the world, learning age-old beauty secrets. She discovered that what you eat is the ultimate beauty product, and she's developed a powerful program that rids the body of toxins so you can look and feel your very best.

The China Study: The Most Comprehensive Study of Nutrition Ever Conducted and the Startling Implications for Diet, Weight Loss and Long-Term Health, T. Colin Campbell, PhD, and Thomas M. Campbell II ~ Referred to as the "Grand Prix of epidemiology" by *The New York Times*, this study examines more than 350 variables of health and nutrition with surveys from 6,500 adults in more than 2,500 counties across China and Taiwan, and conclusively demonstrates the link between nutrition and heart disease, diabetes, and cancer. While revealing that proper nutrition can have a dramatic effect on reducing and reversing these ailments as well as curbing obesity, this text calls into question the practices of many of the current dietary programs, such as the Atkins diet, that are widely popular in the West. The politics of nutrition and the impact of special interest groups in the creation and dissemination of public information are also discussed.

The Ethics of What We Eat: Why Our Food Choices Matter, Jim Mason and Peter Singer ~ Peter Singer, the groundbreaking ethicist whom *The New Yorker* calls the most influential philosopher alive teams up again with Jim Mason, his coauthor on the acclaimed *Animal Factories*, to set their critical sights on the food we buy and eat: where it comes from, how it is produced, and whether it was raised humanely. *The Ethics of What We Eat* explores the impact our food choices have on humans, animals, and the environment. Recognizing that not all of us will become vegetarians, Singer and Mason offer ways to make healthful, humane food choices. As they point out: you can be ethical without being fanatical.

The Food Revolution: How Your Diet Can Help Save Your Life and Our World, John Robbins ~ In 1987, John Robbins published *Diet for a New America*, which was an early version of this book, and he started the food revolution. He continues to work tirelessly to promote conscious food choices more than twenty years later. First published in 2001, *The Food Revolution* is still one of the most frequently cited and talked about books of the food-politics revolution. It was one of the very first books to discuss the negative health effects of eating genetically modified foods and animal products of all kinds, to expose the dangers inherent in our factory-farming system, and to advocate a complete plant-based diet. The book garnered endorsements by everyone from Paul Hawken to Neal Donald Walsch, Marianne Williamson to Julia Butterfly Hill. After ten years in print, *The Food Revolution* is timelier than ever—and a very compelling read. The tenth anniversary edition has an updated, contemporary look and a new introduction by the author.

The McDougall Plan, John McDougall, MD, and Mary McDougall ~ Are Americans the most malnourished people in the world? Are the meat and dairy industries brainwashing us? Is the medical profession ignorant about our nutritional needs? Has our government given us faulty information on proper diets? *Yes* is the answer to all the above.

The Pig Who Sang to the Moon: The Emotional World of Farm Animals, Jeffrey Moussaieff Masson ~ Weaving history, literature, anecdotes, scientific studies, and Masson's own vivid experiences observing pigs, cows, sheep, goats, and chickens over the course of five years, this important book at last gives voice, meaning, and dignity to these gentle beasts that are bred to be milked, shorn, butchered, and eaten. Can we ever know what makes an animal happy? Many animal behaviorists say no. But Jeffrey Masson has a different view: An animal is happy if it can live according to its own nature. Farm animals suffer greatly in this regard. Chickens, for instance, like to perch in trees at night, to avoid predators and to nestle with friends. The obvious conclusion: They cannot be happy when confined twenty to a cage.

Veganist: Lose Weight, Get Healthy, Change the World, Kathy Freston ~ Kathy Freston wasn't born a vegan. The best-selling author and renowned wellness expert actually grew up on chicken-fried steak and cheesy grits and loved nothing more than BBQ ribs and vanilla milkshakes. Not until her thirties did she embrace the lifestyle of a veganist— someone who eats a plant-based diet not just for their own personal well-being, but for the whole web of benefits it brings to our ecosystem and beyond. Kathy's shift toward this new life was gradual—she leaned into it—but the impact was profound. Now Kathy shows us how to lean into the veganist life. Effortless weight loss, reversal of disease, environmental responsibility, spiritual awakening—these are just a few of the ten profound changes that can be achieved through a gentle switch in food choices. Filled with compelling facts, stories of people who have improved their weight and health conditions as a result of making the switch, and Q&As with the leading medical researchers, *Veganist* concludes with a step-by-step practical guide to becoming a veganist ... easily and gradually. It is an accessible, optimistic, and illuminating book that will change the way you eat forever. No less delicious, still hearty and satisfying—just better for you and for all.

Why we Love Dogs, Eat Pigs, and Wear Cows: An Introduction to Carnism, Melanie Joy, PhD ~ This groundbreaking work, voted one of the top ten books of 2010 by *VegNews* Magazine, offers an absorbing look at why and how humans can so wholeheartedly devote ourselves to certain animals and then allow others to suffer needlessly, especially those slaughtered for our consumption. Social psychologist Melanie Joy explores the many ways we numb ourselves and disconnect from our natural empathy for farmed animals. She coins the term "carnism" to describe the belief system that has conditioned us to eat certain animals and not others.

World Peace Diet: Eating for Spiritual Health and Social Harmony, Will Tuttle, PhD ~ Food is our most intimate and telling connection both with the living natural order and with our living cultural heritage. By eating the plants and animals of our Earth, we literally incorporate them. It is also through this act of eating that we partake of our culture's values and paradigms at the most primal levels. It is becoming increasingly obvious, however, that the choices we make about our food are leading to environmental degradation, enormous human health problems, and unimaginable cruelty toward our fellow creatures. Incorporating systems theory, teachings from mythology and religions, and the human sciences, *World Peace Diet* presents the outlines of a more empowering understanding of our world, based on a comprehension of the far-reaching implications of our food choices and the worldview those choices reflect and mandate. The author offers a set of universal principles for all people of conscience, from any religious tradition, that they can follow to reconnect with what we are eating, what was required to get it on our plate, and what happens after it leaves our plates. *World Peace Diet* suggests how we as a species might move our consciousness forward so that we can be freer, more intelligent, more loving, and happier in the choices we make.

Recommended cookbooks:

Forks Over Knives – The Cookbook, Del Sroufe, Isa Chandra Mskowitz

Quick-Fix Vegan: Healthy, Homestyle Meals in 30 Minutes or Less, Robin Robertson

The Engine 2 Diet: The Texas Firefighter's 28-Day Save-Your-Life-Plan That Lowers Cholesterol and Burns Away the Pounds, Rip Esselstyn

Vegan Handbook, Debra Wasserman and Reed Mangels

Veganomicon: The Ultimate Vegan Cookbook, Isa Chandra Moskowitz and Terry Hope Romero

Skinny Bitch in the Kitch, Rory Freedman and Kim Barnouin

The Compassionate Cook, PETA's Ingrid Newkirk

The Native Foods Restaurant Cookbook, Tanya Petrovna

Raw Basics: Incorporating Raw Living Foods Into Your Diet Using Easy and Delicious Recipes, Jenny Ross

The Vegan Table, Colleen Patrick Goudreau

Simply Vegan: Quick Vegetarian Meals, Debra

Wasserman and Reed Mangels

Eat Vegan on $4 a Day and/or *Paleo Vegan: Plant-Based Primal Recipes*, Ellen Jaffe Jones

NEW (and awesome!): Betty Goes Vegan: 500 Classic Recipes for the Modern Family, Dan & Annie Shannon

Recommended viewing:

*** Forks Over Knives (2011) ~ *Forks Over Knives* examines the profound claim that most, if not all, of the so-called "diseases of affluence" that afflict us can be controlled, or even reversed, by rejecting our present menu of animal-based and processed foods. The major storyline in the film traces the personal journeys of a pair of pioneering yet underappreciated researchers, Dr. T. Colin Campbell and Dr. Caldwell Esselstyn. Dr. Campbell, a nutritional scientist at Cornell University, was concerned in the late 1960s with producing "high quality" animal protein to bring to the poor and malnourished areas of the developing world. While in the Philippines, he made a life-changing discovery: the country's wealthier children, who were consuming relatively high amounts of animal-based foods, were much more likely to get liver cancer. Dr. Esselstyn, a top surgeon and head of the Breast Cancer Task Force at the world-renowned Cleveland Clinic, found that many of the diseases he routinely treated were virtually unknown in parts of the world where animal-based foods were rarely consumed. These discoveries inspired Campbell and Esselstyn, who didn't know each other yet, to conduct several groundbreaking studies. One of them took place in China and is still among the most comprehensive health-related investigations ever undertaken. Their research led them to a startling conclusion: degenerative diseases such as heart disease, type 2 diabetes, and even several forms of cancer could almost always be prevented—and in many cases reversed—by adopting a whole-foods, plant-based diet. Despite the profound implications of their findings, their work has remained relatively unknown to the public. The filmmakers travel with Drs. Campbell and Esselstyn on their separate but similar paths, from their childhood farms where they both produced "nature's perfect food," to China and Cleveland, where they explored ideas that challenged the established thinking and shook their own core beliefs. The idea of food as medicine is put to the test. Throughout the film, cameras follow "reality patients" who have chronic conditions from heart disease to diabetes. Doctors teach these patients how to adopt a whole-foods, plant-based diet as the primary approach to treat their ailments—while the challenges and triumphs of their journeys are revealed. (This is the one movie that will change your life and those of your loved ones – buy several copies because you will want to give them away!)

Super Size Me (2004) ~ Documentary filmmaker Morgan Spurlock makes himself a test subject in this documentary about the commercial food industry. After eating a diet of McDonald's fast food three times a day for a month straight, Spurlock proves the physical and mental effects of consuming fast food. Spurlock also provides a look at the food culture in America through its schools, corporations, and politics. *Super Size Me* is a movie that sheds a new light on what has become one of our nation's biggest health problems: obesity.

Mad Cowboy (2004) - The story of Howard Lyman, a fourth-generation brash Montana cattle rancher pressed into running the family farm. Sweeping aside his father's traditional methods in favor of the new, highly industrialized form of agribusiness, Howard jeopardizes the health of his family and himself. When tragedy strikes, he must choose either "business as usual" or open his eyes to a hard truth. Risking everything, this mad cowboy speaks out and takes on billionaire cattle barons who want to destroy him and all he fights for.

Earthlings, Starring Joaquin Phoenix (2007) ~ *Earthlings* is a feature-length documentary about humankind's absolute economic dependence on animals raised as pets, food, clothing, entertainment, and for scientific research. Using hidden cameras and never-before-seen footage, *Earthlings* chronicles the day-to-day practices at some of the largest industries in the world, all of which rely entirely on animals for profit. Powerful, graphic, stomach-turning, informative, and thought-provoking, *Earthlings* is by far the most comprehensive documentary ever produced on the correlation between nature, animals, and human economic interests.

Food, Inc. Starring Eric Schlosser (2009) ~ *Food, Inc.* lifts the veil on our nation's food industry, exposing how our nation's food supply is now controlled by a handful of corporations that often put profit ahead of consumer health, the livelihood of the American farmer, the safety of workers, and our own environment. *Food, Inc.* reveals surprising and often shocking truths about what we eat, how its produced, and who we have become as a nation.

Food Matters, Starring Andrew Saul, Charlotte Gerson (2009) ~ "Let thy Food be thy Medicine and thy Medicine be thy Food," Hippocrates. That is the message from the founding father of modern medicine echoed in the controversial new documentary. With nutritionally depleted foods, chemical additives, and our tendency to rely upon pharmaceutical drugs to treat what's wrong with our malnourished bodies, it's no wonder that modern society is getting sicker. *Food Matters* sets about uncovering the trillion-dollar worldwide sickness industry and gives people some scientifically verifiable solutions for curing disease naturally.

Fresh, Starring Ana Joanes (2009) ~ While *Food, Inc.* raised awareness about the consequences of consolidation, *Fresh* advances the argument by talking about solutions. Both an enlightening documentary and a stirring call to action, *Fresh* outlines the vicious cycle of our current food-production methods, while also celebrating the farmers, thinkers, and business people across America who are reinventing our food system.

Fat, Sick & Nearly Dead, Starring Joe Cross (2010) ~ An inspiring film that chronicles Joe's personal mission to regain his health while traveling across America, juicer in tow, and inspiring others to do the same. Overweight, loaded up on steroids, and suffering from a debilitating autoimmune disease, Joe was at the end of his rope and the end of his hope. With doctors and conventional medicine unable to help, Joe traded in junk food and hit the road with a juicer and generator in tow, vowing only to drink fresh fruit and vegetable juice for sixty days. Across 3,000 miles Joe had one goal in mind: to get off his pills and achieve a balanced lifestyle.

Vegucated, Starring T. Colin Campbell and Brian Flegel (2011) ~ Part sociological experiment and part adventure comedy, *Vegucated* follows three meat- and cheese-loving New Yorkers who agree to adopt a vegan diet for six weeks. Lured by tales of weight lost and health regained, they begin to uncover the hidden sides of animal agriculture that make them wonder whether solutions offered in films like *Food, Inc.* go far enough. This entertaining documentary showcases the rapid and at times comedic evolution of three people who discover they can change the world one bite at a time.

Hungry for Change, Starring Mike Adams & Nick Bolton (2012) ~ We all want more energy, an ideal body, and beautiful, younger-looking skin. So what is stopping us from getting this? From the creators of the best-selling documentary *Food Matters* comes another hard-hitting film certain to rock your world. *Hungry for Change* exposes shocking secrets the diet, weight-loss and food industries don't want you to know about—deceptive strategies designed to keep you coming back for more. Find out what's keeping you from having the body and health you deserve and how to escape the diet trap forever. Featuring interviews with best-selling health authors and leading medical experts plus real-life transformational stories with those who know what it's like to be sick and overweight. Learn from those who have been there before and continue your health journey today.

Planeat, Starring Yvonne O'Grady (2012) ~ The story of three men's lifelong search for a diet, which is good for our health, good for the environment, and good for the future of our planet. Where have we gone wrong? Why has the death rate from heart disease and cancer exploded in recent times? Why are the ice caps melting, the oceans dying, and the forests being cut down as we produce the food necessary to support our burgeoning populations? Against a backdrop of colorful and delicious food grown by organic farmers and prepared in the kitchens of world-famous chefs, *Planeat* for the first time brings together the groundbreaking studies of three prominent scientists who have made it their life's work to answer these questions.

Peaceable Kingdom: The Journey Home (2012) ~ *Peaceable Kingdom* explores the powerful struggle of conscience experienced by several people from traditional farming backgrounds who come to question the basic assumptions of their way of life. A riveting story of transformation and healing, the documentary portrays the farmers' sometimes amazing connections with the animals under their care, while also providing insight into the complex web of social, psychological, and economic forces that have led to their inner conflict. Interwoven with the farmers' stories is the dramatic animal-rescue work of a newly trained humane police officer whose sense of justice puts her at odds with the law she is charged to uphold. With strikingly honest interviews and rare footage demonstrating the emotional lives and intense family bonds of animals most often viewed as living commodities, this groundbreaking documentary shatters stereotypical notions of farmers, farm life, and perhaps most surprisingly, farm animals themselves.

May I Be Frank, Starring Frank Ferrante (2013) ~ Frank Ferrante is a fifty-four-year-old Sicilian from Brooklyn living in San Francisco. A lover of life, great food, beautiful women, and a good laugh, Frank is also a drug addict, morbidly obese, pre-diabetic, and fighting hepatitis C. *May I Be Frank* documents the transformation of Frank's life when he stumbles into a local raw and vegan restaurant, becomes friends with the staff, and strikes an agreement to turn his life over to three twenty-something young men to be coached physically, emotionally, and spiritually. Over forty-two days, the four men go on the ride of their lives. Through Frank's story of love, redemption, and transformation, we witness the power of change in one person's life and its impact on countless others.

Speciesism: The Movie (2013) ~ Modern farms are struggling to keep a secret. Most of the animals used for food in the United States are raised in giant, bizarre factories, hidden deep in remote areas of the countryside. *Speciesism: The Movie* director Mark Devries set out to investigate. The documentary takes viewers on a sometimes funny, sometimes frightening adventure, crawling through the bushes that hide these factories, flying in airplanes above their toxic "manure lagoons," and coming face-to-face with their owners. But this is just the beginning. In 1975, a young writer published a book arguing that no justifications exist for considering humans more important than members of other species. It slowly began to gain attention. Today, a quickly growing number of prominent individuals and political activists are adopting its conclusions. They have termed the assumption of human superiority "speciesism." And, as a result, they rank these animal factories among the greatest evils in our history. *Speciesism: The Movie* brings viewers face-to-face with the leaders of this developing movement, and, for the first time ever on film, fully examines the purpose of what they are setting out to do.

Cowspiracy: The Sustainability Secret (2014) ~ *Cowspiracy* is a groundbreaking feature-length environmental documentary following intrepid filmmaker Kip Andersen as he uncovers the most destructive industry facing the planet today and investigates why the world's leading environmental organizations are too afraid to talk about it. Animal agriculture is the leading cause of deforestation, water consumption, and pollution; is responsible for more greenhouse gases than the transportation industry; and is a primary driver of rainforest destruction, species extinction, habitat loss, topsoil erosion, ocean "dead zones," and virtually every other environmental ill. Yet it goes on, almost entirely unchallenged. As Andersen approaches leaders in the environmental movement, he increasingly uncovers what appears to be an intentional refusal to discuss the issue of animal agriculture, while industry whistleblowers and watchdogs warn him of the risks to his freedom and even his life if he dares to persist. As eye-opening as *Blackfish* and as inspiring as *An Inconvenient Truth*, this shocking yet humorous documentary reveals the absolutely devastating environmental impact large-scale factory farming has on our planet and offers a path to global sustainability for a growing population.

Meet Your Meat Starring Alec Baldwin ~ A documentary about factory farming created by PETA and found on the PETA website, explores the treatment of animals in modern animal agriculture (only 12 minutes long).

Recommended websites to visit:

Happycow.net ~ to find veggie-friendly restaurants anywhere in the world

Cok.net ~ a non-profit animal advocacy organization with tons of helpful info

Mercyforanimals.org ~ a non-profit dedicated to preventing cruelty to farm animals

Meat.org ~ the website the meat industry does not want you to see

Pcrm.org ~ the Physicians Committee for Responsible Medicine

Peta.org ~ largest animal rights group in the world

Farmsanctuary.org ~ animal protection sanctuaries in New York and California

Veganstore.com ~ food, clothing, body and health care items

Veganessentials.com ~ complete online vegan store

Nutritionfacts.org ~ all the info you need about a vegan diet from a nutritional perspective

Gentlebarn.org ~ farm animal rescue, Santa Clarita, CA

Bustersbarn.org ~ farm animal rescue, Acton, CA

Rowdygirlsanctuary.org ~ cattle ranch converted to farm animal sanctuary, Angleton, TX

Kickbuttboots.com ~ vegan cowboy boots

Best Vegan Recipe Websites:

- **Fatfreevegan.com**
- **Choosingraw.com**
- **Allysonkramer.com**
- **Rickiheller.com**

- **kblog.lunchboxbunch.com**
- **ohsheglows.com**
- **veganyumyum.com**
- **viveleveganrecipes.blogpost.com**
- **jlgoesvegan.com**
- **vegkitchen.com**
- **kriscarr.com**
- **thekindlife.com**
- **theppk.com**

Appendix D – Endnotes

1. Dotinga, Randy. "Obesity Has Nearly Doubled Worldwide Since 1980: Report." *Healthday* (Feb. 4, 2011). consumer.healthday.com/circulatory-system-information-7/blood-pressure-news-70/obesity-has-nearly-doubled-worldwide-since-1980-report-649633.html
2. "Adult Obesity Facts." *Centers for Disease Control and Prevention* (Sept. 9, 2014). www.cdc.gov/obesity/data/adult.html
3. "Obesity and Overweight: Fact Sheet." *World Health Organization* (January 2015). www.who.int/mediacentre/factsheets/fs311/en/
4. "Chronic Disease Prevention and Health Promotion." *Centers for Disease Control and Prevention* (May 9, 2014). www.cdc.gov/chronicdisease/overview/
5. Olshansky, S. Jay PhD; Douglas J. Passaro, MD; Ronald C. Hershow, MD; Jennifer Layden, MPH; et al. "A Potential Decline in Life Expectancy in the US in the 21st Century." *The New England Journal of Medicine* (March 17, 2005). www.nejm.org/doi/full/10.1056/NEJMsr043743
6. "Medical costs push millions of people into poverty across the globe." *World Health Organization* (December 5, 2005). www.who.int/mediacentre/news/releases/2005/pr65/en/
7. Ibid.
8. Allan, JD. "New directions for the study of the overweight." *Western Journal of Nursing Research* (February 20, 1998). www.ncbi.nlm.nih.gov/pubmed/9473964
9. Pew Forum on Religion & Public Life, The. *U.S. Religious Landscape Survey: Religious Affiliation.* February 1, 2008. www.pewforum.org/2008/02/01/chapter-1-the-religious-composition-of-the-united-states/
10. Saad, Lydia. "Conservatives Remain Largest Ideological Group in U.S." *Gallup.* January 12, 2012.

www.gallup.com/poll/152021/conservatives-remain-largest-ideological-group.aspx

11. Imhoff, Dan. "Food, Four Ways the Farm Bill Makes Me Crazy." *Huffington Post*, February 20, 2015. www.huffingtonpost.com/dan-imhoff/farm-bill_b_1398135.html

12. Lyman, Howard. *Mad Cowboy: Plain Truth from the Cattle Rancher Who Won't Eat Meat*, August 2, 2001. www.madcowboy.com

13. Physicians Committee for Responsible Medicine. "Meat is the New Tobacco: Exporting a Dangerous Habit." Autumn 2013. www.pcrm.org/media/good-medicine/2013/autumn2013/meat-is-the-new-tobacco-exporting-a-dangerous

14. National Center for Biotechnical Information. "Does low meat consumption increase life expectancy in humans?" *American Journal of Clinical Nutrition* (Sept. 2003). www.ncbi.nlm.nih.gov/pubmed/12936945

15. International Vegetarian Union. "History of Vegetarianism: North America: Early 20th Century: Albert Einstein (1879-1955)." www.ivu.org/history/northam20a/einstein.html

16. Mangels, Reed, PhD, RD. "Protein in the Vegan Diet." *The Vegetarian Resource Group*. www.vrg.org/nutrition/protein.php

17. Mills, Milton R. *The Comparative Anatomy of Eating*. [PDF] The Comparative Anatomy of Eating - Adaptt

18. Chang, Kwen-jen, Eli Hazum, and Pedro Cuatrecasas. "Novel opiate binding sites selective for benzomorphan drugs." *Proceedings of the National Academy of Sciences* 78, no.7 (July 1981): 4141-4145.

19. DeSalle, Rob, and Ian Tattersall. "Do Plants Have Brains?" *Natural History Magazine*. Adapted with permission from *The Brain: Big Bangs, Behaviors, and Beliefs*, Yale University Press, 2012. www.naturalhistorymag.com/features/152208/do-plants-have-brains

20. Dawkins, Marian Stamp. "Animal Minds and Animal Emotions." *Oxford Journals, Integrative & Comparative Biology* 40, no. 6: 883-888. icb.oxfordjournals.org/content/40/6/883.full

21. CDC, NCHS. Underlying Cause of Death 1999-2013 on CDC WONDER Online Database, released 2015. Data are from the Multiple Cause of Death Files, 1999-2013, as compiled from data

provided by the 57 vital statistics jurisdictions through the Vital Statistics Cooperative Program. Accessed Feb. 3, 2015. www.cdc.gov/chronicdisease/resources/publications/AAG/obesity.htm

22. Rizzo, Nico, Karen Jaceldo-Siegl, Joan Sabate, and Gary Fraser. "Nutrient Profiles of Vegetarian and Nonvegetarian Dietary Patterns." *Journal of the Academy of Nutrition and Dietetics* (August 28, 2013). www.andjrnl.org/article/S2212-2672(13)01113-1/abstract

23. Glynn, Sarah. "Vegetarians Live Longer Than Meat-Eaters." *Medical News Today* (June 4, 2013). www.medicalnewstoday.com/articles/261382.php

24. Fuhrman, Joel MD. "Dangers of the Atkins Diet." *Health 101.* health101.org/art_Atkins_diet.htm

25. Organic Consumers Association. "Growth Hormones Fed to Beef Cattle Damage Human Health." May 1, 2007. www.organicconsumers.org/scientific/growth-hormones-fed-beef-cattle-damage-human-health

26. Mayo Clinic. "Dietary fiber: Essential for a healthy diet." Institute of Medicine 2012. www.mayoclinic.org/healthy-living/nutrition-and-healthy-eating/in-depth/fiber/art-20043983

27. Ward, Elizabeth M., MS, RD. "Fast Facts: Good Fats vs. Bad Fats." *WebMD*. October 30, 2008. www.webmd.com/food-recipes/good-fats-bad-fats

28. Neubert, Amy Patterson. "Study: 3 square meals a day paired with lean protein help people feel full during weight loss." *Purdue University*. March 30, 2011. www.purdue.edu/newsroom/research/2011/110330CampbellPork.html

29. Barnard, Neal MD; Joshua Cohen, MD; Gabrielle Turner-McGrievy, MS, RD; Lise Gloede, RD, CDE, Brent Jaster, MD, Kim Seidl, MS, RD, Amber A. Green RD, and Stanley Talpers, MD. "A Low-Fat Vegan Diet Improves Glycemic Control and Cardiovascular Risk Factors in a Randomized Clinical Trial in Individuals with Type 2 Diabetes." *American Diabetes Association, Diabetes Care*, May 15, 2006. care.diabetesjournals.org/content/29/8/1777.full

30. Centers for Disease Control and Prevention. *2014 National Diabetes Statistics Report*. www.cdc.gov/diabetes

31. Harvard School of Public Health, The Nutrition Source. "Simple Steps to Preventing Diabetes." www.hsph.harvard.edu/nutritionsource/diabetes-full-story/

32. Physicians Committee for Responsible Medicine. "The Vegan Diet How-To Guide for Diabetes." Dr. Neal Barnard. www.pcrm.org/health/diabetes-resources/the-vegan-diet-how-to-guide-for-diabetes

33. Centers for Disease Control and Prevention. "Heart Disease Facts and Statistics." Feb. 19, 2015. www.cdc.gov/heartdisease/facts.htm

34. Esselstyn, Caldwell, and Mladen Golubic. "The Nutritional Reversal of Cardiovascular Disease—Fact or Fiction? Three Case Reports." *Experimental & Clinical Cardiology* 20, no. 7: 1901-1908. www.dresselstyn.com/Esselstyn_Three-case-reports_Exp-Clin-Cardiol-July-2014.pdf

35. Esselstyn, Caldwell Jr. "Abolishing Heart Disease." *Center for Nutrition Studies*, October 15, 2013. nutritionstudies.org/abolishing-heart-disease/

36. Centers for Disease Control and Prevention. "Heart Disease Facts and Statistics." Feb. 19, 2015. www.cdc.gov/heartdisease/facts.htm

37. Pendick, Daniel. "New study links L-carnitine in red meat to heart disease." *Harvard Medical School, Harvard Health Publications*, April 17, 2013. www.health.harvard.edu/blog/new-study-links-l-carnitine-in-red-meat-to-heart-disease-201304176083

38. Centers for Disease Control and Prevention. "Cancer Statistics by Cancer Type." Sept. 2, 2014. www.cdc.gov/cancer/dcpc/data/types.htm

39. "Meat Consumption and Cancer Risk." *Physicians Committee for Responsible Medicine*. Dr. Neal Barnard, www.pcrm.org/health/cancer-resources/diet-cancer/facts/meat-consumption-and-cancer-risk

40. Bottemiller, Helena. "Most U.S. Antibiotics Go To Animal Agriculture." *Food Safety News*, Feb. 24, 2011.

www.foodsafetynews.com/2011/02/fda-confirms-80-percent-of-antibiotics-used-in-animal-ag/#.VP4cGkJd0ng

41. Gill ON, Spencer Y., Richard-Loendt A., et al. "Prevalent abnormal prion protein in human appendixes after bovine spongiform encephalopathy epizootic: large scale survey." *thebmj* (Oct. 15, 2013). www.bmj.com/content/347/bmj.f5675

42. "About Dr. Esselstyn." *Dr. Esselstyn's Prevent & Reverse Heart Disease Program.* www.dresselstyn.com/site/about/about-dr-esselstyn/

43. "Dean Ornish, MD." *Preventative Medicine Research Institute.* www.pmri.org/dean_ornish.html

44. "Neal Barnard, M.D." *Physicians Committee for Responsible Medicine.* www.pcrm.org/media/experts/bios/neal-barnard-md

45. "T. Colin Campbell." *Center for Nutrition Studies.* nutritionstudies.org/about/board/dr-t-colin-campbell/

46. "About Dr. Fuhrman." *Dr. Fuhrman: Smart Nutrition. Superior Health.* www.drfuhrman.com/ask/default.aspx

47. "About Dr. Michael Greger." *Michael Greger, MD.* www.drgreger.org/about

48. "John A. McDougall, MD and Mary McDougall." *Dr. McDougall's Health & Medical Center.* www.drmcdougall.com/about/dr-john-mcdougall/

49. Gerbens-Leenes, P.W., M.M. Mekonnen, and A.Y. Hoekstra. "A Compartaive Study on the Water Footprint of Poultry, Pork and Beef in Different Countries and Production Systems." *UNESCO-IHE Institute for Water Education*, December 2011. www.waterfootprint.org/Reports/Report55.pdf

50. Burns, John D. "The Eight Million Little Pigs – a Cautionary Tale: Statutory and Regulatory Responses to Concentrated Hog Farming." The National Agricultural Law Center, University of Arkansas, 1996. nationalaglawcenter.org/publication/comment-the-eight-million-little-pigs-a-cautionary-tale-statutory-and-regulatory-responses-to-concentrated-hog-farming-31-wake-forest-l-rev-851-883-1996-2/wppa_open/

51. Robbins, John. "Our Food, Our World – Choices for a Healthy Environment." *Celsias*, Nov. 3, 2007. www.celsias.com/article/our-food-our-world-choices-for-a-healthy-environme/

52. Cone, Marla. "State Dairy Farms Try to Clean Up Their Act." *Los Angeles Times*, April 28, 1998. articles.latimes.com/1998/apr/28/news/mn-43842

53. Blair, Kathleen, MS. "Cryptosporidium and Public Health." *Water Quality & Health Council*, March 1, 1995. www.waterandhealth.org/newsletter/old/03-01-1995.html

54. "Officials Approve New California Polluted Runoff Program." *United States Environmental Protection Agency*, July 31, 2000. yosemite.epa.gov/opa/admpress.nsf/b1ac27bf9339f1c28525701 c005e2edf/7340a18a132b249c852570d8005e13dd!OpenDocum ent

55. Goodland, Robert, and Jeff Anhang. "Livestock and Climate Change: What if the key actors in climate change are cows, pigs and chickens?" *World Watch* (November/December 2009). www.worldwatch.org/files/pdf/Livestock%20and%20Climate% 20Change.pdf

56. "Press Release No. 1009." *World Meteorological Organization*, December 2, 2014. www.wmo.int/pages/mediacentre/press_releases/pr_1009_en.ht ml

57. Cummins, Ronnie. "How Factory Framing Contributes to Global Warming." *EcoWatch*, January 21, 2013. ecowatch.com/2013/01/21/factory-farming-global-warming/

58. "Grazing systems and tropical rainforests." *Food and Agriculture Organization*. www.fao.org/ag/againfo/resources/documents/Lxehtml/tech/c h2d.htm

59. "Rainforests: Facts About Rainforests." *The Nature Conservancy*. www.nature.org/ourinitiatives/urgentissues/rainforests/rainfor ests-facts.xml

60. Robbins, John. The Food Revolution: How Your Diet can Help Save Your Life and our World. San Francisco: Conari, 2001. P. 257 livestockandtheenvironment.wordpress.com/tag/rainforests/

61. Humane Society International. *An HSI Report: the Impact of Animal Agriculture on Global Warming and Climate Change*. p. 411 www.humanesociety.org/assets/pdfs/farm/hsus-the-impact-of-animal-agriculture-on-global-warming-and-climate-change.pdf

62. "Our Food, Our Future." *VegSource Interactive, Inc.* www.vegsource.com/articles/factoids.htm

63. IUCN 2014. *The IUCN Red List of Threatened Species. Version 2014.3.* www.iucnredlist.org/about/summary-statistics

64. United States General Accounting Office. *Wildlife Services Program: Information on Activities to Manage Wildlife.* November 2001. www.gao.gov/new.items/d02138.pdf

65. Wilson, Edward O. *The Future of Life* (New York: Knopf, 2002).

66. Kirby, Alex. "Hungry world 'must eat less meat.'" *BBC News,* August 16, 2004. news.bbc.co.uk/2/hi/science/nature/3559542.stm

67. Carus, Felicity. "UN urges global move to meat and dairy-free diet." *The Guardian,* June 2, 2010. www.theguardian.com/environment/2010/jun/02/un-report-meat-free-diet

68. Warrick, Joby. "'They Die Piece by Piece'; In Overtaxed Plants, Humane Treatment of Cattle Is Often a Battle Lost." *The Washington Post,* Apr. 10, 2001. www.washingtonpost.com/pb/newssearch/?query=Joby+Warrick

69. "More than 150 Billion Animals Slaughtered Every Year." *Animals Deserve Absolute Protection Today and Tomorrow.* www.adaptt.org/killcounter.html

70. "Chickens." *United Poultry Concerns.* www.upc-online.org/chickens/chickensbro.html

71. "Veal Crates: Unnecessary and cruel." *The Humane Society of the United States,* Feb. 22, 2013. www.humanesociety.org/issues/confinement_farm/facts/veal.html

72. Dawson, Gloria. "No Goat Left Behind: Getting Americans to Eat Goat." *Modern Farmer,* Sept 19, 2013. modernfarmer.com/2013/09/goat-left-behind/

73. Eisnitz, Gail. *Slaughterhouse: The Shocking Story of Greed, Neglect, and Inhumane Treatment Inside the U.S. Meat Industry* (New York: Prometheus Books, 2006).

74. Corbo, Tony. "Time to Clean House at FSIS." *Food Safety News,* August 22, 2013. www.foodsafetynews.com/2013/08/its-time-to-clean-house-at-fsis/#.VQCAIkJd0ng

75. "UK – In the Slaughterhouse, Lovis Corinth, 1893." Meat Trade News Daily, August 8, 2010. www.meattradenewsdaily.co.uk/news/100810/uk__in_the_slaug hterhouse_lovis_corinth_.aspx

76. "Consumers' Section: Macronutrients in Health and Disease." *NutritionMD*. www.nutritionmd.org/consumers/general_nutrition/macro_prot ein.html

77. Craig, WJ, and AR Mangels. "Position of the American Dietetic Association: vegetarian diets." *Journal of the American Dietetic Association* 109, no. 7 (July 2009):1266-1282. www.ncbi.nlm.nih.gov/pubmed/19562864

78. "Amino Acids." *MedlinePlus*, Feb. 18, 2013. www.nlm.nih.gov/medlineplus/ency/article/002222.htm

79. "The Protein Myth." *Physicians Committee for Responsible Medicine*. www.pcrm.org/health/diets/vegdiets/how-can-i-get-enough-protein-the-protein-myth

80. "Kidney Patients: If You're Eating 'Southern' Food, Make It Vegan." *Physicians Committee for Responsible Medicine*, Aug. 4, 2014. www.pcrm.org/health/medNews/kidney-patients-eat-vegan

81. "Carbohydrates." *MedlinePlus*. www.nlm.nih.gov/medlineplus/carbohydrates.html

82. "Making Sense of Foods: Choosing Carbohydrates Wisely." *NutrtitionMD*. www.nutritionmd.org/nutrition_tips/nutrition_tips_understand_f oods/carbs_choosing.html

83. Rodriguez, Diana. "Good vs. Bad Carbohydrates." *Everyday Health*, March 27, 2013. www.everydayhealth.com/diet-nutrition/101/nutrition-basics/good-carbs-bad-carbs.aspx

84. "Fiber." *Harvard School of Public Health*. www.hsph.harvard.edu/nutritionsource/carbohydrates/fiber/

85. "Dietary Fats." *MedlinePlus*. www.nlm.nih.gov/medlineplus/dietaryfats.html

86. "Saturated Fats." American Heart Association. www.heart.org/HEARTORG/GettingHealthy/NutritionCenter/He althyEating/Saturated-Fats_UCM_301110_Article.jsp

87. "Shining the Spotlight on Trans Fats." *Harvard School of Public Health*. www.hsph.harvard.edu/nutritionsource/transfats/
88. "Monounsaturated Fats." *American Heart Association*. www.heart.org/HEARTORG/GettingHealthy/NutritionCenter/He althyEating/Monounsaturated-Fats_UCM_301460_Article.jsp
89. "Polyunsaturated Fats." *American Heart Association*. www.heart.org/HEARTORG/GettingHealthy/NutritionCenter/He althyEating/Polyunsaturated-Fats_UCM_301461_Article.jsp
90. "Essential Fatty Acids." *Physicians Committee for Responsible Medicine*. www.pcrm.org/health/health-topics/essential-fatty-acids
91. Lane, Katie, Emma Derbyshire, Weili Li, and Charles Brennan. "Bioavailability and Potential Uses of Vegetarian Sources of Omega-3 Fatty Acids: A Review of the Literature." *Critical Reviews in Food Science and Nutrition* 54, no. 5: 572-579. www.ncbi.nlm.nih.gov/pubmed/24261532
92. Zelman, Kathleen M., MPH, RD, LD. "Know the Difference Between Fat- and Water-Soluble Nutrients." *WebMD*. www.webmd.com/vitamins-and-supplements/nutrition-vitamins-11/fat-water-nutrient
93. "Food Composition: Vitamins and Minerals." *United States Department of Agriculture: National Agricultural Library*. fnic.nal.usda.gov/food-composition/vitamins-and-minerals
94. "Dr. Weil's Anti-Inflammatory Diet." *Andrew Weil, M.D.* www.drweil.com/drw/u/ART02012/anti-inflammatory-diet
95. Zelman, Kathleen M., MPH, RD, LD. "6 Reasons to Drink Water." *WebMD*, May 8, 2008. www.webmd.com/diet/6-reasons-to-drink-water
96. "Water and Your Diet: Staying Slim and Regular With H20." *WebMD*. www.webmd.com/diet/water-for-weight-loss-diet?page=2
97. Batmanghelidj, F., MD. *The Water Cure*. www.watercure.com
98. "The Power Plate." Physicians Committee for Responsible Medicine. www.pcrm.org/health/diets/pplate/power-plate
99. "Feeling weary? Your body isn't as old as you think." *News.com.au*, January 24, 2013. www.news.com.au/lifestyle/fitness/your-body-isnt-as-old-as-you-think/story-fneuzle5-1226560675662

100.   Larsson, SC, and N. Orsini. "Red meat and processed meat consumption and all-cause mortality: a meta-analysis." *American Journal of Epidemiology* 179, no. 3 (Feb. 1, 2014): 282-289. www.ncbi.nlm.nih.gov/pubmed/24148709

101.   Chan, Doris S. M., Rosa Lau, Dagfinn Aune, Rui Vieira, et al. "Red and Processed Meat and Colorectal Cancer Incidence: Meta-Analysis of Prospective Studies." *PLoS One* 6, no. 6 (June 6, 2011). www.ncbi.nlm.nih.gov/pmc/articles/PMC3108955/

102.   "Salmonella and Chicken: What You Should Know and What You Can Do." *Centers for Disease Control and Prevention*, Oct. 28, 2013. www.cdc.gov/features/SalmonellaChicken/index.html

103.   "Legal Protections for Farm Animals." *ASPCA*. www.aspca.org/fight-cruelty/farm-animal-cruelty/legal-protections-farm-animals

104.   Agency for Toxic Substances and Disease Registry, U.S. Department of Health and Human Services. "Toxicological Profile for Mercury." Chapter 1, Public Health Statement, March 1999. www.atsdr.cdc.gov/toxprofiles/tp46-c1.pdf

105.   National Oceanic and Atmospheric Administration, U.S. Department of Commerce. "Vision 2040: The Future of U.S. Marine Fisheries: Final Report of the Marine Fisheries Advisory Committee," 2012. www.nmfs.noaa.gov/ocs/mafac/meetings/2012 05/docs/vision 2040 final draft.pdf

106.   "Veal: A Byproduct of the Cruel Dairy Industry." *People for the Ethical Treatment of Animals*. www.peta.org/issues/animals-used-for-food/animals-used-food-factsheets/veal-byproduct-cruel-dairy-industry/

107.   "Diet-Induced Precocious Puberty." *The McDougall Newsletter*, November/December 1997. www.drmcdougall.com/newsletter/nov dec97.html

108.   Centers for Disease Control and Prevention, U.S. Department of Health and Human Services. *Antibiotic Resistant Threats in the United States, 2013*. April 23, 2013: 36-37. www.cdc.gov/drugresistance/threat-report-2013/pdf/ar-threats-2013-508.pdf

109.   Watson, Stephanie. "The Truth About Mucus." *WebMD*, April 10, 2014. www.webmd.com/allergies/features/the-truth-about-mucus

110.   Mattar, Rejane, Daniel Ferraz de Campos Mazo, and Flair José Carrilho. "Lactose intolerance: diagnosis, genetic, and clinical factors." *Clinical and Experimental Gastroenterology* 5 (July 5, 2012): 113-121. www.ncbi.nlm.nih.gov/pmc/articles/PMC3401057/

111.   "Breaking the Cheese Addiction: Step 3 Cleansing the Palate." *Physicians Committee for Responsible Medicine*, August 2013. pcrm.org/health/diets/ffl/newsletter/breaking-the-cheese-addiction-step-3-cleansing-the

112.   "The China Study." Wikipedia. en.wikipedia.org/wiki/The_China_Study

113.   "Protecting Your Bones." *Physicians Committee for Responsible Medicine*, April 30, 2014. www.pcrm.org/health/health-topics/calcium-and-strong-bones

114.   "Lurking Beneath the Shell: Health Concerns with Eggs." *Physicians Committee for Responsible Medicine*. www.pcrm.org/health/diets/vegdiets/salmonella-and-other-egg-hazards-cooking-without

115.   "The Egg Industry." *People for the Ethical Treatment of Animals*. www.peta.org/issues/animals-used-for-food/factory-farming/chickens/egg-industry/

116.   Kam, Katherine. "The Truth About Sugar." *WebMD*, August 29, 2011. www.webmd.com/food-recipes/health-effects-of-sugar?page=3

117.   Zelman, Kathleen M., MPH, RD, LD. "The Truth About White Foods." *WebMD*. www.webmd.com/diet/truth-about-white-foods

118.   Downs, Martin, MPH. "The Truth About 7 Common Food Additives." *WebMD*, December 17, 2008. www.webmd.com/diet/the-truth-about-seven-common-food-additives

119.   Kovacs, Betty, MS, RD. "Artificial Sweeteners." *MedicineNet.com*, April 16, 2014. www.medicinenet.com/artificial_sweeteners/article.htm

120.	Chow, Reuben. "Fried foods are more harmful than you think." *Natural News*, January 23, 2014. www.naturalnews.com/043619_fried_foods_trans_fats_whole_bo dy_health.html
121.	"20 Worst Drinks in America 2010." *bmj.com*, Sept. 20, 2010. blogs.bmj.com/bjsm/files/2010/09/20-Worst-Drinks_2010.pdf
122.	"Chlorophyll." *Hippocrates Health Institute.* hippocratesinst.org/Diet/chlorophyll
123.	Gunnars, Kris. "Is Fruit Good or Bad For Your Health? The Sweet Truth." *Authority Nutrition.* authoritynutrition.com/is-fruit-good-or-bad-for-your-health/
124.	Warner, Jennifer. "Drinking Juice May Stall Alzheimer's: Fruit and Vegetable Juice May Cut Alzheimer's by up to 76%." *WebMD*, August 31, 2006. www.webmd.com/alzheimers/news/20060831/drinking-juice-may-stall-alzheimers
125.	"Vegetables and Fruits." *Harvard School of Public Health.* www.hsph.harvard.edu/nutritionsource/what-should-you-eat/vegetables-and-fruits/
126.	Kovacs, Jenny Stamos. "Beans: Protein-Rich Superfoods." *WebMD*, February 26, 2007. www.webmd.com/diet/beans-protein-rich-superfoods
127.	Hennessy, Maggie. "10 ancient grains to watch: from kamut to quinoa." *Food Navigator-USA*, November 14, 2013. www.foodnavigator-usa.com/Markets/10-ancient-grains-to-watch-from-kamut-to-quinoa
128.	"What are the Health Benefits?" *Whole Grains Council.* wholegrainscouncil.org/whole-grains-101/what-are-the-health-benefits
129.	"Soy and Your Health." *Physicians Committee for Responsible Medicine.* www.pcrm.org/health/health-topics/soy-and-your-health
130.	Freedman, Neal D., PhD, Yikyung Park, ScD, Christian C. Abnet, PhD, Albert R. Hollenbeck, PhD, et al. "Association of Coffee Drinking with Total and Cause-Specific Mortality." *The New England Journal of Medicine* 366, no. 20 (May 17, 2012): 1891-1904. www.nejm.org/doi/full/10.1056/NEJMoa1112010

131.   "Red wine and resveratrol: Good for your heart?" *Mayo Clinic*. April 25, 2014. www.mayoclinic.org/diseases-conditions/heart-disease/in-depth/red-wine/art-20048281

132.   Courage, Katherine Harmon. "Why Is Dark Chocolate Good for You? Thank Your Microbes." *Scientific American*, March 19, 2014. www.scientificamerican.com/article/why-is-dark-chocolate-good-for-you-thank-your-microbes/

133.   Elliott, John. "Healing Herbs: The 15 Most Powerful Healing Herbs in Your Kitchen." *Healthy Holistic Living*. www.healthy-holistic-living.com/healing-herbs.html

134.   Aggarwal, Bharat B. "5 Healing Spices." *Experience Life*, Jan/Feb 2012. experiencelife.com/article/5-healing-spices/

135.   "Health Benefits of Matcha Tea." *MatchaSource.com*. www.matchasource.com/matcha-tea-health-benefits-s/14.htm

136.   Dault, Meredith. "7 herbal teas that will make you healthier." *Best Health Magazine*. www.besthealthmag.ca/best-eats/nutrition/7-herbal-teas-that-will-make-you-healthy#AEd22pJTMzYFCdM7.97

137.   "12 Common Toiletries and their chemicals of concern." *CANCERactive*. www.canceractive.com/cancer-active-page-link.aspx?n=223

138.   Healthy Child Healthy World. "13 Dangerous Toxins To Avoid In Your Food." *Mind Body Green*, May 28, 2013. www.mindbodygreen.com/0-9694/13-dangerous-toxins-to-avoid-in-your-food.html

139.   Cancer Nutrition Centers of America, Greening Your Kitchen: Tips to Banish Environmental Toxins www.cncahealth.com/explore/learn/green-living/greening-your-kitchen-tips-to-banish-environmental-toxins#.VQC-W0Jd0ng

140.   "Methylcobalamin: A Potential Breakthrough in Neurological Disease." *ProHealth*, February 1, 1999. www.prohealth.com/library/showarticle.cfm?libid=481

141.   Greger, Michael, MD. "omega-3 fatty acids." *NutritionFacts.org*, March 9, 2015. nutritionfacts.org/topics/omega-3-fatty-acids/

142.   "Dietary Reference Intakes for Calcium and Vitamin D." *Institute of Medicine of the National Academies*. November 2010. www.iom.edu/~/media/Files/Report%20Files/2010/Dietary-

Reference-Intakes-for-Calcium-and-Vitamin-D/Vitamin%20D%20and%20Calcium%202010%20Report%20Brief.pdf

143.　　"Dietary Reference Intakes – RDAs." *Nutrition.gov.* www.nutrition.gov/smart-nutrition-101/dietary-reference-intakes-rdas

144.　　Wolfe, David. *Superfoods: The Food and Medicine of the Future* (Berkeley: North Atlantic Books, 2009).

145.　　"Classical element." *Wikipedia.* en.wikipedia.org/wiki/Classical_element

146.　　"Minority Rules: Scientists Discover Tipping Point for the Spread of Ideas." *Rensselaer Polytechnic Institute*, July 25, 2011. news.rpi.edu/luwakkey/2902

147.　　Casalena, Nina. "How Many Adults Are Vegan in the U.S.?" *The Vegetarian Resource Group*, December 05, 2011. www.vrg.org/blog/2011/12/05/how-many-adults-are-vegan-in-the-u-s/

148.　　Douillard, John. *The 3-Season Diet: Eat the Way Nature Intended: Lose Weight, Beat Food Cravings, and Get Fit* (New York: Three Rivers Press, 2001).

149.　　Halpern, Marc. *Principles of Ayurvedic Medicine* (Nevada City, CA: California College of Ayurveda, 2010), 264-265.

150.　　Ibid., 266

151.　　Ibid.

152.　　Ibid., 266-267

153.　　Ibid., 267

154.　　Ibid., 266

155.　　Ibid., 268

156.　　Ibid.

157.　　Ibid., 269

158.　　Ibid.

159.　　Ramaswamy, Sandhiya. "The Benefits of Ayurveda Self-Massage 'Abhyanga'." *Chopra Centered Lifestyle.* www.chopra.com/ccl/the-benefits-of-ayurveda-self-massage-abhyanga

160.　　"Why Is Sleep Important?" *National Heart, Lung, and Blood Institute, National Institute of Health*, Feb. 22, 2012. www.nhlbi.nih.gov/health/health-topics/topics/sdd/why

161.		"What is acupuncture? What are the benefits of acupuncture?" *Medical News Today*, February 16, 2015. www.medicalnewstoday.com/articles/156488.php

162.		"Chiropractic Care for Back Pain." *WebMD*, Jan. 22, 2015. www.webmd.com/pain-management/guide/chiropractic-pain-relief

163.		"Facial health benefits: Pampering yourself on the outside is beneficial inside." *Examiner.com*, October 14, 2012. www.examiner.com/article/facial-health-benefirs-pampering-yourself-on-the-outside-is-beneficial-inside

164.		"The Health Benefits of Manicures and Pedicures." *Answers.com*. spa.answers.com/manicures-and-pedicures/the-health-benefits-of-manicures-and-pedicures

165.		"Massage: Get in touch with its many benefits." *Mayo Clinic*, Jan. 30, 2013. www.mayoclinic.org/healthy-living/stress-management/in-depth/massage/art-20045743

166.		Davis, Jeanie Lerche. "Detox Diets: Cleansing the Body." *WebMD*, 2002. www.webmd.com/diet/detox-diets-cleansing-body

167.		"Blue Zone." *Wikipedia*. en.wikipedia.org/wiki/Blue_Zone, www.bluezones.com

168.		Maltz, Maxwell. *Psycho-Cybernetics, A New Way to Get More Living Out of Life* (New York: Pocket Books, 1989).

169.		Iliades, Chris. "7 Reasons to Add Strength Training to Your Workout Routine." *Everyday Health*, Jan. 29, 2015. www.everydayhealth.com/fitness/add-strength-training-to-your-workout.aspx

170.		"The Health Benefits of Yoga." *WebMD*, June 24, 2014. www.webmd.com/balance/guide/the-health-benefits-of-yoga

171.		Knight, Madeline. "9 Health Benefits of Dance." *Everyday Health*, July 1, 2011. www.everydayhealth.com/fitness-pictures/health-benefits-of-dance.aspx

172.		Smith, Melinda, and Jeanne Segal. "Laughter is the Best Medicine: The Health Benefits of Humor and Laughter." *HelpGuide.org*, February 2015. www.helpguide.org/articles/emotional-health/laughter-is-the-best-medicine.htm

173.   Waehner, Paige. "Why You Need Cardio Exercise: It's not just for weight loss anymore." *About.com*, December 16, 2014. exercise.about.com/od/cardioworkouts/a/cardio_exercise.htm

174.   Douillard, John. "15 Benefits of Nose Breathing Exercise." *LifeSpa*, May 6, 2014. lifespa.com/15-benefits-nose-breathing-exercise/

175.   Nussbaum, Paul David. "Five Brain-Health Factors." *Aging Today* XXVIII, no. 5 (Sept./Oct. 2007). www.paulnussbaum.com/AT-285-Nussbaum2.pdf

176.   "The Law of Dharma or Purpose in Life." *The Chopra Center*. www.chopra.com/the-law-of-dharma-or-purpose-in-life

177.   Saraswati, Satyananda. "Prana: the Universal Life Force." *Yoga Magazine*, September 1981. www.yogamag.net/archives/1982/emay82/prana582.shtml

178.   Griffin, R. Morgan. "Give Your Body a Boost – With Laughter." *WebMD*, April 10, 2008. www.webmd.com/balance/features/give-your-body-boost-with-laughter

179.   "Sleep." Wikipedia. en.wikipedia.org/wiki/Sleep

180.   McCoy, Krisha. "How to Stay Sharp As You Age." *Everyday Health*, Feb. 19, 2015. www.everydayhealth.com/senior-health/staying-sharp.aspx

181.   McGreevey, Sue. "Eight weeks to a better brain." *Harvard Gazette*, Jan. 21, 2011. news.harvard.edu/gazette/story/2011/01/eight-weeks-to-a-better-brain/

182.   Kingham, Neil. "Chinese Nutrition – The Energetics Of Food." *Positive Health Online*, January 2009. www.positivehealth.com/article/chinese-oriental-medicine/chinese-nutrition-the-energetics-of-food

183.   Roberts, Holly. *Vegetarian Christian Saints: Mystics, Ascetics & Monks* (USA: Anjeli Press, 2004).

184.   "Essenes." *Wikipedia*. en.wikipedia.org/wiki/Essenes

185.   Isaiah 7:14-15. www.biblegateway.com/passage/?search=Isaiah+7%3A14-15&version=NKJV

186.   Hosea 6:6. biblehub.com/hosea/6-6.htm

187.   Akers, Keith. "Was the Last Supper Vegetarian?" *CompassionateSpirit.com*. www.compassionatespirit.com/last_supper.htm

188.   Dysinger, Luke, O.S.B. "Accepting the Embrace of God: The Ancient Art of Lectio Divina." *Saint Andrew's Abbey*, Dec. 9, 2005. www.valyermo.com/ld-art.html

189.   "Origen." *Wikipedia*. en.wikipedia.org/wiki/Origen

190.   "Anthony the Great." *Wikipedia*. en.wikipedia.org/wiki/Anthony_the_Great

191.   "Evagrius Ponticus" *Wikipedia*. en.wikipedia.org/wiki/Evagrius_Ponticus

192.   "Evagrius Ponticus: On Asceticism and Stillness in the Solitary Life." *Hermitary*, 2002. www.hermitary.com/solitude/evagrius.html

193. "Blind men and an elephant." *Wikipedia*. en.wikipedia.org/wiki/Blind_men_and_an_elephant

About the Author

Laura Robinson Oatman

———————•———————

Laura Robinson Oatman is an author, speaker, and Vegan Warrior for Peace. She educates, supports, and empowers individuals and groups toward a sustainable, holistically healthy life rooted in a vegan diet. She offers one-to-one coaching and motivational speaking, leads workshops and group programs, and takes clients on amazing wellness journeys worldwide. She is a Certified Holistic Health Coach from the Institute of Integrative Nutrition in New York, a Certified Ayurvedic Educator from the California College of Ayurveda, and a Certified Plant-Based Nutritionist from eCornell. Her company, Whole Earth Wellness, is an Educational Alliance Partner with the Physician's Committee for Responsible Medicine in Washington, DC. *Whole Earth Diet* focuses mostly on physical health, is the foundation for the holistic Whole Earth Wellness philosophy, and lays the groundwork for many more books to come.

Her ideal clients are folks who refuse to grow old gracefully without fighting back, and who want to shed a few pounds, regain youthful joy and energy, and reduce or eliminate those medications they've been prescribed. They want to simply start eating well, living right, and enjoying a long, healthy life to the fullest. They are positive, proactive idealists from around the world of every age, race, color, religion, sexual orientation, and cultural identity with big passionate hearts, open purposeful minds, and joyous prayerful souls. She is building a tribe of Warriors for Peace who will stop at nothing to create a healthy, peaceful world.

In addition to being a Wellness Warrior, Laura is a licensed architect who specializes in design and development of hotels, spas, and wellness centers that are looking for a unique combination of both luxury and sustainable green design. She is a partner at Newport Beach–based Oatman Architects with her husband, Homer Oatman, who specializes in high-end custom homes. Prior to this, she was Project Director for Viceroy Hotel Group in Los Angeles. She helped develop the Viceroy and Tides brands, managed high-profile projects with interior designer Kelly Wearstler, and was founding director of Viceroy's "sustainable green program." Her career prior to that was with the international hotel design firm WATG Architects.

Homer and Laura met at UCLA Graduate School of Architecture in 1981 while earning their Masters in Architecture, married in 1984, and created their most beautiful work together in the late '80s and early s'90s—Erik Andrew, Annalise Nicole, Dane Cameron, Scott Robinson, and Brett Christian Oatman.

Laura is a Southern California native who enjoys vegan food, red wine, matcha green tea lattes, and dark chocolate. She loves travel, good books, hiking, skiing, and yoga, and she has never met an animal or a person she didn't like. She lives in Newport Beach with her husband, her pit bull Gracie, her mystery mutt Chucho, her old cat Dooey, her African leopard tortoise Sheldon, and her outdoor treehouse full of well-fed wild birds, crows, squirrels, and mice. Their five twenty-something adult children and their friends drift in and out like the tide and are always welcomed home with open arms and warm soup. Two weddings for two of the boys are currently being planned, so perhaps soon one day they will welcome some grandchildren into their lives.

In her free time, Laura is an animal rights' activist who supports PETA, Farm Sanctuary, Mercy for Animals, Compassion Over Killing, and FARM. She is also a women's rights promoter and an active member of NAWBO-OC and eWomen Network, and she volunteers her time as a mentor to young businesswomen at NAWBO-OC. She also enjoys travel, yoga, wine tasting, hiking, line dancing, Motown music, horseback riding, Zumba, being in big cities, and being in the wilderness.

Why does she do what she does? She is passionate about compassion, and about helping people live their best, longest, healthiest, happiest lives. She firmly believes that the road to health and happiness begins when we stop eating animals. World peace begins on our plates by eating the healthy, peaceful energy of plant-based foods instead of the unhealthy, violent energy of flesh-based foods. It is a diet best for our health, best for the planet, and inarguably best for the animals. And it is definitely best for the soul.

Her dream is to purchase land somewhere in California and design and build a wellness spa resort that will include a sustainable green hotel, a spa and yoga pavilion, a wellness center, a farm animal sanctuary, and an organic farm and vineyard for the farm-to-table vegan restaurant—the first Whole Earth Wellness Resort. The business plan is available upon request.

whole earth
·WELLNESS·

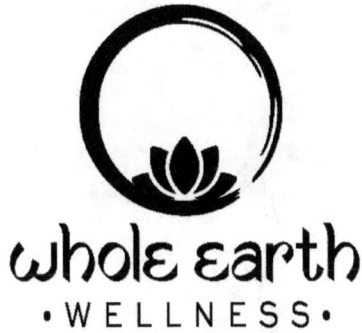

Connect with Laura Robinson Oatman

Facebook: www.facebook.com/laura.oatman

Twitter: twitter.com/Laura_Oatman

Skype: laura.oatman

YouTube Channel: Laura Oatman bit.ly/1OoikKo

Meet Laura Oatman:
www.youtube.com/watch?v=pM_6yk1AaG0

Pinterest: www.pinterest.com/lauraoatman/

Instagram: instagram.com/lauraoatman/

LinkedIn: www.linkedin.com/in/lauraoatman

Connect with Whole Earth Wellness

———●———

Facebook: www.facebook.com/WholeEarthWellnessLLC

Whole Earth Diet Book:
www.youtube.com/watch?v=qQm1fZYjtRQ

LinkedIn: linkd.in/1LCrXHQ

Website: www.whole-earth-wellness.com;
wholeearthdiet.com

Connect Page: wholeearthdiet.com/contact-laura

Mailing Address:

2618 San Miguel Drive, #309
Newport Beach, CA 92660

Phone: 800-208-6303

Email: info@wholeearthdiet.com

In Gratitude to You...

———————————•●•———————————

Thank you for listening to your heart and gut in purchasing **Whole Earth Diet.** I know it's a significant investment of time you're making for your growth and happiness.

Because this book is also an expression of *my* passionate commitment to healthier relationships and families on the planet, the more people that read it, the more impact that can be made.

If you're willing to help that happen, I would be so grateful if you could take a minute or two to share what you loved about this book and provide an honest review on our Amazon sales page.

www.ingramcontent.com/pod-product-compliance
Lightning Source LLC
Chambersburg PA
CBHW062149270326
41930CB00009B/1482